Computers in Critical Care and Pulmonary Medicine

Edited by P. M. Osswald

in Cooperation with

O. Prakash, H.-J. Hartung and H. J. Bender

With 197 Figures and 29 Tables

Springer-Verlag
Berlin Heidelberg New York Tokyo

Priv.-Doz. Dr. Peter Michael Osswald
Priv.-Doz. Dr. H.-J. Hartung
Dr. Dr. H. J. Bender
Department of Anesthesiology and Resuscitation
Mannheim Faculty of Clinical Medicine
(Director: Prof. Dr. H. Lutz)
Univesity of Heidelberg
6800 Mannheim,
Federal Republic of Germany

O. Prakash, M. D.
Thorax Centre
Rijksuniversiteit Rotterdam
Rotterdam
The Netherlands

ISBN-13: 978-3-540-13840-2 e-ISBN-13: 978-3-642-70068-2
DOI: 10.1007/978-3-642-70068-2

Printed and binding: Beltz Offsetdruck, Hemsbach/Bergstraße
2119/3140-543210

Table of Contents

List of Contributors

Aloy, A., Research Center for Intensive Care of the Clinic for Anesthesia and General Intensive Care Medicine, and the II. Surgical Clinic, University of Vienna, A-1090 Vienna, Austria

Arbinolo, M.A., Secondo servizio di anestesia e rianimazione, Ospedale Maggiore San Giovanni Battista di Torino, Turin, Italy

Baehrendtz, S., Medical Intensive Care Unit, Department of Medicine at the South Hospital, Karolinska Institute, Stockholm, Sweden

Balestra, G., Instituto "Giorgio Quazza" per l'informatica e l'elettronica, Formazione e ricerca. Citta' di Torino, Turin, Italy

Ball, P., Institut für Biochemische Endokrinologie, Medizinische Hochschule, D-2400 Lübeck, Federal Republic of Germany

Bekemeyer, U., Klinik für Innere Medizin, Medizinische Hochschule, D-2400 Lübeck, Federal Republic of Germany

Bellero, M.L., Secondo servizio di anestesia e rianimazione, Ospedale Maggiore San Giovanni Battista di Torino, Turin, Italy

Bender, H.-J., Department of Anesthesiology and Resuscitation, Mannheim Faculty of Clinical Medicine, D-6800 Mannheim, Federal Republic of Germany

Bertino, R., Secondo servizio di anestesia e rianimazione, Ospedale Maggiore San Giovanni Battista di Torino, Turin, Italy

Bleicher, W., Dept. of Anaesthesiology, University of Tübingen, Tübingen, Federal Republic of Germany

Brunner, J.X., Division of Cardiothoracic Surgery, Clinical Physiology, Department of Surgery of the University of Basel, Kantonsspital Basel, Basel, Switzerland

Burney, R., University of Massachusetts Medical Center, Worcester, Massachusetts, U.S.A.

Djonlagic, H., Klinik für Innere Medizin, Medizinische Hochschule, D-2400 Lübeck, Federal Republic of Germany

EINHÄUPL, K. M., Department of Neurology, Klinikum Großhadern, University of Munich, D-8000 Munich, Federal Republic of Germany

EKENBÄCK, K., Medical Intensive Care Unit, Department of Medicine at the South Hospital, Karolinska Institute, Stockholm, Sweden

ENGEL, H.-P., Department of Experimental Surgery, Surgical Center, University of Heidelberg, Im Neuenheimer Feld 347, D-6900 Heidelberg, Federal Republic of Germany

EPPLE, E., Department of Anesthesiology, University of Tübingen, D-7400 Tübingen, Federal Republic of Germany

ERDMANN, K., Institut für Anaesthesiologie, Johannes Gutenberg-Universität, Langenbeckstr. 1, D-6500 Mainz, Federal Republic of Germany

ESSIN, D. J., Departments of Anesthesiology and Pediatrics, University of Southern California / Los Angeles County Medical Center, Los Angeles, California 90033, U.S.A.

FAGAN, L. M., Medical Computer Science, Room TC-135, Department of Medicine, Stanford University School of Medicine, Stanford, California 94305, U.S.A.

FELDMANN, U., Division of Medical Statistics, Biomathematics and Information Processings, Klinikum Mannheim, University of Heidelberg, D-6800 Mannheim, Federal Republic of Germany

FORNAI, E., Second Medical Clinic of the University of Pisa, Pisa, Italy

FORSSBLAD, M., Medical Intensive Care Unit, Department of Medicine at the South Hospital, Karolinska Institute, Stockholm, Sweden

FRANCO, C., Secondo servizio di anestesia e rianimazione, Ospedale Maggiore San Giovanni Battista di Torino, Turin, Italy

FRIBERG, B., Medical Intensive Care Unit, Department of Medicine at the South Hospital, Karolinska Institute, Stockholm, Sweden

GAAB, M. R., University Neurological Clinic, General Hospital, Alser Str. 4, A-1090 Vienna, Austria

GARNER, C., Department of Neurology Klinikum Großhadern, University of Munich, D-8000 Munich, Federal Republic of Germany

GEIGER, K., Institute of Anesthesiology, Faculty of Clinical Medicine Mannheim, University of Heidelberg, D-6800 Mannheim, Federal Republic of Germany

GESSA, M., Secondo servizio di anestesia e rianimazione, Ospedale Maggiore San Giovanni Battista di Torino, Turin, Italy

GIUNTINI, C., Second Medical Clinic of the University of Pisa, Pisa, Italy

GUARNACCIA, A., Secondo servizio di anestesia e rianimazione, Ospedale Maggiore San Giovanni Battista di Torino, Turin, Italy

HAASS, A., Universitätsnervenklinik, Homburg/Saar

HANKELN, K., Department of Anesthesiology, Zentralkrankenhaus Links der Weser, D-2800 Bremen, Federal Republic of Germany

HARTUNG, H.-J., Institut for Anesthesiology and Resuscitation, Klinikum Mannheim, University of Heidelberg.

HAUPTMANN, A., Klinik für Innere Medizin, Medizinische Hochschule, D-2400 Lübeck, Federal Republic of Germany

HEIDBÜCHEL, K., Klinik für Innere Medizin, Medizinische Hochschule, D-2400 Lübeck, Federal Republic of Germany

HEITZ, M., Stadtspital Triemli, Zürich, Switzerland

HOARE, M. R., The Thoracic Center, Erasmus University and University Hospital, Rotterdam, The Netherlands

HUGENHOLTZ, P. G., The Thoracic Center, Erasmus University and University Hospital, Rotterdam, The Netherlands

HULTING, J., Medical Intensive Care Unit, Department of Medicine at the South Hospital, Karolinska Institute, Stockholm, Sweden

ISHIHARA, H., Department of Anesthesiology, Hirosaki University, School of Medicine, Hirosaki, Aomori-ken, Japan

ISOZAKI, K., Department of Anesthesiology, Hirosaki University, School of Medicine, Hirosaki, Aomori-ken, Japan

JAGODOWICZ, M., Departments of Anesthesiology and Pediatrics, University of Southern California / Los Angeles County Medical Center, Los Angeles, California 90033, U.S.A.

JANTZEN, J.-P., Institut für Anaesthesiologie, Johannes Gutenberg-Universität, Langenbeckstr. 1, D-6500 Mainz, Federal Republic of Germany

JENSEN, U., Institute for Anesthesiology University of Munich, Klinikum Großhadern, Marchioninstr. 15, 8000 Munich 70, Federal Republic of Germany

JOHANSSON, M., Medical Intensive Care Unit, Department of Medicine at the South Hospital, Karolinska Institute, Stockholm, Sweden

JUNGER, H., Dept. of Anesthesiology, University of Tübingen, D-7400 Tübingen, Federal Republic of Germany

KELLERMANN, W., Institute for Anesthesiology, University of Munich, Klinikum Großhadern, Marchionistr. 15, 8000 Munich 70, Federal Republic of Germany

KERSCHER, G., Department of Neurology, Klinikum Großhadern, University of Munich, D-8000 Munich 70, Federal Republic of Germany

KLOCKE, H., Helmholtz-Institute for Biomedical Engineering, University Hospital, D-5100 Aachen, Federal Republic of Germany

KNAFLITZ, M., Istituto "Giorgio Quazza" per l'information e l'elettronica, Formazione e ricerca. Citta' di Torino, Turin, Italy

Köhler, C. O., Institute of Documentation, Information and Statistics, Department of Central Data Processing, German Cancer Research Center, D-6900 Heidelberg, Federal Republic of Germany

Koller, W., Research Center for Intensive Care of the Clinic for Anesthesia and General Intensive Care Medicine, and the II. Surgical Clinic, University of Vienna, Vienna, Austria

Kopp, M., Dept. of Anesthesiology, University of Tübingen, D-7400 Tübingen, Federal Republic of Germany

Kufner, G., Department of Neurology, Klinikum Großhadern, University of Munich, D-8000 Munich 70, Federal Republic of Germany

List, W. F., Institute of Anesthesiology, University of Graz, Austria

Lutz, H., Institute for Anesthesiology and Resuscitation, Klinikum Mannheim, University of Heidelberg, D-6800 Mannheim, Federal Republic of Germany

Madler, T., Universitätsnervenklinik Homburg/Saar

Maiwald, M., Stress Research Group, Department of Internal Medicine II, University of Heidelberg, Alte Bergheimer Str. 5, D-6900 Heidelberg, Federal Republic of Germany

Mason, J., Department of Neurosurgery, Pinderfields Hospital, Wakefield, England

Matell, G., Medical Intensive Care Unit, Department of Medicine at the South Hospital, Karolinska Institute, Stockholm, Sweden

Matsuki, A., Department of Anesthesiology, Hirosaki University, School of Medicine, Hirosaki, Aomori-ken, Japan

Meij, S. H., The Thoracic Center, Erasmus University and University Hospital, Rotterdam, The Netherlands

Messmer, K., Department of Experimental Surgery, Surgical Center, University of Heidelberg, Im Neuenheimer Feld 347, 6900 Heidelberg, Federal Republic of Germany

Metzler, H., Institute of Anesthesiology, University of Graz, Austria

Michelsen, H., Department of Anesthesiology, Zentralkrankenhaus Links der Weser, D-2800 Bremen, Federal Republic of Germany

Miller, P. L., Department of Anesthesiology, Yale University School of Medicine, New Haven, CT 06510, U.S.A.

Müller-Esch, G., Klinik für Innere Medizin, Medizinische Hochschule, D-2400 Lübeck, Federal Republic of Germany

Müller, M., Department of Anesthesiology, University Clinics, Im Neuenheimer Feld 110, D-6900 Heidelberg, Federal Republic of Germany

Mutz, N., Research Center for Intensive Care of the Clinic for Anesthesia and General Intensive Care Medicine, and the II. Surgical Clinic, University of Vienna, Vienna, Austria

Neto, A. G., Second Medical Clinic of the University of Pisa, Pisa, Italy

Neumeier, D., Institute for Clinical Chemistry, University of Munich, Klinikum Großhadern, Marchioninstr. 15, 8000 Munich 70, Federal Republic of Germany

Ossmer, B., Medical Intensive Care Unit, Department of Medicine at the South Hospital, Karolinska Institute, Stockholm, Sweden

Osswald, P.-M., Institute for Anesthesiology and Resuscitation, Klinikum Mannheim, University of Heidelberg, D-6800 Mannheim, Federal Republic of Germany

Oyama, T., Department of Anesthesiology, Hirosaki University, School of Medicine, Hirosaki, Aomori-ken, Japan

Paoletti, P., CNR Institute of Clinical Physiology, Pisa, Italy

Pauser, G., Research Center for Intensive Care of the Clinic for Anesthesia and General Intensive Care Medicine, and the II. Surgical Clinic, University of Vienna, Vienna, Austria

Peter, K., Institut für Anaesthesiologie der Universität München, Klinikum Großhadern, Marchioninstr. 15, D-8000 Munich 70, Federal Republic of Germany

Peters, A., Klinik für Innere Medizin, Medizinische Hochschule, D-2400 Lübeck, Federal Republic of Germany

Prediletto, R., Second Medical Clinic of the University of Pisa, Pisa, Italy

Price, D. J., Department of Neurosurgery, Pinderfields Hospital, Wakefield, England

Prys-Roberts, C., Sir Humphrey Davy Department of Anaesthesia, University of Bristol, Bristol Royal Infirmary, Bristol, United Kingdom

Ransil, B. J., The Charles A. Dana Research Institute and the Harvard-Thorndike Laboratory of Beth Israel Hospital, Department of Medicine, Beth Israel Hospital and Harvard Medical School, Boston, MA 02215, U.S.A.

Rau, G. Helmholtz-Institute for Biomedical Engineering University Hospital, D-5100 Aachen, Federal Republic of Germany

Rudowski, R., Institute of Biocybernetics and Biomedical Engineering, Polish Academy of Sciences, Warsaw, Poland

Ruschi, S., Second Medical Clinic of the University of Pisa, Pisa, Italy

Schlimgen, R., Department of Anesthesiology, University Hospital, D-5100 Aachen, Federal Republic of Germany

Scriba, C., Klinik für Innere Medizin, Medizinische Hochschule, D-2400 Lübeck, Federal Republic of Germany

SCHIMRIGK, K., Universitätsnervenklinik Homburg/Saar

SCHMIDT, G., Department of Anesthesiology, University Clinics, Im Neuenheimer Feld 110, D-6900 Heidelberg, Federal Republic of Germany

SCHMIEDER, G., Department of Neurology, Klinikum Großhadern, University of Munich, D-8000 Munich, Federal Republic of Germany

SCHOSSER, R., Department of Experimental Surgery, Surgical Center, University of Heidelberg, Im Neuenheimer Feld 347, D-6900 Heidelberg, Federal Republic of Germany

SCHUY, S., Institute of Biomedical Engineering, Technical University, Graz, Austria

STAFFORD, T. J., University of Massachusetts Medical Center, Worcester, Massachusetts, U.S.A.

SIEGL, K., Department of Neurology, Klinikum Großhadern, University of Munich, Munich, Federal Republic of Germany

SHORTLIFFE, E. H., Medical Computer Science, Room TC-135, Department of Medicine, Stanford University School of Medicine, Stanford, California 94305 U.S.A.

SMITH, N. T., Professor of Anesthesiology, University of California, San Diego, VA Medical Center, 3350 La Jolla Village Drive, San Diego, California 92161, U.S.A.

SNOWDEN, S., Department of Neurosurgery, Pinderfields Hospital, Wakefield, England

SPANNE, C., Medical Intensive Care Unit, Department of Medicine at the South Hospital, Karolinska Institute, Stockholm, Sweden

STEEN, S. N., Departments of Anesthesiology and Pediatrics, University of Southern California / Los Angeles County Medical Center, Los Angeles, California 90033, U.S.A.

SUMMA, Y., Institute for Anesthesiology, University of Munich, Klinikum Großhadern, Marchioninstr. 15, D-8000 Munich 70, Federal Republic of Germany

SUZUKI, T., Department of Anesthesiology, Hirosaki University, School of Medicine, Hirosaki, Aomori-ken, Japan

SWOBODA, A., Department of Cardiac Surgery, University Hospital Eppendorf, D-2000 Hamburg, Federal Republic of Germany

TRISPEL, S., Helmholtz-Institute for Biomedical Engineering, University Hospital, D-5100 Aachen, Federal Republic of Germany

TYBUSSEK, R., Klinik für Innere Medizin, Medizinische Hochschule, D-2400 Lübeck, Federal Republic of Germany

URCIUOULI, R., Istituto di Neurochirurgia dell'Universita' di Torino, Turin, Italy

Warner, D. L., Departments of Anesthesiology and Pediatrics, University of Southern California / Los Angeles County Medical Center, Los Angeles, California 90033, U.S.A.

Westenskow, D. R., Division of Bioengineering, Department of Anesthesiology, University of Utah, Salt Lake City, Utah, U.S.A.

Wieczorek, R., Department of Neurology, Klinikum Großhadern, University of Munich, D-8000 Munich, Federal Republic of Germany

Wiedemann, K., Department of Anesthesiology, University Clinics, Im Neuenheimer Feld 110, D-6800 Heidelberg, Federal Republic of Germany

Wiesspeiner, G., Institute of Biomedical Engineering, Technical University of Graz, Austria

Winter, D., Institute for Anesthesiology and Resuscitation, Klinikum Mannheim, University of Heidelberg, D-6800 Mannheim, Federal Republic of Germany

Wolff, G., Division of Cardiothoracic Surgery, Clinical Physiology, Department of Surgery of the University of Basel, Kantonsspital Basel, Basel, Switzerland

Wood, W. G., Klinik für Innere Medizin, Medizinische Hochschule, D-2400 Lübeck, Federal Republic of Germany

Yamashita, M., Department of Anesthesiology, Hirosaki University, School of Medicine, Hirosaki, Aomori-ken, Japan

Zeelenberg, C., The Thoracic Center, Erasmus University and University Hospital, Rotterdam, The Netherlands

Application of Computer Systems in Critical Care

K. Geiger

During the past decade innovations in biomedical computing have produced hardware and software systems that now enable monitoring of critically ill patients on a much more extensive and useful level than was possible before. Intensive care unit computer systems were designed initially for monitoring vital signs such as heart rate and blood pressure from bedside hardware, but increasing numbers of signals are now being demanded and no end is yet in sight. The technological imperative is partially responsible. Advances in electronic monitoring devices have paralleled progresses in information processing and miniaturization of microprocessors. Clinical and experimental medicine has responded by examining new parameters of monitoring which can be employed more efficiently in patient assessment. A great number of intensive care units in Germany are still equipped with noncomputerized monitoring systems. Such systems have some inherent problems which encroach on the efficiency of patient management:

1. They cannot perform quantitative analyses or present the data in a variety of formats. Current noncomputerized monitoring systems have no storage capacity, making trend analysis of any of the patient's physiologic parameters impossible. Such information is important, helping the clinician to assess the patient's status and determine the necessary therapeutic measures.
2. They lack the capability of automated logging and data retrieval. Significant events are recorded solely by manual charting. Such systems do not allow the setting of priority alarm conditions according to previous events. Neither is it possible to recall and display past data in an easy and convenient manner.

Present-day computerized monitoring systems provide continuous or intermittent monitoring of many input data. Clinically relevant ICU data center on cardiopulmonary function. The physiologic parameters commonly monitored nowadays are as follows:

Systolic, diastolic, and mean *blood pressure* are displayed. An automatic calibration system for blood pressure transducers has been described (Martin et al. 1973). A computer algorithm has been developed to detect the distortion of arterial blood pressure wave forms caused by blood clots or air bubbles in the catheter.

ECG is continuously monitored. The ECG wave form can be sampled at a rate of 250 or 300 per second and the R waves identified on the basis of their amplitude and the steepness of the downslope. The data points can subsequently be analyzed to give the R wave widths. A computer program may than sort the beats into various categories such as normal, premature, wide and late. Preprocessing computer programs like the *Aztec* inaugurated by Cox (Cox et al. 1968) have been developed for the efficient sorting of ectopic beats. This system accurately detected 78% of ventricular ectopic beats; however, movements artifacts and/or conduction defects are associated with significant error rates. Most arrhythmia-detecting systems use measurements of QRS width, offset, amplitude, and area to classify complexes into morphological families. Another approach combines the major elements of cross-correlation of QRS signals, as well as grouping of complexes into families and clusters. Westenskow (1982) recently described a system that uses both esophageal and surface electrodes to detect cardiac arrhythmias in the operating room. A strip chart recorder provides a permanent record of ectopic beats and the computer's interpretation of these. He reported a false-positive rate of 0.034% and a false-negative rate of 0.107%. A typical application of such systems could be the monitoring of the efficiency of antiarrhythmic therapy.

Cardiac output is commonly determined by thermal dilution. Warner et al. (1968) developed a method, of measuring cardiac output that was not dependent upon analysis of the indicator dilution method. They attempted to estimate stroke volume from central aortic pressure analysis. This method is based on an application of signal-processing techniques in which the computer is programmed to identify critical points on the central arterial pressure contour. Since the arterial vascular system possesses elements both of resistance and capacitance, only a fraction of the blood expelled from the left ventricle during systole will leave the large vessels of the arterial system during systole. A considerable portion of the blood ejected from the heart stays within the elastic reservoir of the vascular bed and leaves large vessels during diastole. In Warner's analysis the stroke volume can therefore be separated into systolic drainage and diastolic drainage. The final mathematical equation involves a constant which relates pressure to volume in the aorta and is in practice obtained for each individual by a single measurement of cardiac output using the indicator dilution method. In general, this technique appears to be a reasonable measure of cardiac output which can be obtained on a beat-by-beat basis in many clinical situations. However, it has recently been shown that major changes in the constant may occur in individual patients during their postoperative course (Kouchoukos et al. 1969).

When it is required to monitor *cardiac function* apart from cardiac output, a computer can be used to follow changes occuring in systolic time intervals.

Respiratory rate can be monitored directly or indirectly from the pressure fluctuations observed on the central venous pressure or from the variations in the height of the R waves of the ECG. Detailed accounts of computer-based bedside monitoring and respiratory system analysis have been given by Osborn (1975) and by Peters' group (Peters and Hilberman 1971). In their approach a pneumotachograph is placed in the respiratory line. This may be at the endotracheal tube for an intubated patient or in a face mask for a patient breathing spontaneously. This sensor has been modified to permit measurement of airway pressure as well as flow and to allow continuous sampling of the gas mixture passing through the pneumotachograph. In this way respiratory flows, pressures, and gas composition can be continuously monitored, gas analysis being carried out by rapid analyzers carbon dioxide and oxygen. The computer program permits the computation of respiratory mechanics and gas exchange, including oxygen consumption, carbon dioxide production, respiratory quotient, and the physiologic dead space. By manual, digital entry of the arterial and central venous blood gases and hemoglobin it is possible to obtain estimates of the cardiac output (using the Fick method) as well as the percentage of venoarterial admixture across the lung. These data as well as pressure-volume curves can be displayed at frequent time intervals and pulmonary work per minute, compliance and resistance computed along with the ratio of dead space to tidal volume. Such techniques provide the means to identify those points in the chain of ventilatory events at which defects have appeared and to give quantitative information helping to rectify the clinical problems. Peters (Peters and Hilberman 1971) has developed indices that may be used to warn in advance of deterioration of pulmonary function. There is, however, a continuing need for the development of error detection and on-line multivariable pattern recognition algorithms which can delineate significant trends while rejecting artifactual transients.

A new generation of microcomputer-controlled ventilators has just emerged. They incorporate the features of a versatile lung ventilator and a lung function testing unit. Complex breathing maneuvers for a variety of single- and multi-breath lung function tests can be automatically performed. If equipped with a gas analyzer, the devices can function as "demand" ventilators allowing for set-point control of end-tidal PCO_2 and PO_2.

Computer systems have been successfully utilized in the analysis of *blood gases* and *acid-base status* (Maas et al. 1972; Neff et al. 1970; Valbona et al. 1971).

Attempts have been made to analyze the *EEG* with respect to frequency and wave shape. Computer-aided EEG monitoring has been employed in guiding barbiturate therapy in intracranial hypertension (Hjrth 1970; Myers et al. 1973; Sebel et al. 1983).

Enormous efforts are being made to develop new computer systems to fulfill *other functions,* including management of pharmacologic interventions, evaluation of the effectiveness of various modes of therapy, and repeated analyses of patient status. Automated systems have been developed to deliver prescribed and programmed treatment, such as the administration of appropriate and adequate amounts of blood or of a pharmaceutical agent to maintain specific physiologic conditions in a patient. There have been several attempts to computerize the control of specific pathophysiologic situations.

In appraising the use and value of computer technology in critical care, other aspects of patient care must also be considered.

A potentially valuable application of computer technology is in the delineation of physiologic models. The principle behind the application of mathematical modeling to physiologic systems is to obtain more information from the observed data by fitting them with a set of equations that can be used to describe quantitatively particular aspects of the system. Mathematical representations of biological signals have often been developed into true functional models in an attempt to characterize various aspects to the system generating the signal. Such models can be considered as attempts to describe the general biochemical or physiologic functions of the system in circumstances where it is difficult to develop or test sufficiently detailed mathematical expressions of the mechanical or physiochemical properties, or control mechanisms that are aspects of the system. Such techniques have successfully been used in defining compartment models.

Another important area where computer technology may be extremely useful in solving critical care problems is simulation. Simulation has been mainly confined to physical models because of their preciseness in describing biological phenomena. A valuable application of this approach is the description of behavioral models of different body systems. Siegel (Siegel and Farell 1973) has used it to study how changes in cardiac output and alveolar ventilation and their respective distributions interact in the patient with acute post-traumatic pulmonary insufficiency and thus find out how the transitions between the typical pathophysiologic states can take place. The most exciting prospect of this technique is the possibility of effective clinical computer simulation of different forms of treatments in the critically ill patient. This application may help to identify the best therapy with greater sophistication and with a better chance of success.

Computers have also been applied in student instruction and medical education. Computer-assisted learning is a versatile and stimulating means of acquiring knowledge, forming a useful adjunct to traditional methods. However, it should not be used as a substitute for traditional teaching methods, because by its very nature, it tends to provide information in an unqualified, factual form which is often remote from the realities of clinical practice. At present there is only limited experience in the evaluation of such programs in terms of quantitative and qualitative knowledge. It appears, however, that computer-assisted learning offers the opportunity of an earlier introduction to intensive care problems and the possibility of continuing self-evaluation.

Comprehensive automatic monitoring systems have proved to be effective in increasing the efficiency of ICU staff. For example, by relegating routine, well-defined, repetitive tasks of these systems, nurses have been able to concentrate on direct patient care. Compared to the ususal manual methods of measurement, automated measurements are more accurate, more reliable, and more consistent. Furthermore, once these data are stored in the computer memory, they can be retrieved more quickly and can be presented to the personnel to indicate trends in the various measurements, enabling the staff to assess the patient's condition more accurately.

The various applications of computer systems have the potential of providing a better understanding of the patient's clinical problems and a better outcome. The most successful aspect of the use of computer technology in critical care has been its demonstrated capability of assimilating and processing enormous amounts of physiologic data in a short period of time. This may enable the intensive care staff to relate the present pattern of patient response to past experiences in a quantitative manner. By using new types of data correlation it may contribute to enhancement of diagnostic ability and recognition of clinical patterns and their therapeutic implications.

There are, however, still many problems regarding the application of a useful and efficient monitoring system in the intensive care unit environment. The most significant ones do not involve available technology. The establishment of prescribed medical procedures that can be programmed and turned over to an automated approach is the greatest challenge of all. Successful application of computer technology to the monitoring of critically ill patients requires definitive, quantitative descriptions of signal characteristics and specific conditions that must be detected. It is the explicit nature of programming the computer that imposes such demanding specifications. The development of computer programs with sufficient sophistication to recognize specific life-threatening patterns reliably has proved extremely difficult. The ability of the human observer to correlate an observed pattern with previous experience or training and to identify the event is not understood well enough to allow precise description and quantitation of the pattern recognition procedure that would permit the appropriate computer programs to be written. Computer systems for patient maintenance can only be used in clearly defined situations in which the treatment protocol is well established.

Other pressing problems remaining to be solved are those having to do with computer interpretation of quantitative data and the genesis of reports about the patient's condition that are meaningful to the intensive care staff and helpful in decision-making.

An absolute prerequisite for achieving this goal is that the information gathered is reliable and relevant. If the signals measured are incorrect, the information derived is deceptive and the decision based on it may be detrimental to the patient. Most sensor devices are tested at the workbench, and there is no doubt that they perform to specification. However, the question arises of whether the conditions for the proper functioning of these devices are indeed met. They are connected to a biological system rather than to a clearly defined laboratory model. Exact knowledge of the possible influence of technical physical artifacts on measurements is the prerequisite for reliable interpretation of them. Otherwise, technical artifacts are mistaken for biological observations.

Brunner and Wolff (Brunner et al. 1983), for example, have shown that the conditions for accurate flow measurement are not met if the resistant flow meter (Fleisch pneumotachograph or screen pneumotachograph) is attached directly to the mouth or endotracheal tube and the breath flows directly through it, firstly because gas composition, temperature, and humidity change radically even within the course of one respiratory cycle, secondly because the expiratory peak flow of the patient being ventilated rapidly tends to become too high, and thirdly because the entire system is sensitive to turbulence. By employing methods which compensate continuously for the influence of the changing gas concentrations and which reduce expiratory peak flow without increasing resistance, the authors were able to reduce the error from 20% to approximately 2%. With the help of suitable mathematical models, systemic errors can be analytically and quantitatively assessed and then corrected. Computers should help to improve the accuracy and reliability of measured variables.

A key question is which physiologic variables are relevant for description of the patient's condition and should therefore be measured or derived from primary data by computation. Systems currently in use allow the measurement and computation of an astonishing number of variables. Free-format data collection can well be a detriment, as potentially useful information can be overlooked in the mass of variables. It is unlikely that dozens of variables are all equally important; some must be more important than others. Therefore, data collection protocols need to be established so that data can be collected in a quick and organized way. The data have to be assembled into a descriptive form so that this discription can be used for the care of the patient. Assembly and utilization of those data involve the application of clinical judgement and knowledge to formulate a description of the physiologic condition of the system. The purpose of the application of computer techniques to patient monitoring activities must be to extract more information than is currently obtained by the ordinary measurement of cardiac, respiratory, and metabolic paramenters. The computer should provide an analysis of various physiologic systems and their interrelationship in the critically ill. It should elucidate the adequacy of the performance of physiologic subsystems, as well as the reserve capacity of these systems, and describe and predict system failures.

Recently, attempts have been made to utilize the computer to delineate physiologic patterns that may have diagnostic or prognostic significance. The approach used is multivariate analysis, a technique of extracting information from the measurement of several variables, including the information contained in the relationship between them. Sometimes this latter information is a very small part of the total, sometimes the important information is contained entirely in the relationship between variables. The application of various multivariable statistical techniques may provide the intensive care staff with means for quantitative characterization of the nature of the specific system failures and their interactions. In addition, this quantitative information should furnish the input for appropriate statistical and other types of mathematical models by which the computer may assist the clinician in evaluating the probability that a given individual will move into a crisis situation. If such a condition can be corrected, the onset of crisis will be prevented. The ultimate goal of computerized monitoring systems is to predict problems before they occur, rather than to raise the alarm as difficulties arise.

The technology is available to carry out comprehensive patient monitoring, but despite this fact, advanced computerbased monitoring is confined to only a few places. In the places where such computer systems are in operation and function efficently, they were implemented by physicians who worked in this field for many years and had their primary interest in research. The reasons for the lack of widespread use of modern computer technology in critical care, or for that matter in medicine as a whole, are the insufficient knowledge and competence in this area, which lead to feelings of inadequacy. These feelings also seem to be the cause for the fears expressed by many physicians that they are losing control of their domain. Regardless of cause, when physicians do not utilize available technology, progress is inhibited. It is unlikely that new techniques will be put into operation unless the physician vigorously encourages their application. Physicians will not urge the use of the new systems unless they are personally convinced, through utilization, of safety and clinical usefulness. Thus, for the future there seem to be more problems with people than with technology. Current technologic advances in mathematics, engineering, electronics, and computer science are too rapid and too complex to be adapted to medicine without much additional training for physicians. Even though physicians can tell competent programmers what is wanted, they often lack the background and skill to provide crucial input and become creative collaborators. The current medical education does not produce the kind of physicians needed to apply and implement modern technology in critical care. If there is no change, the medical education may be a rate-limiting step in the realization of future that the inventors and researchers are planning. Physicians need more knowledge about the aspects of electronic instruments and computers that are relevant to medicine. Mathematics and physics must be given a greater place in the curricula of medical schools. At least one computer language course should be required, and formal courses in programming should be offered during the medical years. In my opinion, modern computer technology will enter medicine and will play an ever-increasing role in patient care in the years to come. If we do not acknowledge this fact and take steps to be prepared for this process, somebody else may take over our job. Thus, the challenge for the deans and faculties, of medical schools is to propose models and methods for initiating these changes. So far, medicine has not been taught or applied as a strictly quantitative science. The future will show if we can approach this goal.

References

Brunner J, Langenstein H, Wolff G (1983) Direct accurate gas flow measurement in the patient: compensation for unavoidable error. Med Progr Technol 9: 233

Cox JR Jr, Nolle FM, Fozzard HA et al. (1968) AZTEC, a pre-processing program for real time ECG rhythm analysis. IEEE Trans Biomed Eng 15: 128

Hjorth B (1970) EEG analysis based on time domain properties. Electroencephalog, Clin Neurophysiol 29: 206

Kouchoukos NT, Sheppard LC, McDonald DA et al. (1969) Estimation of stroke volume from the central arterial pressure contour in postoperative patients. Surg Forum 20: 180

Maas AHJ, Kreuger JA, Hoelen AJ et al. (1972) A computer program for calculating the acid base parameters in samples of blood using a minicomputer. Pflügers Arch 334: 264

Martin RW, Weil MH, Shubin H et al. (1973) Automated calibration of blood pressure signal conditioners. IEEE Trans Biomed Eng 20: 60

Myers RR, Stockard JJ, Fleming NJ et al. (1973) The use of on-line telephone computer analysis of the EEG in anaesthesia. Br J Anaesth 45: 664

Neff GW, Radke WA, Sambucetti CJ et al. (1970) A computer-assisted electrode system for measuring blood pH, PO_2, PCO_2, sodium and potassium. Clin Chem 16: 566

Osborn JJ (1975) Monitoring respiratory function. Crit Care Med 2: 217

Peters RM, Hilbermann M (1971) Respiratory insufficiency diagnosis and control of therapy. Surgery 70: 280

Sebel PS, Maynard DE, Major E et al. (1983) The cerebral function analysing monitor (CFAM). Br Anaesth 55: 1265

Siegel JH, Farell EJ (1973) A computer simulation model to study the clinical observability of ventilation and perfusion abnormalities in human shock states. Surgery 73: 898

Valbona C, Penny E, McMath F (1971) Computer analysis of blood gases and acid-base status. Comput Biomed Res 4: 623

Warner HR, Gardner RM, Toronto AF (1968) Computer based monitoring of cardiovascular functions in postoperative patients. Circulation (Suppl 2) 37: 68

Westenskow DR (1982) 4th Annual IEEE EMB Society Conference, Philadelphia

On-line Cardiovascular Applications of Microcomputers in Intensive Care

C. PRYS-ROBERTS

Introduction

Computer solutions to the processing of electrical signals derived from the cardiovascular system have been available for many years; however, minicomputers in the operating theatre or land-lines to main-frame computers have not been overwhelmingly successful except in those intensive care units dealing with a high turnover of patients requiring critical cardiovascular care (Sheppard et al. 1968). Microcomputers, despite some disadvantages, have the major advantage of size and portability, allied to speed of operation, and storage capabilities that are quite adequate for most of the functions required of them in the medical field.

Microprocessor systems are particularly valuable in critical care areas for the processing of physiological signals to provide information that cannot easily be derived by other means. This review will cover the application of microcomputers in the acquisition of signals derived from the cardiovascular systems of patients in critical care areas, and their processing to provide displays for medical and nursing staff. Because events in the cardiovascular system change on a beat-to-beat basis, most processing has to be done on the same basis, or in epochs of a few seconds, providing results at intervals of 30 s to 1 min. In this sense the demands on the microprocessor system are rather greater than those posed by signals related to pulmonary, renal or cerebrospinal function. Perhaps the greatest advance in the application of microprocessors is in the servocontrol of physiological variables such as arterial pressure or heart rate.

Although this subject is dealt with elsewhere in this symposium, certain aspects of cardiovascular control will be dealt with in this review.

Table 1 identifies those applications to be dealt with in this review.

Table 1. Cardiovascular signals suitable for computer processing

Electrocardiogram
Aterial pressure wave (central)
Pulmonary arterial pressure (balloon occluded pressure)
Echocardiogram
Pulsed Doppler aortovelogram
Thoracic impedance cardiogram

Signals Suitable for Computer Processing

Electrocardiogram

In the recovery room and intensive care unit two aspects of electrocardiographic interpretation are particularly amenable to microprocessor identification. Recognition of dysrhythmia is an important pattern recognition process for which there are numerous commercial software packages available. By contrast, the detection and quantification of ST-segment changes is less well served.

ST Segment Matrix Processing

Subendocardial ischemia is associated with depression of ST segments in the appropriate ventricular leads. Detection of such ventricular muscle ischemia can be enhanced by the use of a matrix of precordial leads each multiplexed by a microprocessor giving a sequential or programmed display of each lead. By suitable programming, the degree of ST segment depression in each sampled lead can be quantified and those leads showing predetermined degrees of depression (e. g., 1, 2 or >2mm) can be displayed on a VDU screen as a matrix map.

Arterial Pressure Wave

The arterial pressure wave is created by the interaction of the flow wave, generated by the left ventricular ejection of blood into the arterial system, and the impedance, which is the complex parameter which represents the combined inductance, capacitance and resistance of the arterial system to a pulsatile flow wave (Mc.Donald 1974). Thus the arterial pressure wave contains a wealth of information above and beyond the numerical values of systolic and diastolic pressures which are usually derived.

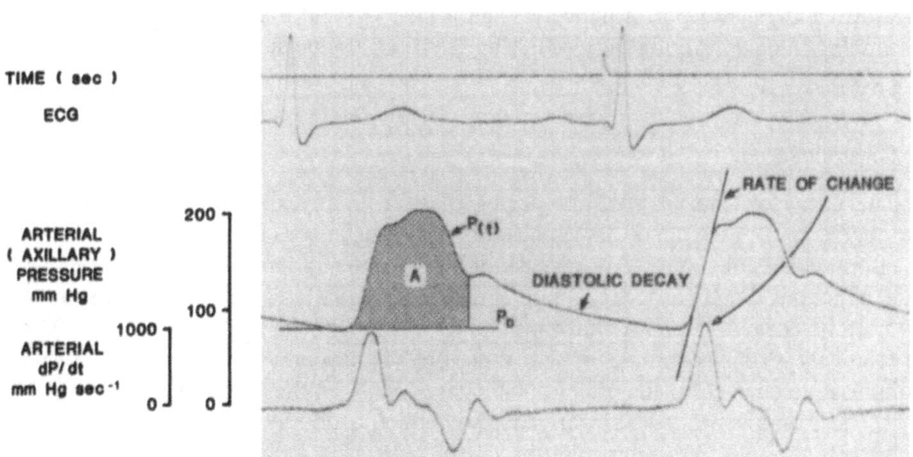

Fig. 1. Arterial pressure waves, showing the methods for deriving: area under the systolic ejection curve; rate of change of pressure (dP/dt); and exponential decrease of diastolic pressure. Prys-Roberts 1981

Derivation of Stroke Volume

The area under the systolic ejection curve of the central (aortic) pressure wave (Fig. 1) is proportional to the stroke volume which created the pulse wave (Prys-Roberts and Curnow 1982). However, the proportionality constant *(k)* in Eq. (1) is the reciprocal of the characteristic impedance (Z_0) of the arterial bed, in accordance with the Uniform Transmission Line theory:

$$\text{stroke volume} = \text{k} \times \text{area} = (1/Z_0)\,\text{area} \tag{1}$$

Numerous attempts have been made in the past to find a way to predict the value of Z_0 on the basis of mean arterial pressure, age, and other factors (Wesseling et al. 1974). This was the basis of a commercial instrument based on a hybrid analog/digital computer. The values for stroke volume and cardiac output produced by this system have been shown to be very accurate when changes of cardiac output were not associated with simultaneous changes of systemic vascular resistance (SVR). When changes of stroke volume and cardiac output accompany major changes of SVR, k in Eq. (1) changes, diminishing the strength of the correlation between the derived and true values of stroke volume. The microprocessor can easily be programmed to measure the areas under each pressure wave (Fig. 1), and these can be multiplied by a different value for k derived from the exponential decay of arterial pressure during diastole (see section below on diastolic decay). The method is valuable in that it can provide beat-by-beat information about stroke volume under conditions when rapid changes are occurring (Fig. 2). Simultaneous values of cardiac output by other methods (dye or thermodilution, Fick) can be used to scale the pressure-pulse values on an intermittent basis.

Arterial dP/dt

The rate of rise of pressure at the onset of the ejection phase of the central aortic pressure is directly correlated with the maximum LV dP/dt, and is a good index of ventricular muscle performance. While a beat-by-beat value can be derived by a simple analog differentiating circuit (Fig. 1), it can also be derived digitally as part of a package for processing the wave.

Diastolic Decay

The decay of arterial pressure during diastole is an exponential function which represents the product of the capacitance and resistance (CR) of the arterial system (Bourgeois et al. 1974). An increase of SVR causes an increase in the slope of the exponential diastolic decay, while a decrease of SVR causes a flattening of the diastolic decay. Assuming that the changes of capacitance in the arterial system are relatively small by comparision with those of SVR, the value of R from CR above can be used to correct for the effect of changes of SVR on the value of k in Eq. (1).

These on-line procedures were computed by a purpose built microcomputer based on a NASCOM Z80 8-bit microprocessor with a 64 Kbyte memory. The system incorporated a 4-channel 8-bit ADC and a 2-channel 8-bit DAC. The computer used a CP/M operating system and the programs were written in FORTRAN and assembler code.

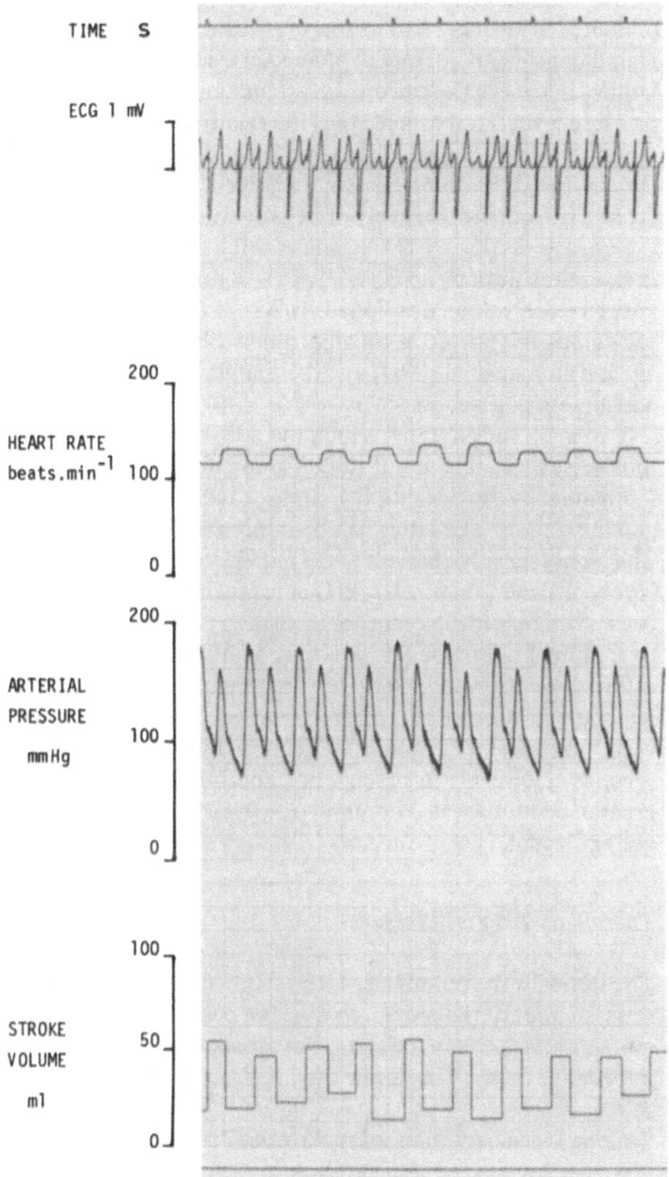

Fig. 2. Sequence of supraventricular dysrhythmia (coupled junctional extra-systoles), showing the ability of the stroke volume computer to derive stroke volumes from adjacent beats of disparate size. (Prys-Roberts and Curnow 1982)

On-line Control of Arterial Pressure

Several methods have been available for the automatic control of arterial pressure by computerised infusion of vasoactive drugs. Sheppard and his colleagues (1968) pioneered the application of PID control systems in the maintenance of arterial pressure following cardiac surgery. Others have used the same systems for the maintenance of deliberate hypotension using sodium nitroprusside (Low et al. 1983). Under many circumstances, the attainment and maintenance of the desired arterial pressure level is not urgent, thus the relatively slow attainment of the desired arterial pressure by a PID controller is no great disadvantage, and the stability of pressure control (MAP ± 1mmHg) is impressive. However, there are many patients whose arterial pressure is positively or negatively perturbed by factors outside the control of the anaesthesiologist. Under these conditions, a more rapid restoration of arterial pressure than can be achieved by PID control is desirable. Progressing from the non-adaptive controllers developed by Koivo (1980), our current preoccupation is with self-tuning adaptive control algorithms (Slate and Sheppard 1982; Arnsparger et al. 1983; Kaufman et al. 1984) and their application for induced hypotension for middle-ear surgery and neurosurgery.

Two main considerations limit the adequacy of control with a PID system, and are thus more amenable to self-tuning minimum variance control: firstly the sensitivity of the patient to the drug (SNP), and secondly the "dead-time" of the system for drug administration. The latter can be minimized by central venous infusion of the drug. The highly sensitive patient (>30 mmHg decrease of arterial pressure per ml-h-SNP) is very difficult to control by PID because of the large swings of arterial pressure which occur, whereas the average less sensitive patient (10 mmHg ml-h-) can be controlled to ± 1 mmHg. Provided there is time to allow the self-tuning system an initial low-gain estimation phase, in order to characterize the patient's response to SNP, the subsequent application of full minimum variance law enables the pressure to be controlled with a dead-beat response to achieve the desired arterial pressure within a few seconds. However, in practice we and others (Kaufman et al. 1984) have found a greater peak-to-peak variation of arterial pressure and especially the controlling voltage signal.

Pulmonary Arterial Pressure

Theoretically the pulmonary arterial pressure wave can be treated in the same way as the systemic arterial pressure wave, but because the pulmonary vasculature is so much more distensible than the systemic vasculature, much greater changes of characteristic impedance occur. This limits the application of the methodology described above.

Balloon Occluded Pulmonary Arterial Pressure

When the balloon-tipped pulmonary artery catheter is correctly positioned in a main branch of the right or left pulmonary artery, inflation of the balloon replaces the phasic pulmonary arterial pressure wave with a reflected wave from the left atrium which should show the characteristic A-C-V pattern. It is customary to identify and measure the "wedge" pressure at the end of the expiratory phase. For computer registration we have chosen to register a suitable epoch of the "wedged" pressure wave form, and to identify the appropriate point for measurement with a cursor. After such a registration, the user-friendly program reminds the operator to deflate the balloon. Failure to identify a subsequent phasic pressure wave triggers an alarm system.

The Sarnoff Diagram

The relationship between LV stroke work and LV end-diastolic pressure was emphasized by Sarnoff and Berglund (19) as the best representation, in the intact animal or man, of Starling's Law of the Heart. As the balloon occluded PA pressure, under most circumstances, accurately reflects the mean left atrial pressure, it is now customary to use a graphical representation of stroke work (or stroke volume) and PA wedge pressure as a means of plotting trends of LV performance (Barash et al. 1980). The microcomputer is ideal for producing a visual display of such sequential measurements. To achieve this, each time a registration of PA wedge pressure is made, a value for stroke work is calculated from the systemic arterial pressure and a measurement of cardiac output. The latter can be derived from thermodilution measurements if the appropriate thermistor-tipped catheter has been inserted. Alternatively cardiac output can be measured by dye-dilution (using the microprocessor to calculate the area under the curve and process the data), pulsed Doppler aortovelography, or thoracic impedance cardiography.

To emphasize the fallibility of using PA wedge pressure in lieu of measurements of left ventricular end-diastolic volume, the VDU display relates the Sarnoff diagram to the compliance curve for a normal and hypertrophic ventricle. Use of colour graphics on the BBC microcomputer makes this registration particularly impressive. Alternatively the envelopes for different ventricular function groups (Barash et al. 1980) can be superimposed.

Echocardiography

The main applications of echocardiography in critical care are: estimation of end-systolic and end-diastolic dimensions; derivation of ventricular ejection fraction; estimation of contractile element velocity; and measurement of aortic diameter

M-mode Echocardiography

Pulsed echo imaging of the heart and its chambers can yield useful information about ventricular function by a non-invasive method. In particular the time-position B-scan, commonly known as M-mode echocardiography, is amenable to microcomputer processing to yield specific dimensions and their rates of change.

The derivation of true ventricular ejection fraction requires estimation of the end-systolic and end-diastolic volumes. To achieve such values from single-plane echocardiography demands too many assumptions about left ventricular geometry (Linhart et al. 1975). Alternatively linear dimensions (end-systolic, D_S, and end-diastolic D_d, diameters) may be substituted to yield a value for shortening fraction (SF):

$$SF = D_D - D_S / D_D \qquad (2)$$

Microcomputers can be used to derive these dimensions from the continuously displayed M-mode echocardiogram, either by a cursor identification and registration procedure, or by a more complex pattern recognition or spectral edge detection algorithm.

The mean velocity of circumferential fiber shortening (V_{cf}), analogous to contractile element velocity in the isolated cardiac muscle preparation, can be derived by a further simple calculation:

$$V_{cf} = SF/LVET \tag{3}$$

Pulsed Doppler Aortovelography

A beam of ultrasound directed from the suprasternal notch toward the ascending aorta will be reflected by the blood moving toward the beam. The velocity v of the moving blood can be estimated from the Doppler frequency shift, FD between the incident and reflected beams:

$$f_D = 2v(\cos\theta) f/c \tag{4}$$

where θ is the angle between the moving reflector and the incident beam, f is the ultrasonic frequency of incident wave (usually 2 MHz) and c is the velocity of ultrasound in the appropriate medium.

If the incident beam is pulsed (as opposed to a continuous wave (Light and Cross 1972) it can be range gated in such a way that the velocity of the blood stream can be measured at a fixed and repeatable position in the aorta (Wells and Skidmore 1982). The analog signal representing the velocity of blood in the ascending aorta (Fig. 3) can be processed on-line by a microcomputer to yield the area under each velocity curve. If an estimate of aortic diameter has previously been obtained by M-mode echocardiography, the flow signal (velocity × aortic cross-sectional area) can be integrated to give beat-by-beat estimate of stroke volume. In this respect the role of the microcomputer is simply to perform repeated rapid calculations, and provide a display of the results either on a VDU or as a reprocessed analog signal. At present, the deficiencies of this non-invasive method are less to do with the computer processing than the problems of ensuring consistent alignment of the incident ultrasonic beam.

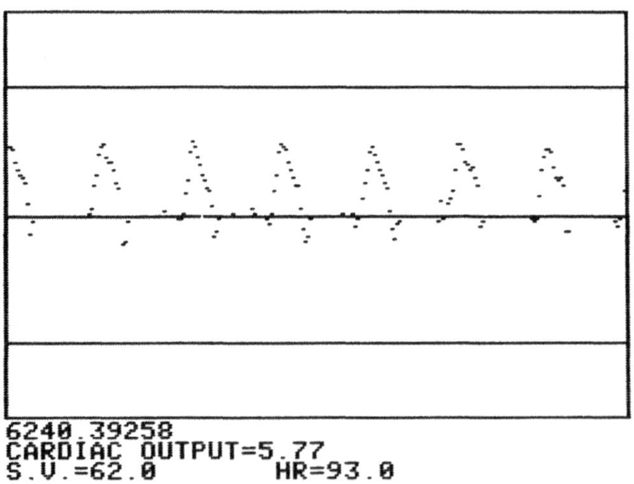

Fig. 3. Microprocessor computer screen showing aortic velocity signals for seven heart beats derived by A–D conversion. Stroke volume was derived by integration of each waveform, and multiplication by the aortic cross-sectional area derived from a previous B-scan image of the aorta

In addition to the stroke volume, the aortic velocity signal can be differentiated to yield the accèleration of blood in the aorta, an index of left ventricular performance (Noble et al. 1973). While this latter derivation can be achieved by a simple analog differentiation circuit, the use of digital filtering enables a rather cleaner acceleration signal to be achieved. A limitation of the pulsed Doppler method is that the maximum velocity which can be measured is determined by the pulse-repetition frequency, or Nyquist effect. This effect may limit the accuracy of acceleration derived by differentiation, especially at high values associated with sympathetic nervous overactivity.

Thoracic Impedance Cardiography

If a constant current (4 mA rms at 100 kHz) is applied across four disposable Mylar strip electrodes, two of which are applied around the neck and the other two around the lower thorax, the electrical impedance across the thoracic cage varies in a pulsatile manner with a characteristic waveform. Kubicek et al. (1974) described an equation which related the stroke volume of the left ventricle, SV, to the change of impedance, dZ/dt, the ejection time, T, and a constant relating the blood resistivity, P, the mean thoracic impedance Z_0 and the distance L between the upper and lower electrodes:

$$SV = \varrho \, (L/Z_0)^2 \, T(dZ/dt)_{max} \tag{5}$$

Values of stroke volume can be derived continuously from the impedance signal by a microcomputer, and these can be useful as a means of cardiovascular trend recording in the ICU (Bleicher 1982). However, credence can be given to the results only when they are scaled against values derived by methods which give better absolute accuracy (Mohaptra 1981). The greatest problem with this method is the interbeat variation. Chilcoat and colleagues (Mapleson et al. 1977) found that the standard Kubicek equation gave results which varied from 51% to 196% of the correct value, and introduced the possibility of applying correction factors to decrease the interbeat variation, a task as well suited to on-line processing by a microcomputer. Based on an analysis of the impedance waveform they derived an expression for SV as calculated above:

$$SV \propto P^{2.05} T_W{}^{1.25} A_W{}^{-1.25} A_N{}^{0.4}$$

This expression (based on amplitudes P, times T and areas A associated with the impedance waveform) decreased the variability of the measured stroke volume to 17%.

References

Arnsparger JM, McInnis BC, Glover JR, Normann NA (1983) Adaptive control of blood pressure. IEEE Trans Biomed Eng 30: 168–176

Barash P, Chen Y, Kitahata LM, Kopriva CJ (1980) The hemodynamic tracking system: A method of data mangagement and guide for cardiovascular therapy. Anesth Analg 59: 169–174

Bleicher W (1982) Possibilities and limitations of thoracic impedance cardiography. In: Prys-Roberts C, Vickers MD (eds) Cardiovascular measurement in anaesthesiology. Springer, Berlin Heidelberg New York

Bourgeois MJ, Gilbert BK, Donald DW, Wood EH (1974) Characteristics of aortic diastolic pressure decay application to the continuous monitoring of changes in peripheral vascular resistance. Circ Res 35: 55–66
Kaufman H, Roy R, Xu X (1984) Model reference adaptive control of drug infusion rate. Automatica 20: 205–209
Koivo AJ (1980) Automatic continuous-time blood pressure control in dogs by means of hypotensive drug injection. IEEE Trans Biomed Eng 27: 574–581
Kubicek WG, Kottke FJ, Ramous MU, et al. (1974) The Minnesota impedance cardiograph – theory and applications. Biomed Eng 9: 410–416
Light H, Cross G (1972) Cardiovascular data by transcutaneous aortovelography. In: Roberts C (ed) Blood flow measurements. Sector, London, pp 60–60
Linhart JW, Mintz GS, Segal BL, et al. (1975) Left ventricular volume measurements of echocardiography. Am J Cardiol 36: 114–118
Low JM, Hutton P, Curnow JSH, Millard RK, Prys-Roberts C (1983) Induced hypotension by servo-control of sodium nitroprusside infusion. Br J Anaesth 44: 219
Mapleson WW, Chilcoat RT, Blewett MC, Lunn JN (1977) Analysis of the thoracic impedance waveform for estimation of cardiac output. Br J Anaesth 49: 185
McDonald DA (1974) Blood flow in arteries, 2nd ed. Arnold, London
Mohapatra SN (1981) Non-invasive cardiovascular monitoring by electrical impedance technique. Pitman, Bath
Noble MIM, Trenchard D, Guz A (1973) Left ventricular ejection in conscious dogs. 1. Measurement and significance of the maximum acceleration of blood from the left ventricle. Circ Res 19: 139–147
Prys-Roberts C (1981) Cardiovascular monitoring in patients with vascular disease. Br J Anaesth 53: 767–776
Prys-Roberts C, Curnow JSH (1982) Direct measurement of arterial pressure and derived variables. In: Prys-Roberts C, Vickers MD (eds) Cardiovascular measurement in anaesthesiology. Springer, Berlin
Sarnoff SJ, Berglund E (1944) Ventricular function 1. Starling's law of the heart studied by means of simultaneous right and left ventricular function curves in the dog. Circulation 9: 706–713
Sheppard LC, Kouchoukos NT, Kurtts MA, Kirklin JW (1968) Automated treatment of critically ill patients following operation. Ann Surg 168: 596–600
Slate JB, Sheppard LC (1982) Automatic control of blood pressure by drug infusion. IEEE Proc 129: 639–645
Wells PNT, Skidmore R (1982) Physical principles of ultrasonics in cardiovascular measurements. In: Prys-Roberts C, Vickers MD (eds) Cardiovascular measurement anaesthesiology. Springer, Berlin
Wesseling KH, Purschke R, Smith NT, et al. (1974) A beat-to-beat cardiac output computer for clinical monitoring. In: Payne JP, Hill DW (eds) Real time computing in patient management. Peregrinus, Stevenage
Westenskow DR, Meline LJ, Pace NL, Bodily NM (1984) Sodium nitroprusside induced hypotension with computer adjustment for varying drug sensitivity. Anesth Analg 63: 281

Organizing and Analyzing Clinical Information Using Table-Based, Graphics-Oriented, Interactive Computer Systems

B. J. RANSIL

Introduction

In the late 1960s, in response to a widely perceived need, there began to develop in the United States a specialized class of computer system which would enable computer-naive clinicians and investigators to organize and analyze data without large investments in computer hardware, software and of personal time. One focus of such activity was the Division of Research Resources of the National Institutes of Health (NIH) under whose auspices this system concept has evolved over the past decade into three operating systems, PROPHET, CLINFO and ANALYZER.

PROPHET is a national shared-timed, DEC PDP10-based national computer resource sponsored by DRR, NIH, under development since 1970 by Bolt, Beranek and Newman (BBN), Cambridge, MA. It includes over 40 sites across the United States organized as a telephone network system. CLINFO, a DEC PDP11 or VAX-based distributed system, sponsored by the Clinical Research Centers program, DRR, NIH, originated by Rand Corporation, but now also under development by BBN, is in use at a number of Clinical Research Centers (CRC) in the United States. ANALYZER, an HP9845-based system designed by the author, and serving the research community at the Beth Israel Hospital, Boston, MA, has been envolving since 1966 on successive generations of Hewlett-Packard (HP) desktop computers, supported by the Clinical Research Center Program of the DRR, NIH.

Design Features

The three systems share several design features in varying degrees:
1. A table file structure for organizing and analyzing data.
2. Simplicity of operation ("friendliness").
3. An interactive operating mode that makes extensive use of graphics.

Of the three, the PROPHET system is the most highly developed, the most versatile, flexible and powerful tool for the extraction of information implicit in a data base. Hence, in this communication we will focus on the PROPHET system as the paradigm of these tablebased, graphics oriented, interactive computer systems which are quietly revolutionizing the way those who use them to organize and analyze data.

Exploitation of the table as a system design feature did not originate with, nor is it unique to, these three systems. OMNITAB (Hilsenrath et al. 1966) began development in 1956 at the National Bureau of Standards; Minitab (Ryan et al. 1980) currently has many enthusiastic users in the U.S. and many commercial software packages of relatively recent design in the U.S. exploit the table in one form or another. But PROPHET (Raub 1972; Castleman et al. 1974; Ransil 1974) is the only system which has taken the analytic power implicit in the table structure, developed it to the greatest extent of any contemporary system, and incorporated it into an operating system with the following properties:

1. Low hardware profile with minimal on-site system overhead and management.
2. Easy to learn and use; activated by unambiguous, terse English commands which generate interactive dialogues and menus of items from which the user makes a selection by typing or pointing.
3. Extensive use of graphics so that one may visualize every step along the analytical pathway.
4. Preprogrammed; analysis performed by calling appropriate commands in appropriate sequences.
5. Camera-ready hard copy of suitable quality for slides and submission to journals.
6. Interactive and batch modes of operation.
7. Multiple levels of communicating.

PROPHET derives its organizational and analytic power from two design features; its highly developed and versatile table structure, and multiple levels of communication which activate a comprehensive mathematical/statistical library. We consider each of these in turn.

PROPHET Table Structure

The PROPHET table is organized by numbered row and column, each of which can also be identified by a "Row Name" and "Column Heading". The data to be analyzed is identified by the table name and the appropriate row or column numbers, or by the column heading. The PROPHET table may also carry a title (for identification purposes) and text footnotes.

Each column of a named PROPHET table may contain one of several possible data types: numerial data, text, descriptor characters, graphs and molecules. A single table can therefore contain a wide variety of information relating to a patient or research project, providing an extremely powerful format for organizing and correlating data, and detecting patterns.

Data processing and analysis is accomplished on PROPHET by typing the desired command, and specifying the table name and respective columns (or rows) upon which it is to operate. This may be accomplished in a single sentence, or by the initiation of an interactive dialogue which, if the operation is complex, like graph editing, may involve menus. Numerial data is operated on by an extensive library of mathematical and of univariate and multivariate, parametric and nonparametric statistical programs. Nominal (text) data and descriptors can be sorted and analyzed by frequency analysis. Graphs and molecules may be stored in a table for economy and retrieval convenience.

Once numerical data is stored in a PROPHET table, columns containing numerical data may be algebraically combined to yield a derived column. The derivation can be anything from a simple arithmetical operation or transform (log, exponential, sin, cos etc.) to complex derivations involving multiple mathematical operations and columns. It will be realized that a derived column in PROPHET, is the equivalent of a program in any other data analysis system. The significant difference here is that to construct a derived column in PROPHET, the computer-naive user need know only the mathematics of his field and how to write an algebraic statement. He does not need to employ a programming language, and the I/0 is automatically handled by the table format.

The derived column concept receives further generalization in PROPHET in the form of the table transform. The simplest transform is the row-column transpose wherein rows and columns are interchanged. The transform command converts all numerial data (X) in a table to some specified function of X, $X \rightarrow f(X)$, where $f(X)$ can be the algebraic statement for percentages, differences, ratios, or any closed-form algebraic function or equation yielding finite, real values.

Once tables are made by the MAKE TABLE command they are readily edited and manipulated by a variety of ADD, DELETE, INSERT, FILLIN, CLEAR, ENTER and EDIT commands. Subtables are readily made from existing tables by variations of the MAKE TABLE command employing "qualifier" phrases which select the desired subset of columns and rows. The same qualifier phrases may also be used with any other command to operate on selected columns and rows rather than the entire table.

The PROPHET graph is not a separate structure but a graphical image produced from three stored tables each time it is displayed. These tables (called AXES OF Graph-Name, CURVES OF Graph-Name and POINTS OF Graph-Name) can be edited and manipulated like any other table using appropriate table commands, to give the investigator complete control over all the cosmetic features of his graph. The EDIT GRAPH command incorporates this process into one rapid, interactive, highly visual operation employing menus and a light pen or keyboard entries.

Level of Communication

The user may communicate with PROPHET at several levels. Most of the system features can be activated and implemented at "top level", that is, by a simple English command. Should the user wish to employ any of these commands in a custom-designed program, he may incorporate them into a procedure using PL/PROPHET, a programming language based on PL/1. Or he may write conventional programs, employing PROPHET table I/0 and any language that is compatible with the PDP10 monitor. Thus, even though this class of analytical instrument is designed with the computer-naive user in mind, the computer-sophisticate soon discovers it to be an instrument that challenges his computer science and analytical skills while producing an n-fold increase in analytical productivity over other system designs.

The Interactive Dialogue

When the prototype development of ANALYZER began in 1966, and of PROPHET in the late 1960s, interactive dialogue was a design feature much discussed, but generally unavailable in commercial software or in standard data analysis software packages available at the time. However, it has recently come into its own with the development of the home and personal computer (PC) market. As many naive computer purchasers have learned to their chagrin, hardware doesn't work without software. And manufacturers for the home market have learned that neither hardware nor software will sell unless the products are designed to meet the needs of computer-naive users. Consequently, designers of contemporary PC systems are learning, as the designers of PROPHET and ANALYZER did a decade and more ago, that system „friendliness" in its complete sense, interactive dialogue, menus, visualization by computer graphics and the use of "pointing" or other locating devices are obligatory rather than optional features in the design of contemporary computer systems.

Impact of Design on Data Analysis

While the interactive dialogue, in the form of a logical progression of questions answered by a yes *(Y)*, no *(NO)*, a number, or a word from a menu, found natural application in making PROPHET tables, graphs and molecules, a major advance in statistical analysis was made when the technique was applied to statistical operations such as testing distribution properties computing complete descriptive statistics profiles, comparing samples, and performing complete regression analysis.

Because column-organized data is a congenial and heuristic format for data analysis, it was realized in the early days of ANALYZER that the output of descriptive statistics would benefit from the same structured format; and further, that because the computer could quickly calculate the approximately 20 measures associated with a normal distribution, that any or all of these could be obtained with the use of an interactive menu. In this manner the STATS command, which computes up two twenty measures associated with a normal distribution, was conceived and developed in the late 1960s on the author's desktop calculators in the Clinical Research Center at the Boston City Hospital, and later incorporated in an amplified form on PROPHET.

Very soon the same thinking was applied to the complex and (for most nonstatistically trained analysts) perplexing task of comparing samples (distribution comparison). It was evident that the comparison process could be reduced to a decision tree and implemented by a suitable interactive quiz requiring the user to response yes *(Y)*, no *(N)* or undecided *(U)*, or with specific information concerning the distribution properties of the data and the experimental design. In this manner the interactive dialogue COMPARE (for comparing 1, 2 and multiple samples) was born on PROPHET in the middle 1970s and, as "compare 2" and "compare *n*", reincarnated on ANALYZER in 1980.

PROPHET Features

Once the prototype of a table-based, interactive, graphics oriented system was operational and being used by scientists representing a wide variety of disciplines, the requirements of data analysis and user needs converged to suggest the design and development of other analytical tools which would operate in the same mode. This user-driven impetus has, over the past 12 years produced an extensive set of interactive mathematical, analytical and graphical tools with which clinician or researcher can now explore his data and extract information to a degree never before possible in so brief a time. These analytical tools include:

1. *Basic structures and operations*

Tables	Digitizing
Plots in 2 and 3 dimensions	Text editing
Molecules: stick and space filled	Data base management

2. *Statistical operations*

STATS (20 measures associated with statistical distributions)
Testing for normality and other distribution types
Comparing samples (parametric and non-parametric), 2-sample and multi-sample
Analysis of variance with multiple designs
Access to BMDP, a statistical package from UCLA (Dixon and Brown)

3. *Other*

Protein, DNA, RNA sequencing
Fitting functions and modeling with MLAB (Knott)
Pharmacokinetics
CELLISM, simulating cell populations and their behavior under specified conditions (Donaghey)
HUMAN, physiological modeling (Coleman)
Making molecules and molecular manipulations

Documentation

The PROPHET documentation for users is extensive. It consists of multiple indexed loose leaf volumes with subject tabs and marginal locators. The manuals include:
1. User Manual
2. Statistics Manual
3. Mathematical Procedures
4. Programming Manual
5. Molecules Manual
6. PROPHET Primer
7. Miscellaneous manuals (BMDP, MLAB, CELLISM, HUMAN)

Conclusion

Until recently clinicians and researchers have been constrained by the lack of adequate computing tools to confine themselves to the simplest (that is, the most easily calculated) data analysis operations and therefore, to the simplest experimental designs. The advent of the modern high speed computer thirty years ago heralded the dawn of a new age which today is being realized in terms of easily operated, easily maintained computer systems with the capacity for solving most data analysis problems encountered in clinical and research medicine. Armed with this new computing power, the clinician and researcher can employ more efficient experimental designs, analyze his data with optimal methodologies and bring much greater rigor to the fitting and modeling of his data. With the design and development of the type of system described in this brief overview, the bottleneck in data analysis is no longer computer power but how proficient the user is in the mathematics of his field, and the limitations of the mathematical and statistical methodologies themselves.

Postcript. Further information about PROPHET can be obtained from PROPHET Project Officer, Chemical-Biological Information Handling Program, Division of Research Resources, National Institutes of Health, Bethesda, MD. 20014

ANALYZER'S software is modeled after PROPHET, and offers the user a selected subset of its functions. It is a prototype of PROPHET as a laboratory and personal computer. Further information can be obtained from the author.

References

Castleman PA, Russel CH, Webb FN, Hollister CA, Siegel JR, Zdonik SR, and Fram DM (1974) The implementation of the PROPHET System, AFIPS Conf Proc43: 457–468

Coleman TG HUMAN: A mathematical model of the human body in health, disease and during treatment. University of Mississippi Medical Center, 2500 North State St., Jackson, MO, 39216, USA

Dixon WJ, Brown MB BMDP biomedical computer programs. Health Sciences Computing Facility, U. of California, Los Angeles, CA 90024, USA

Donaghey C CELLSIM: Computer simulation of cell kinetics models. Industrial Engineering Dept., University of Houston, Houston, TX, USA

Hilsenrath J, Ziegler GG, Messina CG, Walsh PJ, Herbold RJ (1966) OMNITAB: A computer program for statistical and numerical analysis. National Bureau of Standards Handbook 101. U.S. Government Printing Office, Washington, D.C.

Knott G MLAB: An on-line modeling laboratory. Division of Computer Research and Technology, National Institutes of Health, Bethesda, MD 20205, USA

Ransil BJ (1974) Use of table file structures in a clinical research center. Proc Fed Am Soc Exp Biol 33: 2384–2387

Raub WF (1972) The role of specialized data structures in computerbased management, analysis, and communication of pharmacological information. Fourth International Biophysics Conference, Moscow

Ryan TA Jr, Jolner BL, Ryan BF (1980) Minitab reference manual. Minitab Project, Pennsylvania State University, University Park, PA 16802.

An Attempt to Solve the "Information Explosion" in an Intensive Care Ward

D. J. PRICE, J. MASON, and S. SNOWDEN

In the last decade we have seen an increase in the volume of data generated by electronic monitors, ventilators, the laboratory and in particular the nurses in their recording of observations and therapeutic interventions. The number of parameters recorded in our own primarily neurosurgical intensive care ward has increased in those 10 years from 20 to 65. The time taken to record this data set has increased proportionately; and the nurses admit that both their clerical and mathematical duties distract their attention from direct patient care.

With the advent of "intelligent" monitors capable of sampling a signal and displaying derived variables every few seconds, the nurses are bombarded with even more information. They can often only resolve that particular dilemma by reading and recording a sample every 15 or 30 min and they usually do not even attempt to average that signal during such a time epoch. As our data set increased, so did the size and number of bedside charts, but no more than 8 of the 65 parameters could ever be displayed on one chart alone and even then, cross correlation was made difficult by the necessity to use differing time scales. The remaining data were recorded as a matrix of numbers from which trend recognition was very difficult.

Automated data acquisition from bedside monitors has unfortunately generated too much information. If a trending capability of these monitors is used, this merely diverts the nurses' attention from their main data displays on their comprehensive bedside charts and many people would admit that this represents a retrograde step. Computers are ideally suited for data compression by averaging and trend displays do become more meaningful with this simple signal smoothing.

Some 8 years ago, we first attempted to display this smoothed signal at the bedside and found that a 15-s averaging epoch for intracranial pressure was very satisfactory for showing events over the last 2 or 3 h, although it was only necessary to store long-term archiving averages, standard deviations, and pulse wave information (related to intracranial compliance) for 15-min epochs. We soon found that the display of a physiological signal on its own was meaningless unless we could also display with it information about those drugs and factors influencing that signal (Fig. 1).

Automated data acquisition and averaging of physiological signals has now been well established and is perhaps the easiest problem in intensive care computing. However, unless these data are integrated with all those derived directly from the nurses in their recording of oberservations about the patients and their therapeutic interventions, then this results in each patient having two divergent data bases (automated and manual).

ICP MONITORING SYSTEM --- 24-HOUR DATA SUMMARY

PATIENT NAME............CAROL F
DATE.... 24 HOURS TO 0800 9/ 7/ 82

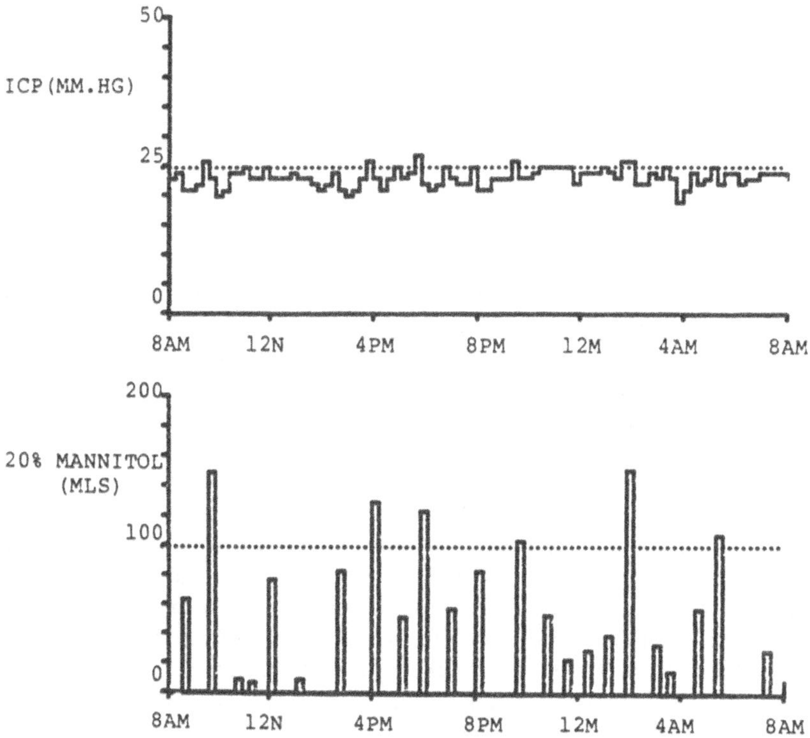

ICP ABOVE 25MM.HG FOR 1.5 HOURS
ICP ABOVE 30MM.HG FOR 0.0 HOURS
ICP ABOVE 35MM.HG FOR 0.0 HOURS

TOTAL 24 HOUR MANNITOL DOSE = 1524MLS

Fig. 1. A printout of intracranial pressure and the dosages of mannitol used to control it

The Bedside Chart

A high proportion of the nurses' time and effort is spent controlling the bedside "data explosion" by transferring and reviewing information from the bedside and laboratory and charting it in numerical or analogue form for subsequent evaluation of short- and long-term trends, interparameter cross correlations and simple mathematics to generate derived variables. The normal bedside chart record may contain all the information required but updating it is tedious and trend recognition is usually restricted to no more than 10% of the parameters. Most clinical decisions and management instructions are made at the bedside and recorded on the chart.

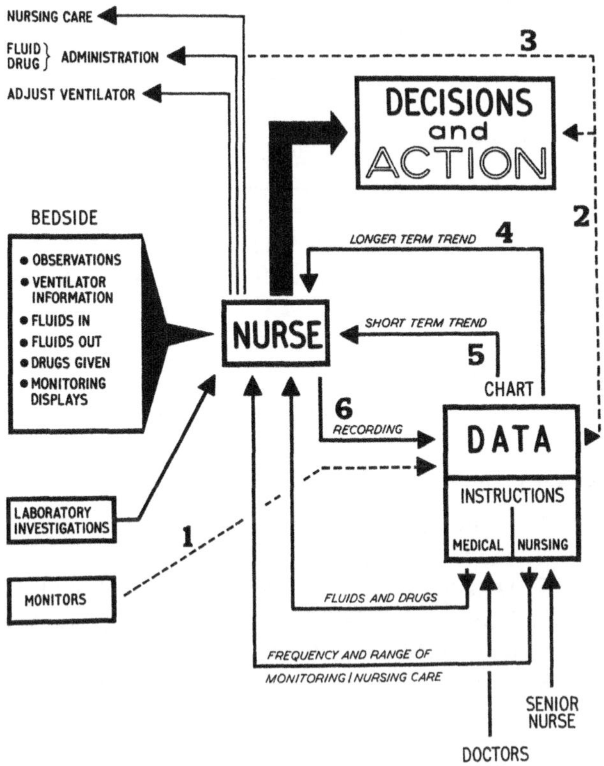

Fig. 2. The simplified flow chart emphasises the nurses' central involvement and the lines 4, 5 and 6 represent conventional data transfers. If a chart is replaced by a computer system, lines 1, 2 and 3 indicate the possibility of effort-saving activity enhancements or even replacements

The simplified flow chart (Fig. 2) emphasises the nurses' central involvement and the lines 4, 5 and 6 represent conventional data transfers. If a chart is replaced by a computer system, lines 1, 2 and 3 indicate the possibility of effort-saving activity enhancements or even replacements.

On reviewing 65 parameters recorded in our own intensive care unit, we found that only a maximum of 10 could be collected automatically by on-line data processing and the remainder could only be logged manually. The nurses would not tolerate two data bases or a transfer of derived data from the monitors to a chart and they would only accept a concept of having their records all manually charted or all recorded on to a computer system. We considered that the only way we could include the bulk of the data originating from the nurses was to design a data input terminal for the bedside.

A Computerised System

After several unsuccessful attempts to produce a bedside terminal which would break through the "prototype barrier" and become an indispensable replacement to the conventional chart, our nurses provided a list of their minimum requirements. By now, by rather bitter experience, they knew exactly what they needed but the list was formidably demanding and necessitated a complete hardware and software redesign and a replacement of the ward minicomputer which would provide longer term database management. Their requirements are listed below:

A. Function

1. To merge all the data generated from whatever source to a single data base which would replace the bedside monitoring chart.
2. Full entry and retrieval facilities should be available at all the beds.
3. All the tedious calculations of derived variables should be delegated to the system.

B. Appearance

4. Bedside equipment should be neat, unobtrusive and waterproof.

C. Data input

5. A new nurse should find it much easier to use the system than the conventional handwritten chart.
6. Data logging should take less than half the time of that of a manual system.
7. Parameter visual displays should be updated during manual input for immediate trend recognition.
8. Event logging, retrograde data input and correction facilities should be simple to use.
9. Both range and intelligent input validation are essential features.

D. Display

10. Recent data should be visualised both graphically and digitally for display of short-term trends.
11. Longer term trends with multiparameter graphic correlations require the use of colour.
12. Graphic printers for hard copy summaries should be of good quality and should not be heard in the ward.

E. Data storage

13. Data protection with duplicate storage and uninterruptible power supplies is mandatory.
14. Inexpensive and easily accessible longer term storage is necessary for research purposes.

The time-saving demands alone excluded the use of a conventional ASCI keyboard with menu-driven software as data-logging time then becomes greater than that for a handwritten chart. This may well explain why virtually all commercially available systems have failed in most countries as the nurses quite rightly insist that any new system should relieve them of these more tedious duties.

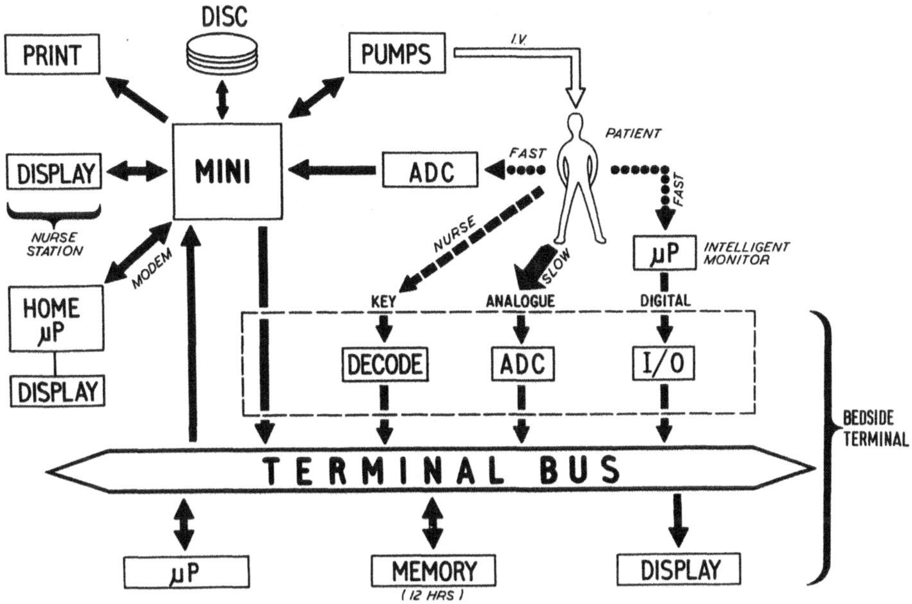

Fig. 3. A diagrammatic representation of the four data pathways from the patient and the integration of the data bases held at the bedside and in the ward minicomputers

The Bedside Terminal

Some 4 years ago we created a team of physicists, nurses, ergonomists, anaesthetists and neurosurgeons to design a bedside data input and trend display device. The prototype bedside terminal was designed around an "Acorn" microprocessor with 8 k of RAM (Fig. 3). The software is written in 6502 machine code and is stored in 12 k of EPROM. A single touch of any of the dedicated parameter buttons of the membrane keyboard display a histogram trend graph of the last 12 h of that parameter, with the last recording also shown in digital form. Displayed data may be updated with new observations or measurements and a new detailed numerical review of the graph is accessed by using a horizontal scanning cursor. The cursor position is identified in real time on the display and allows for retrospective input of laboratory data and correction.

The results and calculations of derived variables are displayed in the same format as the raw data accessed either manually or automatically from the monitors and provide such information as running fluid balances and hourly electrolyte inputs which are too tedious to calculate manually. In addition to the histogram trend graphs, fluid balances for the last 24 h are presented in tabular form.

Data from the bedside terminal are transmitted every 15 min to the ward PDP 11/23 minicomputer running under the RSX 11M operating system. This host computer with its uninterruptible power supply and Winchester disc provides data security, more complex calculation for closed-loop algorithms and archiving. The complete data base on each patient will be stored on the disc to provide immediate availability as a colour display for cross-parameter correlations at the nurses' station or slaved to the Mennon bedside terminals.

The prototype has now been fully tested and it meets all the essential requirements of the nursing and medical staff. The only real proof as to whether we will succeed in controlling the data explosion at the bedside will be when we can show that it has been in use at each of the seven beds in the ward consistently for a year with the nurses wishing to use this system only, in preference to the manual charts.

Towards a Coherent Structure of the Anesthetist – computer Interface

S. Trispel, H. Klocke, G. Rau, and R. Schlimgen

Introduction

The challenge of creating an anesthesia monitoring and information system which is both efficient and manageable for the anesthesiologist led us to develop an Anesthesia Information System (AIS). This system is operational in the laboratory of our "ergonomics in medicine" research group. The emphasis of the continuing development work is on the design and improvement of the human-computer interface. Fig. 1 schematically shows the work environment of the anesthesiologist using our touch-sensitive AIS monitor. The monitor displays all diagnostic and therapeutic data gathered during the operation (organized in "pages") as well as "virtual control elements", such as keys and sliders for data input, data retrieval, and system control procedures. For extensive numeric data input tasks, such as recording blood transfusion data, we provide a bar code reading device (reader in Fig. 1), although there also exists a manual mode whereby this data may be entered with the help of a numeric keyboard displayed on the monitor screen.

The purpose of this paper is to discuss the fundamental considerations that led to the design of the anesthetist-AIS interface and to describe some of its basic features.

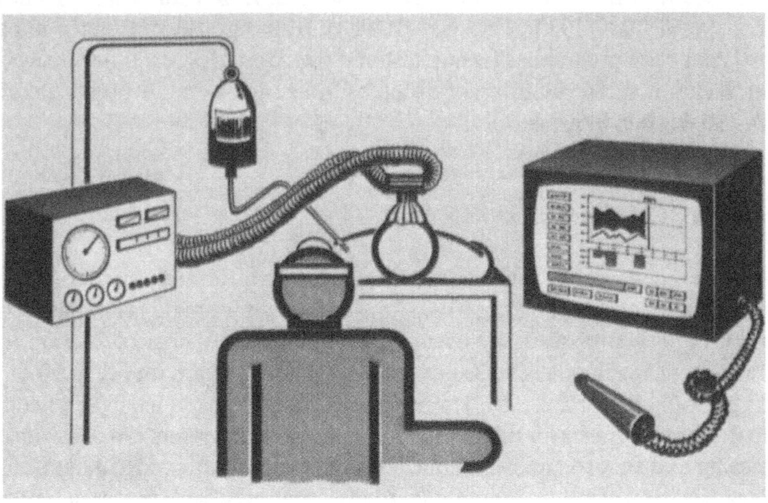

Fig. 1. The AIS work station environment

Prior to the evaluation of the system in the operating room we are presently testing the AIS in the laboratory with a special operation simulation technique which opens up new perspectives as a side-effect.

The Anesthetist-Computer Interface

"Whenever the anesthesia work place is discussed, someone draws an analogy to an airplane cockpit" (Gravenstein 1980). The complexity of the anesthesiologist's task in the operating room has found increased recognition by those researchers and developers who have created computerized data acquisition, processing, display, and/or recording systems (Zollinger et al. 1977; Mitchell 1982a; Meigler et al. 1983; Bender et al. 1983; Ream et al. 1983) or integrated gas delivery and monitoring systems (Newbower et al. 1981; Anthony 1982) within the past 10 years. Whereas in the case of cockpit instrumentation design much effort and money is spent on the human engineering side (as in the case of the new Airbus A310, to give an example), little is done for the anesthesiologist's "cockpit." This in spite of the fact that the mission called "anesthesia" is hazardous and demanding, that decision-making processes take place under time constraints and psychological stress, and that uncertainty in respect of a multitude of variables is ever-present (measurement reliability, patient state predictability, medical knowledge and experience, instrument control).

Contrary to the airplane pilot, the anesthesiologist primarily has his hands and eyes on the patient – a human being – and not machinery. This is why the installation of computerized data processing equipment in the operating room nowadays tends to create additional work unless the new equipment renders old procedures obsolete and provides new decision-making support. The design of new kinds of anesthetist-computer interfaces is one of the approaches to tackle this problem. In recent years the human factors issue has gained more weight in the general discussion (Mitchell 1982b; Arnell and Schulz 1983; Saunders and Jewett 1983) and through special data input technique developments (speech recognition (Sarnat 1983), keypad (Apple et al. 1982), graphics tablet (Cooper et al. 1982), and our own AIS development (Trispel et al. 1982, 1983; Klocke et al. 1984). By integrating the data input and output interface between the anesthesiologist and the computer, as in our AIS concept, the simplification and structuring of different tasks such as monitoring, record keeping, and system control is possible.

What is a "Coherent Structure"?

The term "coherency" suggests attributes like conformity, similarity, consistency, simplicity, reliability, and the like. Confronted with a single monitor interface to the computer (as in our case), the user expects to locate and inspect relevant information with ease and to handle data input and control functions without "further thinking." This can only be achieved by designing self-explaining and user guidance capabilities into the system. The user understands and accepts the system if it consistently exhibits the same and easy to grasp dynamic behavior (among other attributes like reliability, relevance, etc.). In this sense a coherently structured interface to a complex system will mediate a special purpose machine to the user instead of a universal, "everything-can-be-done" system.

In other words: although it is now possible to make everything appear on the screen (trends, tables, input keys, messages, alarms – in all shapes, sizes, colors, and dynamics) it is wise from an ergonomic design point of view to step back, analyze the work and task situation thoroughly, and implement basic information presentation modes as well as basic interaction modes, of which both support the notion of a sophisticated machine. One of the greater problems is the functional expansion of the system without violating the once formulated basic definitions in respect to the user interface. Therefore a sound, task-related interface design is necessary to achieve the coherency wanted by the system user.

In this context it is of interest to reflect on how the user perceives the hierarchy of system attributes.

System attributes as perceived at the user interface:	*Cognitive perception of:*
Graphical appearance	Appearance
Allocation of information to "pages"	Structure
Availability of virtual control elements	Functionality
Purpose and functions of control elements	Control
Dynamics of the system	Behavior
Intelligence quotient (IQ) of the system	Power

At the monitor screen the system should match these cognitive levels. Frustration with computer systems often results from ill-designed interfacing to the user; for examples: system CONTROL may be difficult to understand, system BEHAVIOR may sometimes be unpredictable, and worst of all, the POWER of the system (what can it do for me?) may be overestimated.

The design of the user interface must take all cognitive levels into consideration, starting from the expected power of the system down to its structure and its appearance. Furthermore, it is helpful to separate four logical planes at the monitor interface as depicted in Fig. 2: The process plane, where all automatically measured data from the process (patient, on-line laboratory) appear in a type of "window"; the interactive data plane, where all user-generated data appear; the virtual control elements plane, where data input and system control elements are displayed and the touch frames plane, which contains the touch-sensitive areas individually for each page of the AIS. Of course, the four planes merge within the display.

Summing up, a coherent structure of the anesthetist-computer interface is one of the important design issues in respect of the acceptance of the system by the user – the interface should support the cognitive perception of preferably all of the six above-mentioned system attribute levels.

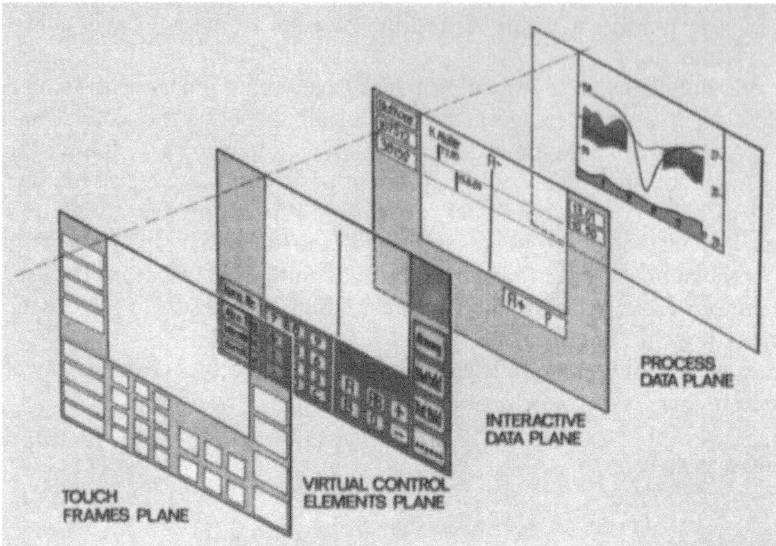

Fig. 2. The "logical planes" of an AIS screen page

Data Input and Output Integration

The step from pure monitoring (data acquisition, preprocessing, and display) to an information system (further data processing, recording, background data accessing, modelling) requires system operation features which resemble those of modern computer operation systems. In particular, certain editing functions are necessary. If these are implemented properly, record keeping as one of the anesthesiologist's activities becomes an integral part of the interaction with the system. Fig. 3 schematically shows the basic structure of an AIS page. Central parts are two display windows for the presentation of measurement data (upper window: vital parameters; lower window: ventilation parameters). Grouped around these windows are input keys. A typical drug data input (recording) sequence consists of three or four steps, as shown in Fig. 3:

1. Touching a drug-related term *(hand 1)*
2. Setting the time by moving the vertical time line horizontally across the measurement window *(hand 2)* (this step is not necessary if data input occurs at real time)
3. Specifying a quantity by moving the horizontal quantity slider *(hand 3)*
4. Terminating the sequence by touching the ⟨return⟩ key *(hand 4)*

The input can be "undone" by performing step 1 instead of step 4. A three-state color (intensity) code indicates to the user which of the virtual keys on the screen are: "disabled" / "enabled" / "activated" (a user guidance feature). Thus at each input step the actually relevant subset of input keys (and sliders) is mediated to the user.

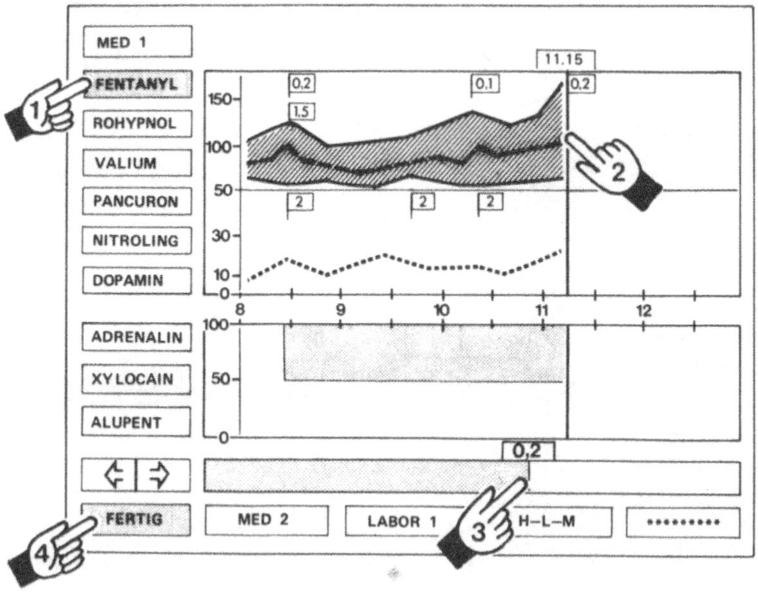

Fig. 3. Typical interaction sequence for drug data input

Looking at step 2 of this input sequence, it becomes clear what Saunders and Jewett (1983) meant by the instinctive "pointing" system in reference to our AIS. Manual data entry to the system always takes place in relation to the displayed measurement data, drug data, or event data, i. e. by pointing at a certain situation that has occurred, e. g. "start of operation," "distinct rise of blood pressure," "shortly before cut," etc. Considering that the majority of parameters to be recorded take the form of term-time-quantity it is obvious that the data input mechanism discussed is a powerful tool that is also useful for machine control (setting ventilator parameters, see next section), for manual entry of vital parameter readings (in case the automatic measurement fails – in fact, it is a trivial task to switch between automatic and manual recording mode with the AIS), and for manual laboratory data entry (reading from paper slips).

Figure 4 shows a page which has been "configured" by the user to contain a set of drugs, the administered quantities of which are displayed within the data windows as "flags." The horizontal slider below the ventilation parameter window serves as the quantity input potentiometer which adjusts its range and scale to the term chosen. But the slider can do more for the user: upon touching a drug term the slider itself graphically shows minimum and maximum quantities (and possibly a recommended range) based on patient data (age, weight, surface) and (possibly) on patient and operation state. Thus the slider may also be used for inquiries.

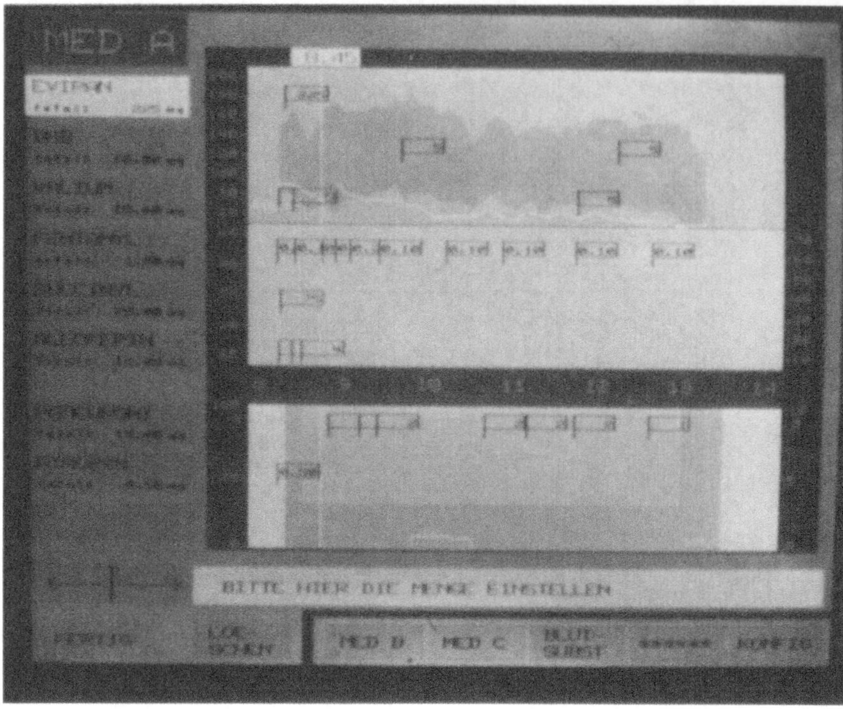

Fig. 4. Entering drug data (Evipan)

Further Integration: Machine Control

Similar to the control of industrial processes via monitor terminal, the anesthesiologist might control the ventilator, infusion pumps, blood analysis devices, and other instruments via the AIS interface. Implementing these possibilities would certainly constitute an expansion of the anesthesia information system towards a control system, a development which introduces many new and unsolved problems. We have nevertheless designed a ventilator control page, shown in Figs. 5 and 6. There are two reasons for doing this: firstly we want to show how machine control can be integrated into the AIS-user interface without violating the basic information display and interaction principles, and secondly we need a ventilator interface for the operation simulation as discussed in the next section.

Adapted to the Siemens (Elema) Servoventilator, the ventilation page (Fig. 5) displays terms related to the independent ventilation parameters (minute, volume, etc.). The procedure of setting any of these parameters is identical with the drug entry procedure described in the previous section. The actual settings are likewise displayed in flags over the time axis. Figure 5 shows how the lower and upper limits for expired minute volume (as one of the measured variables) are being set with the horizontal slider. Again, the user may configure additional terms onto this page; here these are three blood gas parameters. This display space may, however, be superposed up on user request by an on-line display of the pressure or flow curve (Fig. 6).

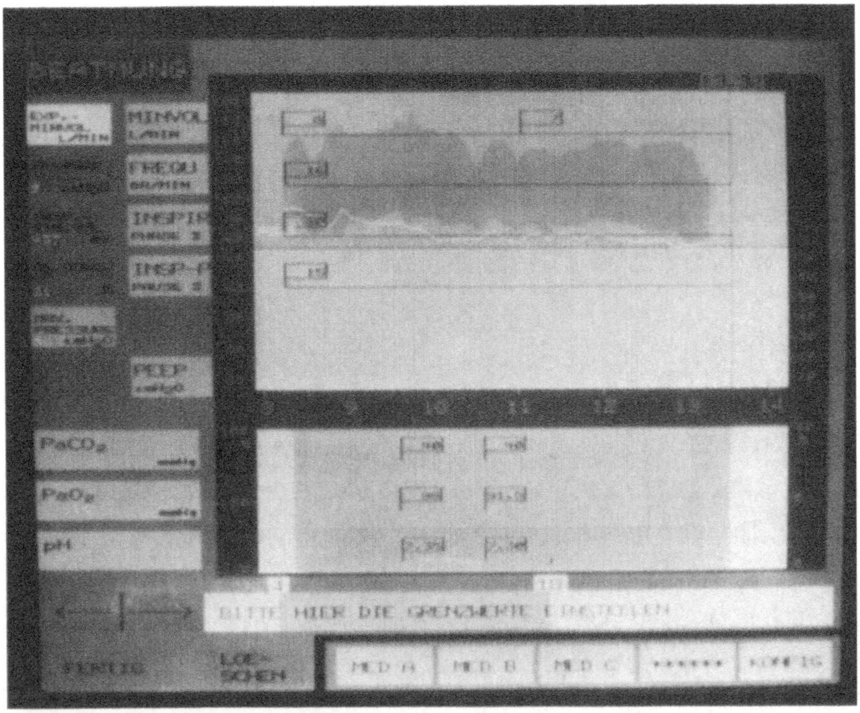

Fig. 5. The ventilation page during the act of setting variable limits

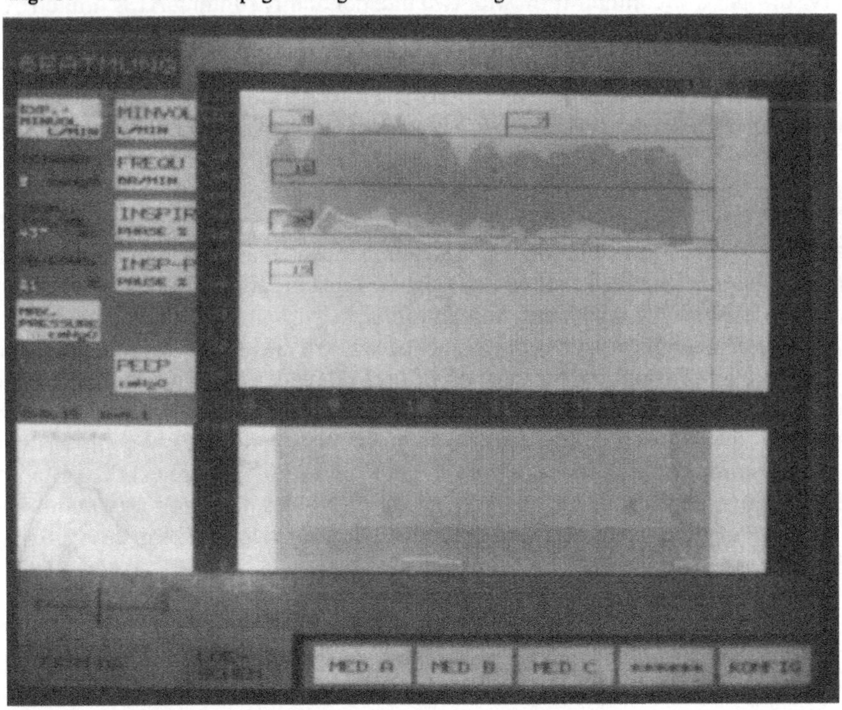

Fig. 6. The ventilation page with the air pressure curve display

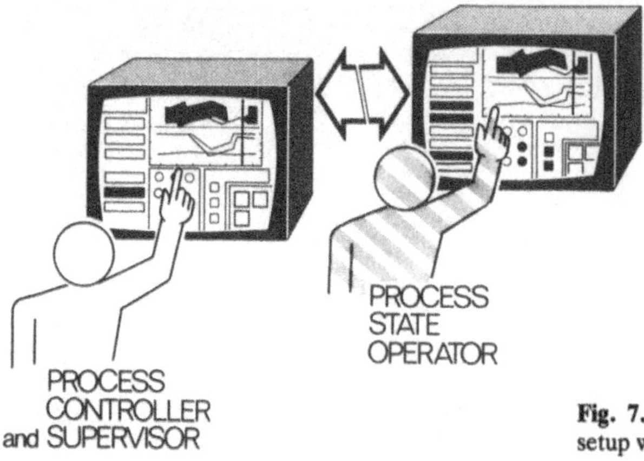

Fig. 7. The AIS simulator setup with two work stations

Our design is by no means final. Many additional control functions could be integrated. The value of this approach has not yet been assessed.

Simulation, Evaluation, and Training

Development and evaluation of a system such as the AIS requires adequate test methods. We have set up a simulator configuration as shown in Fig. 7. It is a supervisor/operator configuration with two independently running AISs, linked over two-way asynchronous serial communication line. The supervisor (left in Fig.7) "models" the patient status by generating patient data in the manual input mode. The supervisor work station sends the patient data to the operator work station, where it is processed as if it were automatically sampled data. Vice versa, the data generated by the operator (drugs, infusions, events, etc.). are transmitted to the supervisor work station. The data base contents on both sides are thus identical.

This is a two-person play with several purposes: (a) it is possible to investigate the system's capabilities in a situation which is more realistic than simple function test (b) users can learn to operate the system outside the operating room, and (c) many aspects of decision-making training are feasible.

This kind of simulation is possible mainly because the AIS-user interface functions as a data throughput medium for most of the data relevant to decision making (except for direct patient inspection, a shortcoming which can be alleviated by certain techniques but which inevitably leads to debate about simulation fidelity). We intend to put one AIS monitor into the operating room by the end of 1984, connect the system to data acquisition devices, display and record the measured data, and use the interactive features of the system in a parallel mode with our own staff for the first-stage evaluation.

Summary

The anesthetist-computer interface tends to be a problem for the utilization of computer systems for anesthesia. Ergonomic interface design with an emphasis on the coherency of the interface's static and dynamic structure may improve this situation. To investigate this proposition we developed an Anesthesia Information System (AIS) with a touch-sensitive monitor as the hardware-user interface. Basic data input and system control techniques were defined and implemented. Record keeping is integrated into the user interface. Ventilator control from the same interface is an additional feature for laboratory simulations. The system is being evaluated using a technique that simulates live operations.

References

Anthony J (1982) BAS – A major change coming in delivery. IEEE EMB 1 (1): 36–42

Apple HP, Schneider AJL, Fadel J (1982) Design and evaluation of a semiautomatic anesthesia record system. Med Instrum 16 (1): 69–71

Arnell WJ, Schultz DG (1983) Computers in anesthesiology – a look ahead. Med Instrum 17 (6): 393–395

Bender HJ, Osswald PM, Hartung HJ, Lutz H (1983) On line – Erfassung haemodynamischer und respiratorischer Größen in der Anaesthesie. Anaesth Intensivther Notfallmed 18: 37–40

Cooper JB et al. (1982) A graphics-tablet for data entry in computer assisted recordkeeping Proc. AAMI 17th Ann. Meet, Arlington, VA, p 26

Gravenstein JS (1980) Failure to monitor (summary). In: Essential noninvasive monitoring in anesthesia Gravenstein JS (ed), Grune and Stratton, New York, 3045–310

Klocke H, Trispel S, Rau G (1984) Entwicklung einer Mensch-Rechner-Schnittstelle für ein Anaesthesie-Informationssystem unter Berücksichtigung ergonomischer Gesichtspunkte. Angew Informatik 5: 197–208

Meijler AP, Beneken JEW, Nandorf A, van Kessel HM, Spierdijk J (1983) A data acquisition and display system for improved medical pattern recognition. Proc Symposium: objective medical decision making, Veldhoven, Springer, Heidelberg

Mitchell, MM (1982) Automated anesthesia data management and recordkeeping. Med Instrum 16 (6): 279–282

Mitchell MM (1982b) Computers key to future progress. IEEE EMB 1(1): 19–22

Newbower RS, Cooper JB, Trautman ED (1981) A microprocessor-based anesthesia delivery system. In: Microcomputers in patient care. Noyes, Park Ridge

Ream AK, Robinson DJ, Nelson PE, Portner PM, Oyer PE (1983) A computer operating system for patient monitoring. Proc 2nd Int. Symp.: computing in anesthesia and intensive care, Rotterdam, p 28

Sarnat AJ (1983) Computerized speech recognition for anesthesia record-keeping. Med Instrum 17(1): 25–27

Saunders RJ, Jewett WR (1983) System integration – the need in future anesthesia delivery systems. Med Instrum 17(6): 389–392

Trispel S, Klocke H, Guenther K, Rau G (1982) Operation simulation for the evaluation and improvement of a medical information system. Proc IFAC conf.: analysis, design, evaluation of man-machine-systems, Baden-Baden, pp 233–239

Trispel S, Klocke H, Rau G (1983) Ergonomic design of the interface between anesthetist and computer system. Proc. 2nd Int. Symp.: computing in anesthesia and intensive care, Rotterdam, p 29

Zollinger RM, Kreul JF, Schneider AJL (1977) Man-made versus computer-generated anesthesia records. J Surg Res 22: 419–424

Effect of Different Ventilation Patterns on the Intracranial Pressure in Neurologic Patients with Mechanical Ventilation

K. M. Einhäupl, C. Garner, G. Schmieder, G. Kerscher, and R. Wieczorek

Since mechanical ventilation in cerebrally injured patients is a frequent problem in intensive care units, the best method of ventilation in respect of cerebral function has been investigated in several studies. Nevertheless, the influence of different ventilation patterns on ICP is still a matter of controversy. In the past most interest was focused on simple monitoring of intracranial pressure (ICP) and its dependence on the positive end-expiratory pressure (PEEP). Most textbooks of neurology warn against using PEEP, because of a possible elevation of the ICP. However, the available evidence regarding this problem is still controversial. Several investigators could not find an increase of ICP during PEEP ventilation either in man (Forst 1977) or in animals (Huseby et al. 1981) – or even in patients with increased baseline ICP (Forst 1977). However, others found ICP elevations in certain patients (Appuzzo et al. 1977). These contradictory results may partly be due to the complexity of the involved mechanism. For further investigations a more sophisticated approach is needed.

Since simple ICP monitoring is of limited use because of its great variation and its late response to different stimuli, the pressure volume index (PVI) has been used in order to estimate the cerebral elastance, which is considered to be a better parameter of the intracranial condition than the ICP itself. However, the required volume injection is sometimes dangerous, may increase ICP, and should be done only a few times a day.

In the last few years the relationship between pulse wave amplitude (PA) and the mean ICP has been used to estimate cerebral elastance. As long as the elastance remains constant, there is a linear relationship between ICP and PA. With increasing elastance the slope of the regression line becomes steeper. Thus this slope, called the pulse pressure/pressure relationship (PPPR), can be used as an estimate of intracranial elastance.

A microcomputer – assisted monitoring system provides a tool for continuous monitoring of changes in cerebral elastance. By this method it is possible to recognize a worsening of the cerebral situation caused by different types of ventilation.

Method

To measure the relevant parameters (e.g., ICP, CVP, MAP, PEEP) and to record them on a data base for real-time on-line as well as later off-line analysis, we

Table 1. Example of an on-line computer printout. MAP, mean arterial pressure; CPP, cerebral perfusion pressure; CVP, central venous pressure; MPAP, mean pulmonal aterial pressure, ICP-pulswave-amplitude (PA), AWP, mean airway pressure; PPPR, pulse pressure/pressure relationship. The PPPR is calculated every 10 min from the slope of the regression line of the ICP/PA Correlation

Time interval	ICP MEAN	MAP	CPP	CVP	MPAP	PA	AWP	PPPR
16.30–16.31	16.3	110.9	94.6	6.5	9.6	8.4	2.8	
16.31–16.32	15.9	112.1	96.2	5.7	8.8	9.1	2.0	
16.32–16.33	15.2	117.4	102.2	6.5	9.9	6.1	3.6	
16.33–16.34	14.6	119.8	105.5	6.2	9.8	5.3	2.6	
16.34–16.35	16.2	121.7	105.5	6.4	10.1	6.2	3.3	
16.35–16.36	17.8	123.0	105.2	7.0	11.1	5.9	4.8	
16.36–16.37	16.3	110.6	94.3	5.6	8.9	6.0	1.0	
16.37–16.38	17.4	121.3	103.9	6.3	10.2	8.4	2.7	
16.38–16.39	16.4	115.4	99.0	6.1	9.3	8.2	2.6	
16.39–16.40	15.5	114.4	98.9	6.7	9.3	6.0	3.7	
16.30–16.40	16.1	117.4	98.8	6.2	9.6	6.9	2.8	0.18
16.40–16.41	17.8	123.0	105.2	7.0	10.2	5.9	4.8	
16.41–16.42	16.3	110.6	94.3	5.6	8.9	6.0	1.0	
16.42–16.43	17.4	121.3	103.9	6.3	10.2	8.4	2.7	
16.43–16.44	16.4	115.4	99.0	6.1	9.3	8.2	2.6	
16.44–16.45	15.5	114.4	98.9	6.7	9.3	6.0	3.7	
16.45–16.46	14.6	119.8	105.5	6.2	9.8	5.3	2.6	
16.46–16.47	16.2	121.7	105.5	6.4	9.1	6.2	3.3	
16.47–16.48	17.8	123.0	105.2	7.0	11.1	5.9	4.8	
16.48–16.49	16.3	110.9	94.6	6.5	9.6	8.4	2.8	
16.49–16.50	15.9	112.1	96.2	5.7	8.8	9.1	2.0	
16.40–16.50	15.9	120.2	104.3	6.3	8.5	7.1	2.9	0.21

developed a microcomputer-assisted system for data acquisition, calculation, and documentation which enables us to monitor and analyze any available biological signals which are available on-line. The system is explained in greater detail elsewhere in this book (Schmieder et al. this volume).

Table 1 shows part of a typical computer protocol of one patient. In the left-hand column the time interval of the measured data is listed, followed by ICP and so on. Each line represents data acquisition over a 10-s period from 1 min. Analysis of the collected data is possible at appropriate intervals. In this example we did it at 10-min intervals. At the end of the interval the PPPR is calculated automatically using these ten points and is printed on the following line.

The different pressures were measured with usual arterial or venous catheters or a Swan-Ganz catheter. ICP was monitored via an indwelling ventricular cannula. All patients were on controlled ventilation and in a 30° head-up position. Each patient was measured for at least 15 min to obtain a baseline recording. Then a period of 15 min with PEEP ventilation (PEEP level, 10 mmHg) was monitored, followed by a 15-min period again without PEEP. Blood gas analysis was done in each period, as were cardiac output and pulmonary artery-wedge pressure measurements when using a Swan-Ganz catheter.

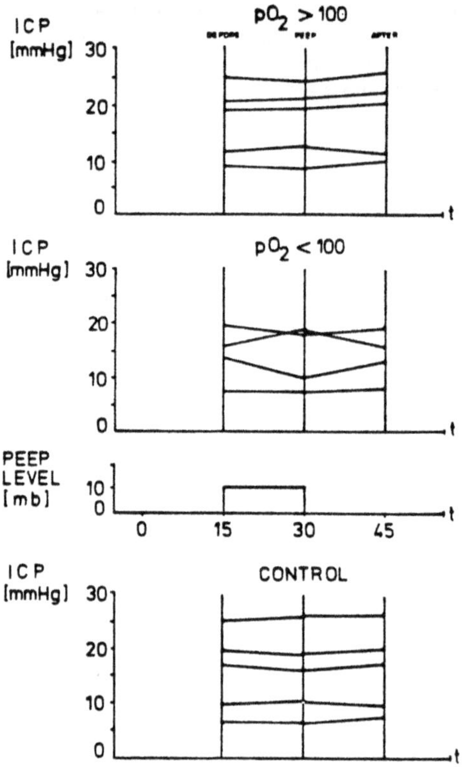

Fig. 1. Influence of PEEP on ICP. Mean ICP per patient before, during, and after PEEP

Results

The patients were divided into two groups. The first group included patients without pulmonary disease and with an arterial oxygen level (PO_2) greater than 100 mmHg. In this group no significant change in ICP occurred despite an average increase of CVP from 6.2 to 10.3 mmHg (Fig. 1). It has been speculated that this lack of ICP response is due to a low elastance. If that were true, the elastance should increase as a result of compensation.

Figure 2 shows the ICP-PA diagram of one patient from the first group. The elastance, estimated as PPPR from the slopes of the regression lines, did not change. (The slopes were 0.19, 0.24, and 0.23 before, during, and after PEEP ventilation, respectively.) Nor was there any change of PPPR in the other patients of his group. The second group included four patients with low PO_2 levels (mean 53 mmHg) before PEEP. Although the changes in ICP did not reach significance, lowering of ICP during the PEEP period was seen in two patients which returned to the previous level after discontinuation of PEEP. In these two and in another patient, who did not show any change in ICP, PEEP caused a marked increase in PO_2 to a mean level of 80 mmHg. The PPPR in these three patients did not change.

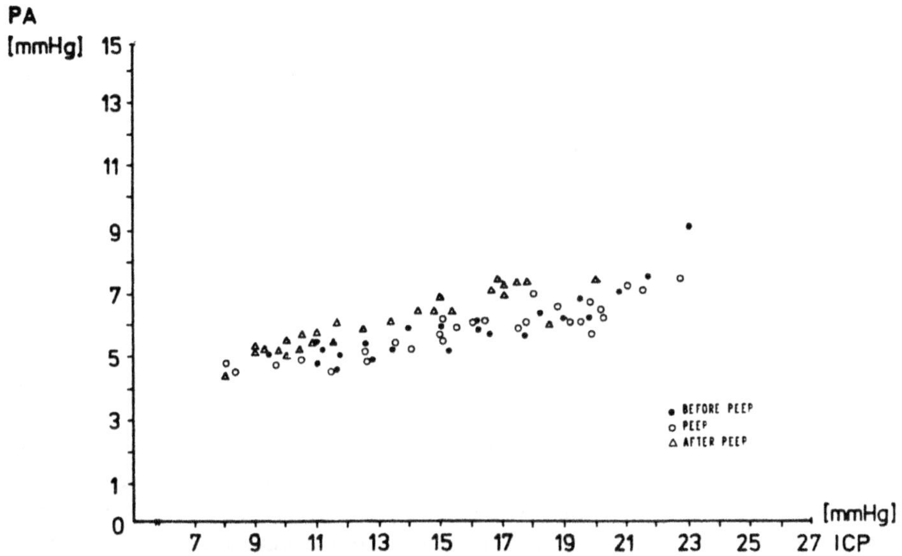

Fig. 2. Pulse pressure/pressure relationship in a single patient with normal PO_2. There is no change in the slope of the three regression lines representing the PPPR

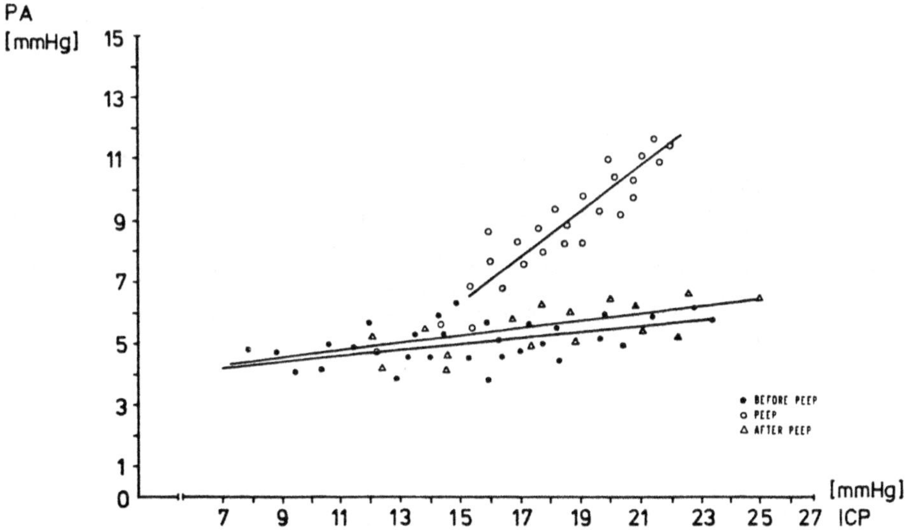

Fig. 3. Pulse pressure/pressure relationship in a single patient with reduced PO_2. During PEEP the slope of the regression line is increased, indicating an elevated elastance. The ICP itself remained fairly constant

More interesting is the observation of one patient who had an increase in PPPR with only a mild elevation in ICP during PEEP. This must be considered as an increase in elastance, where ICP remained compensated. A similar observation has been reported by Forst (1977). This patient showed only a mild response in respect of PO_2. The increase of PPPR preceded the ICP elevation by 5 min.

Ventilation with inversed ratio did not alter ICP nor PPPR in the first group and produced only a mild decrease in ICP in one patient in the second group, while PO_2 increased from 62 to 71 mmHg (mean data).

The number of our patients is as yet too small for us to draw any serious conclusions. Therefore these results must be considered preliminary.

Summary

1. A PEEP level of 10 mmHg does not elevate ICP despite an increase of CVP in patients with normal oxygenation. This is independent of the ICP level.
2. In this group of patients with normal oxygenation the cerebral compliance, estimated from PPPR, is not altered. The compensation of impaired venous outflow in these patients is probably not due to increased elastance.
3. In patients with bad oxygenation, PEEP may even decrease ICP without a change in PPPR. The underlying physiological explanation for this phenomenon migth be a decrease in cerebral blood flow due to better oxygenation.
4. In certain patients PPPR may be a more sensitive parameter for recognizing onset of cerebral deterioration caused or at least supported by PEEP ventilation, than ICP alone.
5. The advantage of microcomputer-assisted multiparameter analysis in respect of ICP is its safety compared with the bolus injection method and the possibility of continuous observation.

References

Apuzzo MLJ, Weiss MH, Peterson V, Small RB, Kurze T, Heiden JS (1977) Effect of PEEP ventilation on intracranial pressure in man. J Neurosurg 46: 227–232

Forst EAM (1977) Effects of PEEP on intracranial pressure and compliance in brain-injured patients. J Neurosurg 47: 195–200

Huseby JS, Luce JM, Cary JM, Pavlin EG, Butler J (1981) Effects of PEEP on intracranial pressure in dogs with intracranial hypertension. J Neurosurg 55: 704–707

Van Eijndhoven JHM, Avezaat CJJ (1981) The analogy between CSF-puls-pressure and volume-pressure response. ICP 4: 173–176

Computer Applications in Pulmonary Function Testing

M. HEITZ

Introduction

During the past few years computers have become important tools in pulmonary medicine. They have applications in lung function testing (lung volumes, gas exchange, mechanics) and in image processing (nuclear medicine, CT, nuclear magnetic resonance). This review concentrates on computer applications in conventional pulmonary function testing (PFT).

Figure 1 demonstrates where computers may be helpful in PFT. The first step in data acquisition is analog to digital (AD) conversion. In the workup of raw data, digital filters are useful to eliminate noise. Under program control a selection or reduction of raw data may be performed. The computer also permits calibration of an analog instrument with a nonlinear output, e.g., a pneumotachograph (Hart et al. 1981; Johns et al. 1982; Minken et al. 1982). In connection with a mass spectrometer, specific conversion factors may be selected according to the gas content.

After data acquisition and workup of primary signals, calculations of secondary parameters are done. This can happen either while further data acquisition is con-

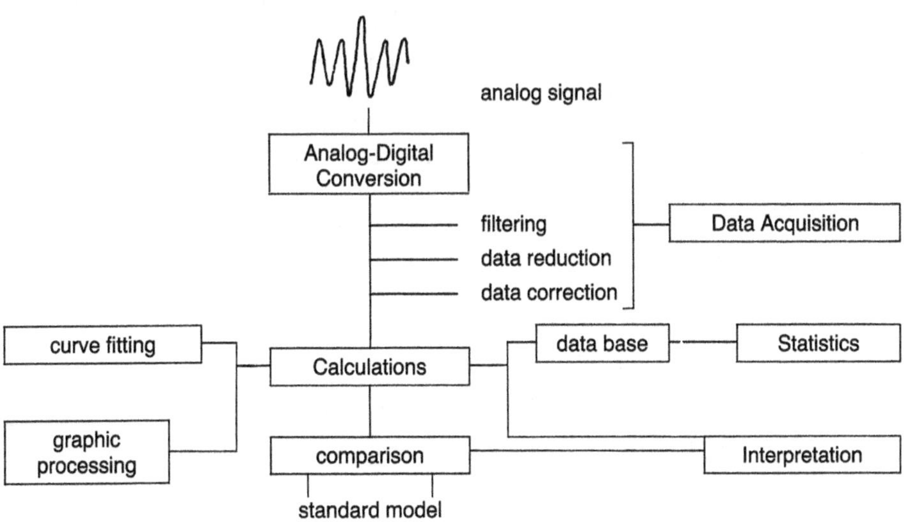

Fig. 1. Application of computers in PFT. For details see text

tinued, or in a free interval, for instance after the end of a forced expiratory maneuver. A curve-fitting procedure could then be applied to the calculated values, for example, a monoexponential function fitter to the pressure volume curve (Colebarch et al. 1978; Pare et al. 1982; Pengelly 1977). The results obtained may be illustrated by graphic documentation (Heise 1982; Heise and Trendelenburg 1979; Lisboa et al. 1979, 1980). Results may be compared to reference values or to a model. To some extent, test results may also be interpreted under computer control. Finally, statistical analysis of a data base is possible.

The computer may also be used for simulation of respiratory mechanics, gas distribution, gas exchange, or control of respiration.

Equipment

AD Converters

Today mainly AD converters (ADCs) with 10 or 12 bits are used. An ADC with 10 bits has a resolution of 0.1%, which means it is able to separate the amplitude of a given analogue signal into 1024 units. If, for instance, we have a spirometer of 7 l, 1 unit would correspond to a volume of 6.8 ml, provided the gain is optimally adjusted. A 12-bit ADC would have a resolution of 0.025%, corresponding to a volume of 1.7 ml. For details see Table 1.

For forced maneuvers, conversion rates of 100–250 Hz are normally sufficient. For breath by breath analysis of gas exchange and respiratory mechanics, conversion rates of 50–60 Hz are considered adequate.

Hardware

Table 2 summarizes typical hardware configurations. The E-prom program microprocessor is typically seen in small automated spirometric systems. Further examples are the dedicated microprocessor with floopy disk stations, possibly very soon the general-purpose personal computer, and the minicomputer based multi-user system. On-line data acquisition is possible with all four types. However, for some of the most popular personal computers there are at present no ADCs and corresponding software commercially available. Real-time data processing with microprocessor-based systems generally requires programs to be written in assembler language. The excellent and now inexpensive graphic features existing for the personal computers can be used for PFT as soon as the interfaces are available.

Table 1. Resolution of ADCs

Bits	Units	Resolution in %	Volume in ml (7000 ml)	Flow in l/s (12 l/s)
8	256	0.4	2.7	0.047
10	1024	0.1	6.8	0.011
12	4096	0.025	1.7	0.003

Table 2. Hardware requirements for PFT

Type of computing	E-prom micro-processor	Floppy disc micro-processor	Personal-computer	Mini-computer
On-line data acquisition	+	+	(+)	+++
Real-time data processing	–	+ (assembler)	+	+++ (HLL)
Graphics, curve fitting	–	+	++	++
Program change, program development	–	+	+	+++
Database	–	+	+	+++
Multi-user support	–	–	?	+++
Statistics on database	–	–	–	++

Suitability of equipment for task: +++, highly suitable; ++, moderately suitable; +, suitable with restrictions; –, unsuitable

Program change and software development are not possible with E-prom programmed systems. For this purpose the minicomputer in combination with a mass-storage device is best qualified. Multiple test stations in parallel require a multi-user operating system with interrupt capabilities. This, to my knowledge, has so for only been implemented on minicomputer based systems. Statistical work on an extensive data base requires large core memories. This work was, until recently, performed on large main-frame systems, for which large statistical program packages are available.

Today, computerized equipment and software are commercially available for spirometry, including flow-volume curve, carbon monoxide diffusion, body plethysmography, forced oscillation, exercise testing, total pulmonary resistance, and static and dynamik compliance. Some manufacturers computerize each major piece of equipment with its own dedicated microprocessor, but there are larger minicomputer based multi-user systems with data management on the market as well. In the following, an overview of computer application in standard PFT will be given. For convenience, PFT may be divided into three groups (Table 3).

Table 3. The three categories of PFT

		Spirometry	
Lung volumes	←	Body plethysmography	
		X-ray	
		Esophageal balloon	
Lung mechanics	←	Body plethysmography	
		Forced oscillation	
		Gas distribution ←	SB N_2 closing volume
Gas exchange	←	Diffusion, blood flow, tissue volume	
		Exercise testing	

Lung Volumes

Spirometry

The first publication on computer-based spirometry came from Schonfeld of Washington in 1964. Dickman (1969) described the first on-line spirometry. Early work was realized on large computers or time-sharing systems (Dickman et al. 1969; Moser et al. 1969; Naimark et al. 1971; Young et al. 1971). Data were entered either off-line (Moser et al. 1969; Naimark et al. 1971; Rosner et al. 1971), or by magnetic tape (Ayers et al. 1969 a, b; Shonfeld et al. 1964; Young et al. 1971). Real-time data entry and analysis in these earlier studies was done by only a few investigators (Boyhuys et al. 1970; O'Brien and Kass 1970; Dickman et al. 1969; Earle and Domizi 1969). With the arrival of the microprocessor the number of publications greatly increased (Black et al. 1980; Bunn et al. 1979; Chang 1972). The flow-volume loop was included (Aikins et al. 1983; Buss et al. 1979; Hankinson 1981; Krumpe et al. 1982; Soto et al. 1975; Sulotto et al. 1983; Tanser 1982). Recently, some work was published on the combination of spirometric equipment with generally available micro- or personal computers (Hansen et al. 1983; Tanser 1982). Table 4, modified and completed after Krumpe, et al. (1982) summarizes the historic development of computerized spirometry. The computer also permits complicated mathematical processing, such as digital filtering of spirometric curves (Peslin and Jardin 1983). Flow characteristics of pneumotachographs may be determined very exactly (Minken et al. 1982).

Computerized Interpretation of PFTs

The first computerized interpretation of spirometric data was reported by Ayers et al. (1969, a, b). Early reports were generally restricted to comparison of individual parameters to predicted values, and did not correlate different types of PFT data with each other (Ellis et al. 1975; Hoffer et al. 1973; Protti et al. 1973). Aikins and Kunz (Aikins et al. 1983) presented at the first symposium a program for interpretation of PFT data. They found agreement between the judgment of the computer and that of the developer of the program in 91% of cases, and between the computer and an independent expert in 88%. Geddes et al. (1978) found disagreement between computerized and manual interpretation in 4.6%. The most recent work in this field, with excellent reviews of earlier publications, came from Krumpe et al. (1982) and Sulotto et al. (1982). Several methods are in use for interpretation of PFT data. The most popular approach is a branching decision tree following the same logic as the evaluative process of the physician reading a set of PFT data (Bunn et al. 1979; Ellis et al. 1975; Hoffer et al. 1973; Pack et al. 1977; Sulotto et al. 1982). Decision trees have some serious disadvantages. The number of parameters which can be simultaneously evaluated are limited and difficult to modify. Other approaches are based on a last-square procedure (Krumpe et al. 1982) or discriminant functions (Tsai et al. 1979). The program of Krumpe (Weigt and Krumpe 1980) and the PUFF-expert program are available in BASIC.

Table 4. Computer management of PFT

		System characteristics				Computer analysis		
Author	Year	Data entry method	Types of data	Measures curves	Type of computer	Computer language	Descriptive statements	Correlates data as interpretation
Shonfeld	1964	T	S	Yes	Lg	Assembler	No	No
Moser	1969	M	S, V, D, O	No	TS	–	No	No
Dickman	1969	RT	S	Yes	TS	–	No	No
Earl	1969	RT	S	Yes	Lg	–	Yes	No
Bouhuys	1970	RT	S	Yes	Lg	–	Yes	No
O'Brien	1970	RT	S	Yes	Lg	–	Yes	No
Naimark	1971	M	S, B, V, D	No	TS	–	Yes	No
Rosner	1971	M	S, V, D, ABG	No	Lg	FORTRAN	Yes	No
Young	1971	T	S	Yes	TS	–	No	No
Chaing	1972	M	S	No	Micro	BASIC	Yes	No
Ellis	1975	M	S, B, V, D	No	Micro	BASIC	Yes	Yes[a]
Soto	1975	T	FV	Yes	L	FOCAL 12	No	No
Guy	1976	T	S, B, V, D, O	Yes	TS	–	No	No
Pack	1977	M	S, B, V, D, O	No	L	FORTRAN IV	Yes	Yes
Bunn	1979	RT	FV, V, O	Yes	H	BASIC	Yes	Yes
Freiherr	1979	RT	FV, B	Unkn.	H	FORTRAN	Yes	Yes
Tsai	1979	M	S	No	–	–	No	No
Krumpe	1982	RT	FV, B, V, D	Yes	Micro	BASIC	Yes	Yes
Sulotto	1982	M	FV, 8, V, D, O	No	Lg	–	Yes	Yes
Tanser	1983	RT	S, FV	Yes	Micro	BASIC	Yes	Yes
Aikins	1983	RT	S, FV, B, V, D, O	Yes	Lg	BASIC + other	Yes	Yes
Hauser	1983	RT	S, FV	Yes	Micro	BASIC	–	–
Verbraak	1984	RT	S, FV, B, V, D, O	Yes	H	FORTRAN	Yes	Yes

M, manual; T, tape storage for AD signal processing; RT, real-time AD processing; S, spirometry; FV, flow-volume curve; B, postbronchodilator FV; V, subdivisions of lung volume; D, diffusion capacity of lung for carbon monoxide; ABG, arterial blood gas data; O, other; Lg, large computer (such as PDP 8, PDP 11/65, CDC 160, or IBM 160); H, hybrid of several computers; TS, time-sharing on a large computer; Micro, microprocessor-based desk-top computer

[a] Utilizes a branching decision tree type of program

Most interpretation programs for PFT data have one or more of the following limitations: limits are arbitrary. Mixed defects may be misinterpreted. The data are not related to the clinical situation. Inspiratory maneuvers are rarely considered.

Plethysmography

Sykes et al. (1977) published a computerized on-line method for plethysmographic determination of lung volumes. Thoracic gas volume is calculated by a linear regression analysis through the mouth pressure vs. box pressure points obtained from a panting maneuver. Most authors fix boundaries within which the points will be accepted for regression (Gradins et al. 1967; Heise and Trendelenburg 1979). Chowienczyk et al. (1981 a, b) accept a pair of points for regression analysis only if they exceed a fixed minimal interval compared to previous points. This avoids cluster building, especially in the turn-points of the curve, and guarantees a more regular spacing of data used for the regression.

Estimation of Lung Volume from Chest Radiographs

Radiological methods for calculation of total lung capacity (TLC) have also been computerized (Barret et al. 1976; Bencowitz and Shigeoka 1980; Channing Rodgers and Tanner 1983; Peacock et al. 1984; Pierce et al. 1979). The first report was by Barrett (1976). Further reports came from the group of Denison (Peacock et al. 1984; Pierce et al. 1979). Channing Rodgers and Tanner (1983) published the implementation of the Barnhard method (Barnhard et al. 1960) on an HP 41-C pocket calculator.

Two methods are in use. The first, termed the ellipsoid method, divides the lung into several cylindroid discs. AP and lateral diameters are calculated from chest radiographs. The volume of the individual discs is then calculated and summed. A correction is made for heart, mediastinum, diaphragm, pulmonary blood, and tissue volumes.

The second method calculates the surface area by planimetry from the AP and lateral chest X-ray. Lung volume is then obtained from a regression equation of surface area vs. TLC measured by body plethysmography. Both methods correlate fairly well with gas dilution methods for calculation of TLC.

Light Plethysmography

If a structured light (e.g., a grid) is projected onto a torso, the regular structure of the grid is distorted. From the distortion on the surface, one can calculate the volume of the underlying thorax. Denison and Peacock (Denison et al. 1982; Morgan et al. 1984; Peacock et al. 1984) have recently computerized this completely non-invasive method for calculation of lung volumes which can also be used in an intensive care area.

Respiratory Mechanics

Compliance

The earliest papers on computerized measurement of dynamic compliance came from Peters and Stacey (1964), Lewis et al. (1966), Osborn et al. (1968), Wald et al. (1969), and Hilberman et al. (1969). These programs were designed to monitor respiratory parameters in postoperative surgical patients.

The static pressure-volume curve provides an excellent example of how the computer greatly enhances the diagnostic possibilities in PFT. While manual analysis of the pressure-volume curve is usually confined to compliance and recoil pressure at TLC, the computer allows fitting of an exponential function to the curve. The constant in the exponent provides a much better parameter for lung elasticity, especially in early emphysema, than static compliance (Parc et al. 1982) Pengelly (1977) published the

Table 5. Computerized methods for calculation of airway resistance

Body plethysmography	– Tangents
	– Integral pressure-volume/flow-volume
Esophageal balloon	– Isovolume method
	– Phase angle
	– Curve fitting
Forced oscillation	– Phase angle

first program for off-line curve fitting on a desk calculator. Colebatch et al. (1978) reported the first on-line system.

Pulmonary Resistance

For calculation of total pulmonary or airway resistance during quiet breathing, the esophageal balloon technique, body plethysmography (Lorino et al. 1978) and the forced oscillation technique (Landser et al. 1976) have been computerized (see Table 5).

There are two methods to calculate airway resistance in on-line body plethysmography. The first follows the manual method, where resistance is calculated from the angle of the turupoints of the pressure-flow curve. Due to variation in breathing patterns, values obtained by this method show considerable variation. While an experienced technician knows which curve to select, out of several trials, as the one representative for the patient under study, this experience is very difficult to program. For computerized analysis, the integral method, as described by Smidt et al. (1975) and Smidt (1979) is more suitable. In this procedure, an integral is calculated from the pressure-volume curve and then divided by the integral of the flow-volume curve. The result represents an average inspiratory or expiratory resistance with little variation. Recently, several improvements to the standard methods, such as drift correction (Soohoo and Brown 1983), numerical BTPS compensation (Rafalsky et al. 1982), correction for nonlinearity of the box pneumotachograph (Hart et al. 1981), and calculation of resistance from differential equations (Chowienczyk et al. 1981a, b), have been published. Heise and coworkers use computerized three-dimensional graphic plots for presentation of resistance and pressure-flow curve (Heise 1982; Heise and Trendelenburg 1979). We have ourselves developed a program for on-line analysis of resistance during forced expiration. By means of an intrabronchial catheter, resistance can be separated into peripheral and central parts. The results can be presented either graphically or numerically. Dierkesman et al. (1980) published a method for on-line calculation of isovolume pressure-flow curves.

Three methods are in use for calculation of pulmonary resistance from transpulmonary pressure obtained from an esophageal balloon (Table 5). The oldest one is termed the isovolume method and corresponds to the one already applied by von Neergard and Wirz in 1927, where from mid-inspiration to mid-expiration the transpulmonary pressure difference is divided by the flow difference (Lewis et al. 1966). Another method which is used by many authors is called the phase-angle method

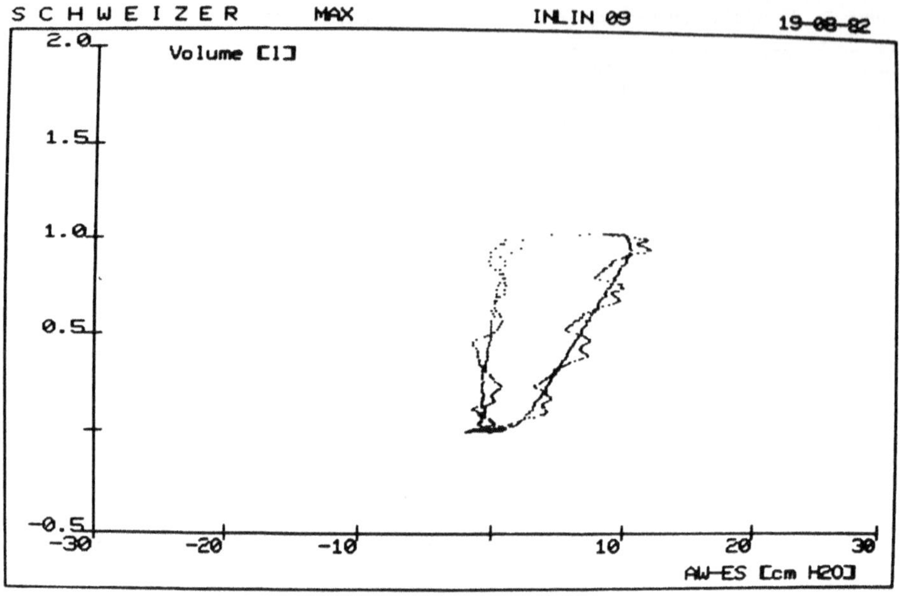

Fig. 2. Dynamic pressure-volume diagram from a ventilated patient. *Curve with oscillation* represents original curve, *smoothed curve* represents fitted curve used for calculation of mechanics. (Courtesy of G. Wolff)

(Hilberman et al. 1969). A Fourier transformation is done on the transpulmonary pressure and flow signal. From the measured phase angle of the two curves, resistance can be calculated by trigonometry. A similar procedure is also used with forced oscillation imposed by a random noise generator. This technique has been computerized by Landser et al. (1976). The third method applies a least-square curve fitting to the pressure-flow-volume curve, by modifying initial estimates of resistance and compliance (Drebes et al. 1979; Uhl and Lewis 1974; Wald et al. 1969). Brunner et al. (1985) use this method for calculation of mechanics in ventilated patients (see Fig. 2). An interesting modification of the esophageal balloon technique came from Lisboa and Macklem (Lisboa et al. 1979, 1980). They combined the "electrical subtraction method" of Mead and Whittenberger with a data-averaging circuit, a typical example of digital noise reduction. The curvelinearity of the resulting pressure-flow curve, which is free of any artefacts, readily allows identification of different flow patterns.

Gas Exchange

Gas Distribution

The combination of a computer with an instrument such as a mass spectrometer for rapid analysis of several different gases tremendously increases the possibilities for investigation of pulmonary gas exchange.

Single-Breath Nitrogen Washout Curve. Craven et al. (1976) and Hankinson (1981) described on-line calculation of closing volume from single-breath nitrogen curves. This has proven to be quite difficult. The single-breath nitrogen test has been incorporated into automated routine pulmonary function testing by other authors (Buss et al. 1979; Grohs et al. 1983). Sophisticated calculations of ventilatory efficiency, various dead spaces (Cummings 1982), moment analysis (Jafar et al. 1979) have been performed on data from single-and or multi-breath nitrogen washout data. These procedures are now implemented by Wolff's group in the intensive care unit on ventilated patients (Wolff (1985)).

Diffusion

On-line determination of single-breath or steady-state diffusing capacity for carbon monoxide belongs today to the standard programs of nearly all commercially available equipment. Computerized algorithms for on-line calculation of diffusing capacity, pulmonary tissue volume, and blood flow have also been published (Kung et al. 1980; Petrini et al. 1982; Sackner et al. 1975).

Guy et al. (1976) described a computerized continous calculation of RQ during a prolonged expiration from the oxygen and carbon dioxide curve which allows interesting physiological conclusions. We use a similar procedure in our exercise test for estimation of mixed venous to arterial oxygen difference according to the method of Farrel and Siegel (1976).

Ventilation-Perfusion Ratio

The enormous progress brought into pulmonary function testing by computers, is probably best demonstrated by the fascinating work of Wagner and West on the ventilation-perfusion ratio (Arnold and Wilson 1971; Olszowka and Wagner 1980; Wagner and West 1972, 1980; Wagner et al. 1974; Wagner 1981). While Riley used a three-compartment model, Wagner enlarged to 50 compartments for analysis of multiple soluble inert gas elimination. This allows calculation of a distribution curve of ventilation/perfusion ratios, which shows quite different configurations depending on the underlying pathological process.

Recently, modifications of the original technique have been described (Evans et al. 1977; Stewart and Mastenbrook 1983a, b) Mertens (1983) reduced the number of compartments to 12, which resulted in great reduction of computing time. Stewart and Mastenbrook (1983b) .use a log-normal distribution of ventilation and perfusion ratios.

Exercise Tests and Blood Gases

Early reports on computerized exercise testing in the German literature came from Rittel et al. (1977). Beaver et al. (1973) published the first on-line program for breath by breath calculation of oxygen uptake and other important respiratory parameters. Many other reports followed (Darryl et al. 1980; Mitchell 1979; Nacamura et al. 1982;

Pearce et al. 1977; Saluminen et al. 1982; Sodat et al. 1983; Wessel et al. 1979). In conjunction with the graphic capabilities of digital plotters and graphic terminals, new possibilities were opened for investigation of exercise physiology. Today a whole range of equipment, from the small dedicated microprocessor calculating oxygen uptake and RQ up to the free programmable system with full graphics, is commercially available. Breath by breath measurements of gas exchange has become important for ventilated patients in the intensive care unit (Wolff (1985)).

There are numerous reports in the literature on calculation of acid-base parameters and of oxygen saturation of hemoglobin from primary blood gas data (Kelman 1966, 1967). Computerized interpretation and graphic presentation of blood gas parameters is also available and incorporated into other diagnostic programs (Osswald et al. 1981; Vallbona et al. 1971).

Computer Simulations

As this review focuses on computerized PFT, space does not allow a detailed description of computer simulations in pulmonary physiology. Fascinating work has been published on respiratory mechanics (Jackson and Milhorn 1975; Kelman 1970), control of respiration (Gomez 1963; Milhorn and Brown 1971; Milhorn et al. 1965; Yamamoto and Hari 1971), gas transport (Fry 1968; Kaneko 1978; Piava and Demeester 1971), ventilation/perfusion ratio (Wagner 1981; Wagner and West 1980; Wagner et al. 1974; West 1969), and diffusion (Kelman 1966, 1967; Wagner and West 1972). Some work has concentrated on the influence of specific conditions: shock, atelectasis, etc. (Farrell and Siegel 1973a, b, 1976; Siegel and Farrell 1973; Siegel et al. 1973)

References

Aikins JS, Kunz JC, Shortliffe EH (1983) Puff: An expert system for interpretation of pulmonary function data. Comput Biomed Res 16: 199–208

Arnold JE, Wilson BC (1981) Computer processing of perfusion, ventilation and V/Q images to highlight pulmonary embolism. Eur J Nucl Med 6: 209–315

Ayers WR, Ward SA, Weihrer AL, Abraham S, Caceres CA (1969a) Description of a computer program for analysis of the forced expiratory spirogram. I. Instrumentation and programming. Comput Biomed Res 2: 207–219

Ayers WR, Ward SA, Weihrer AL, Abraham S, Caceres CA (1969b) Description of a computer program for analysis of the forced expiratory spirogramm. II. Validation. Comput Biomed Res 2: 220–228

Barnhard HJ, Pierce JA, Joyce WW, Bates JH (1960) Roentgenographic determination of total lung capacity. Am J Med 28: 51

Barret WA, Clayton PD, Lambson CR et al (1976) Computerized roentgenographic determinations of total lung capacity. Am Rev Respir Dis 113: 239–244

Beaver L, Karlman, Wasserman, Whipp BJ (1973) On-line computer analysis and breath-by-breath graphical display of exercise function tests. J Appl Physiol 34 (1): 123–132

Bencowitz HZ, Shigeoka JW (1980) Radiographic total lung capacity determination aided by a programmable calculator. Am Rev Respir Dis 122: 791–794

Black KH, Petusevsky ML, Gaensler EA (1980) A general purpose microprocessor for spirometry. Chest 78: 605–612
Bouhuys A, Gulesian PJ (1970) Electronic data processing of flow and volume data from forced expiratory maneuvers. Am Rev Respir Dis 101: 1000 A
O'Brien LE, Kass I. (1970) "On line" computer analysis of flow volume loops: a rapid mass screening system for early chronic obstructive pulmonary disease. Am Rev Respir Dis 101: 1000 A
Brunner J, Langenstein H, Wolff G (1985) A simple method for estimating compliance critical care medicine.
Bunn AE, Vermaak JC, DeKock MA (1979) A comprehensive on-line computerized lung function. Respiration 37: 42–51
Chaing ST (1972) Application of desk-top computer in clinical spirometry: an automatic calculation and diagnosis program. Am Rev Respir Dis 106: 346–351
Channing Rodgers RP, Tanner R (1983) Rapid and accurate determination of total lung capacity (TLC) from routine chest radiograms using a programmable hand-held calculator. Comput Biol Med 13 (2): 125–140
Chowienczyk PJ, Rees PJ Clark TJ (1981 a) Automated system for the measurement of airways resistance, lung volumes and flow-volume loops. Thorax 36: 944–949
Chowienczyk PJ, Rees PJ, Payne J, Clark TJ (1981 b) A new method for computer assisted determination of airways resistance. J Appl Physiol 50 (3): 672–678
Colebatch HJH, Nail BS, CKY Ng (1978) Computerized measurement of pulmonary conductance J Appl Physial 44 (4): 611–618
Crapo RO, Morris AH, Gardner RD, Schaap RN (1982): Computation rechniques for rebreathing lung tissue volume and pulmonary capillary blood flow. J Appl Physiol. Respirat. Environ. Exercise Physiol. 52, 1375–1377
Craven N, Sidwall G, West P, et al. (1976) Computer analysis of the single-breath nitrogen washout curve. Am Rev Respir Dis 113: 445–449
Cumming G (1982) The pathophysiology of airways disease in computers. In: Prakash O (ed) critical: care and pulmonary medicine, vol 2. Plenum, New York, pp 3–14
Darryl SY, Hansen JE, Blais M, Wasserman K (1980) Measurement and analysis of gas exchange during exercise using a programmable calculator. J Appl Physiol 49 (3): 456–461
Denison DM, Peacock AJ, Morgan DL et al. (1982) Shedding light on the subject. Br J Dis Chest 76: 20–34
Dickman ML, Schmidt CD, Gardner RM, Marshall HW, Day WC, Warner HR (1969) On-line computerized spirometry in 738 normal adults. Am Rev Respir Dis 100: 780–789
Dierkesmann R, Deffner D, Markof D, Meier-Sydow J (1980) On-line determination of isovolume-pressure-flow curves, measurement in antigen induced airway obstruction. Bull Physiopathol Respir 16: 173–174
Drebes CB, Minh VD, Shephard JW (1979) Interval estimation of respiratory parameters using least-squares techniques, Comput Biomed Res 12: 149–166
Earle RH, Domizi D (1969) On-line computer analysis of pulmonary function. Dis Chest 56: 247–248
Ellis JH Jr, Perera SP, Levin DC (1975) A computer program for calculation and interpretation of pulmonary function studies. Chest 68: 209–213
Evans JW, Peter D, Wagner PD (1977) Limits on V $^{A}\!/_{Q}$ distributions from analysis of experimental inert gas elimination. J Appl Physiol 42 (6): 889–898
Farrell EJ, Siegel JH (1973 a) Investigation of cardiorespiratory abnormalities through computer simulation. Comput Biomed Res 6: 161–186
Farrell EJ, Siegel JH (1973 b) Simulation of respiratory regulation of blood gases in the critically ill patient. Trans ASME Ser G 95: 321–323
Farrell EJ, Siegel JJ (1976) Estimation of blood gas contents from expired air under normal and pathologic conditions. Respir Physiol 26: 303–325
Freiherr G (1979) Mycin: a medical and education aid. Res Resource Repr 111: 1–6
Fry DA (1968) A preliminary lung model for simulating the bronchial tree. Comput Biomed Res 2: 111
Geddes DM, Green M, Emerson PA (1978) Comparison of reports on lung function tests made by chest physicians with those made by a simple computer program. Thorax 33: 257
Gomez DA (1963) Mathematical treatment of the distribution of tidal volume throughout the lung. Proc Nat Acad Sci USA 49: 312

Grodins F, Buell J, Bart A (1967) Mathematical analysis and digital simulation of the respiratory control system. J Appl Physiol 22: 260
Grohs H, Heise D, Trendelenburg F (1983) Methode zur Simultananalyse von Atemtechnik und Gasaustausch. Prax Klin Pneumol 37: 1073–1075
Guy HL, Gaines RA, Hill PM, Wagner PD, West JB (1976) Computerized, noninvasive tests of lung function. A flexible approach using mass spectrometry. Am Rev Respir Dis 113: 737
Hankinson JL (1981) Automated pulmonary function testing: interpretation and standardization. Ann Biomed Eng 9: 633–643
Hansen DJ, Toy VM, Deininger RA, Collopy TK (1983) Computer assisted spirometry. Am Ind Hyg Assoc J 44 (6): 419–424
Harf A, Atlan G, Lorino H et al. (1981) Correction for nonlinearity of body flow phlethysmograph. J Appl Physiol 50 (3): 658–662
Heise D, Trendelenburg F (1979) Computer-aided measurements in body plethysmography. Prog Respir Res II: 179–187
Heise D (1982) Analysis of body plethysmographic pressure-flow-loops by digital computer. In: Prakash O (ed) Computers in critical care and pulmonary medicine, vol 2. Plenum, New York, pp 71–74
Hilberman M, Sehill JP, Peters RM (1969) On-line digital analysis of respiratory mechanics and the automation of respirator control. J Thorac Cardiovasc Surg 5: 821–828 (1969)
Hilberman M, Stacy RW, Peters RM (1972) A phase method of calculating respiratory mechanics using a digital computer. J Appl Physiol 32 (4): 535–541
Hoffer EP, Kanarek D, Kazemi H, Barnett GO (1973) Computer interpretation of ventilatory studies. Comput Biomed Res 6: 347–354
Jackson AC, Milhorn HT Jr (1973) Digital computer simulation of respiratory mechanics. Comput Biomed Res 6: 27
Jafar S, Saidel GM, Chester EH (1979) Real-time moment analysis of pulmonary nitrogen wash-out. J Appl Physiol 46 (6): 1184–1190
Johns DP, Pretto JJ, Streeton JA (1982) Measurement of gas viscosity with a Fleisch pneumotachograph J Appl Physiol 53 (1): 290–293
Kaneko K (1978) Simultaneous helium and nitrogen singlebreath washout: lung model simulation. J Appl Physiol 44 (4): 499–506
Kelman GR (1966) Digital computer subroutine for conversion of oxygen tension into saturation. J Appl Physiol 21: 1375–1376
Kelman GR (1967) Digital computer procedure for the conversion of P_{CO2} into blood CO_2 content. Respir Physiol 3: 111–115
Kelman GR (1970) new lung model: an investigation with the aid of a digital computer. Comput Biomed Res 3: 241
Krumpe P, Weigt G, Martinez N, Marcan R, Cumariskey JM (1982) Computerized rapid analysis of pulmonary function test: use of a least mean squares correlation for interpretation of data. Comput Biol Med 12 (4): 295–307
Kung M, Tochmes L, Birch SJ, Fernandez RJ, Abraham WM, Sackner MA (1980) Hemodynamics at rest and during exercise in comfortable, hot and cold environments. Measurements with a rebreathing technique. Bull Eur Physio-Pathol Respir 16: 429–441
Lándsér FJ, Nagels J, Demedts M, Billiet L, Van de Woestijne KP (1976) A new method to determine frequency characteristics of the respiratory system. J Appl Physiol 41 (1): 101–106
Lewis FJ, Shimizu T, Scofield AL, Rosi PS (1966) Analysis of respiration by an on-line digital computer system: clinical data following thoracoabdominal surgery. Ann Surg 164: 547
Lisboa C, Ross DWR, Jardim J, Macklem PT (1979) Pulmonary pressure-flow curves measured by a data-averaging circuit. J Appl Physiol 47 (3): 621–627
Lisboa C, Wood LD.H., Jardim J, Macklem PT (1980) Relation between flow, cuvelinearity, an density dependence of pulmonary pressure-flow curves. J Appl Physiol 48 (5): 878–885
Lorino H, Brault Y, Harf A, Atlan G, Lorino AM, Laurent D (1978) On-line calculations of pulmonary mechanics by digital computer. Methods Inf Med 17 (4): 261–711
Mertens Ph (1983) A simple model of V_A/Q distribution for analysis of inert gas elimination data. J Appl Physiol 55 (2): 562–568 (1983)
Millhorn HT Jr, Brown DR (1971) Steady-state summation of the human respiratroy system. Comput Biomed Res 3: 604

Millhorn HT, Benton R, Ross R, Guyton A (1965) A mathematical model of the human respiratory control system. Biophys J 5: 27

Minken YP, Gardner RM, Adams TD, Yanowitz FG (1982) Computerized determination of pneumotachometer characteristics using a calibrated syringe. J Appl Physiol 53 (1): 280–285

Mitchell RR (1979) Incorporation the gas analyzer response time in gas exchange computations. J Appl Physiol 47 (5): 1118–1122

Morgan DL, Gourlay AR, Denison DM (1984) An optical method of studying the shape and movement of the chest wall in recumbent patients. Thorax 39: 101–106

Moser KM, Torzewski DF, Nubla LW (1969) Practical computer program for routine spirometric testing using the "time-sharing" concept. Dis Chest 56: 92–97

Naimark A, Cherniack RM, Ptorri D (1971) Comprehensive respiratory information system for clinical investigation of respiratory disease. Am Rev Respir Dis 103: 229–239

Nakumura T, Miyamoto Y, Sakakibara K, Tamura T, Takahashi M, Hiura T, Mikami T (1982) An on-line computer system for monitoring respiratory and cardiac functions of patients. Biotelem Patient Monit 9: 49–62

Olszowka AJ, Wagner PD (1980) Numerical analysis of gas exchange. In: West JB (ed) Pulmonary gas exchange vol. 1. Academic, New York, pp 263–306

Osborn JJ, Beaumont JO, Raison JCA, Russell J, Gerbode F (1968) Measurement and monitoring of acutely ill patients by digital computer. Surgery 64: 1057

Osswald PM, Bernauer J, Bender MJ, Hartung HJ (1981) Graphic presentation of blood gas data in computers. In: Prakash O (ed) Critical care and pulmonary medicine vd 1. Plenum, New York, pp 343–353

Pack AI, McCusher R, Moran F (1977) A computer system for processing data from routine pulmonary function tests. Thorax 32: 333

Paiva M, Demeester M (1971) Gas transport in the air phase of the lung simulated by a digital computer. Comput Biomed Res 3: 675

Pare PD, Books LA, Bates J, Lawson LM, et al. (1982) Exponential analysis of the lung pressure-volume curve as a predictor of pulmonary emphysema. Am Rev Respir Dis 126: 54–61

Peacock AJ, Morgan MDL, Gourlay S, Tucton C, Dension DM (1984) Optical mapping of the thoraco abdominal wall. Thorax 39: 93–100

Pearce DH, Milhorn HT Jr, Holloman GH Jr, Reynolds WJ (1977) Computer-based system for analysis of respiratory responses to exercise. J Appl Physiol 42 (6): 968–975

Pengelly LD (1977) Curve-fitting analysis of pressure-volume characteristics of the lungs. J Appl Physiol 42 (1): 111–116

Peslin R, Jardin P (1983) Influence of second-order data filtering on common forced expiration indices. Clin Physiol 3: 123–130

Peters M, Stacy RW (1964) Automated clinical measurement of respiratory parameters. Surgery 56 (1): 44–51

Petrini MF, Dwyer TM, Phillips M (1982) A computerized timing algorithm for determination of pulmonary tissue volume. J Appl Physiol 55 (1): 258–262

Pierce RJ, Brown DJ, Holmes M et al. (1979) Estimation of lung volumes from chest radiographs using shape information. Thorax 34: 726–734

Protti DJ, Craven N, Naimark A, Cherniack RM (1973) Computer assistance in the clinical investigation of pulmonary function studies. Methods Inf Med 12: 102–107

Rafalsky D, Sieverts H, Schwindke P (1982) Exact BTPS-compensation: a new concept realized with a microcomputerized system. In: Prakash O (ed) Computers in critical care and pulmonary medicine, vol 2. Plenum, New York, pp 131–137

Rittel H-F, Waterloh E, Rössmann K, Schön FA (1977) Klein- und Großrechner-Einsatz bei Lungenfunktionsuntersuchungen. Prax Pneumol 31: 1–24

Rosner SW, Palmer A, Caceres CA (1971) A computer program for computation and interpretation of pulmonary function data. Comput Biomed Res 4: 141–156

Sackner MA, Greeneltch D, Heiman MS, Epstein S, Atkins N (1975) Diffusing capacity, membrane diffusing capacity, capillary blood volume, pulmonary tissue volume and cardiac output measured by a rebreathing technique. Am Rev Respir Dis 111: 157–65

Saluminen R, Amola S, Malkiä E, Vuori I (1982) Computerized breath-by-breath analysis of respiratory variables during exercise. Med Progr Technol 9: 27–32

Shonfeld EM, Kerekes J, Rademacher CA, Wiehrer AL, Abraham S, Sivler H, Caceres C (1964) Methodology for computer measurement of pulmonary function curves. Dis Chest 45: 427–434
Siegel JH, Farrell EJ (1973) A computer simulation model to study the clinical observability of ventilation and perfusion abnormalities in human shock. Surgery 73: 898–912
Siegel JH, Farrell EJ, Miller M, Goldwyn RM, Friedman HP (1973) Cardiorespiratory interactions as determinants of survival and the need for respiratory support in human shock states. J Trauma 13: 602–619
Smidt U (1979) EDV-unterstützte Auswertung von Lungenfunktionsprüfungen. Prax Pneumol 33: 139–149
Smidt U, Finkenzeller, Remming C (1975) On-line-Computereinsatz in der Ganzkörperplethysmographie zur Berechnung der mittleren Resistance. Pneumologie 151: 223–231
Sodal IE, Swanson GD, Micco AJ, Sprague F, Ellis DG (1983) A computerized mass spectrometer and flowmeter system for respiratory gas measurements. Ann Biomed Eng II: 83–99
Soohoo SL, Brown HV (1983) Computerized body plethysmography: an algorithm for minimizing drift and hysteresis. Comput Biol Med 13 (1): 1–6
Soto RJ, Forster HV, Rasmussen B (1975) Computerized method for analyzing maximum and partial expiratory flow-volume curves. J Appl Physiol 39: 315
Stewart WE, Mastenbrook MS Jr (1983a) Graphical analysis of multiple inert gas elimination data. J Appl Physiol 55 (1): 32–36
Stewart WE, Mastenbrook MS Jr (1983b) Parametric estimation of ventilation-perfusion ratio distributions. J Appl Physiol 55 (1): 37–51
Sulotto F, Romano C, Guazzotti T (1982) A computerized interpretation of standard pulmonary function tests. Bull Eur Physiopathol Respir 18: 983–999
Sykes TW, Haynes RL, McFadden ER Jr (1977) On line determination of lung volumes by plethysmography and digital computer. Am Rev Respir Dis 115: 581–585
Tanser AR (1982) The use of a micro computer system in a lung function testing laboratory. Br J Dis Chest 76: 130–134
Tsai MJ, Pimmel RL, Donohue JF (1979) Automatic classification of spirometric data. IEEE Trans Biomed Eng 26: 293–298
Uhl RR, Lewis FJ (1974) Digital computer calculation of human pulmonary mechanics using a least squares fit technique. Comput Biomed Res 7: 489–495
Vallbona C, Pevny E, McMath F (1971) Computer analysis of blood gases and acid-base status. Comput Biomed Res 4: 623–633
Verbraak AFM, Bogaard JM, Jansen FRC et al: Automatic data processing in the clinical lungfunction laboratory. In computers in critical care and pulmonary medicine. 2, 85–90. Edited by O Prakash. Plenum press (1982)
Wagner PD (1981) Ventilation-perfusion relationships. Clin Physiol 1: 437–451
Wagner PD, West JB (1972) Effects of diffusion impairment on O_2 and CO_2 time courses in pulmonary capillaries. J Appl Physiol 33 (1): 62–71
Wagner PD, West JB (1980) Ventilation-perfusion relationships. In: West JB (ed) Pulmonary gas exchange vol I. Academic, New York, pp 219–259
Wagner PD, Saltzman HA, West JB (1974) Measurement of continuous distributions of ventilation-perfusion ratios: theory. J Appl Physiol 36: 588–599
Wald A, Jason D, Murphy TW, Mazzia VDB (1969) A computer system for respiratory parameters. Comput Biomed Res 2: 411
Weigt G, Krumpe PE (1980) Computerized rapid analysis of pulmonary function tests: complete computer programs, documentations and instructions. National Technical Information Service, No. PB-82. 5285 Port Royal Road, Springfield. VA
Wessel HU, Stout RL, Bastanier Ch K, Paul MH (1979) Breath-by breath variation of FRC: effect on Vo_2 and Vco_2 measured at the mouth. J Appl Physiol 46 (6): 1122–1126
West JB (1969) Ventilation-perfusion inequality and overall gas exchange in computer models of the lung. Respir Physiol 7: 88–110
Wolff G (1985) Series deadspace. Clin Physiol (in press)
Yamamoto W, Hari T (1971) Phasic air movement model of respiratory regulation of carbon dioxide balance. Comput Biomed Res 3: 699
Young RC, Pennix WG, Ewell MJ (1971) Pulmonary function compatibility of the time sharing computer system. J Am Med Assoc 63: 346–351

The Assessment of Gas Exchange by Automated Analysis of O_2 and CO_2 Alveolar to Arterial Differences: 3 Years Experience in Respiratory Clinical Physiology

P. Paoletti, E. Fornai, A. G. Neto, R. Prediletto, S. Ruschi, and C. Giuntini

Introduction

The determination of alveolar to arterial differences (AaD) is a simple and available method to determine the overall efficiency of gas exchange. AaD are strongly related to the measurement of alveolar gas, and the different methods commonly used to measure alveolar gas concentrations are not able to give an estimate of the "mean alveolar gas". Alveolar gas concentrations are commonly measured by

1. end-tidal determinations of expiratory gases using fast analyzers, especially mass-spectrometer; and
2. indirect determinations of alveolar gas by Bohr and ideal alveolar air equations, based on measurements of mean expired fractions, tidal volume, and anatomical dead space.

In 1949 the "mean alveolar gas" was defined by Rahn, using the "V/Q lines" in the O_2-CO_2 diagram, as the gas mixture where the instantaneous respiratory quotient is equal to the mean respiratory quotient, measured previously by mixed expired gas concentrations. Few determinations of alveolar gas concentrations and AaD by Rahn's definition have been performed in clinical studies, essentially because of the complexity of manual determinations.

We developed a computer-based system which allowed the simultaneous determination of alveolar gas concentrations by the traditional methods [end-tidal (ET), Bohr (BE), and ideal alveolar air (ID) equations] and by Rahn's definition (RD), with the aim of studying the pattern of alveolar pressures and AaD measured by different methods in patients with different pulmonary diseases.

This study reports the results of the application of this automated technique in patients with respiratory failure due to chronic obstructive lung disease (COLD) and in patients with acute pulmonary embolism (PE).

Material and Methods

Experimental Setup

The experimental setup is shown in schematic form in Fig. 1. The measurement of gas exchange was performed in steady-state conditions: the patient, in sitting or semi-

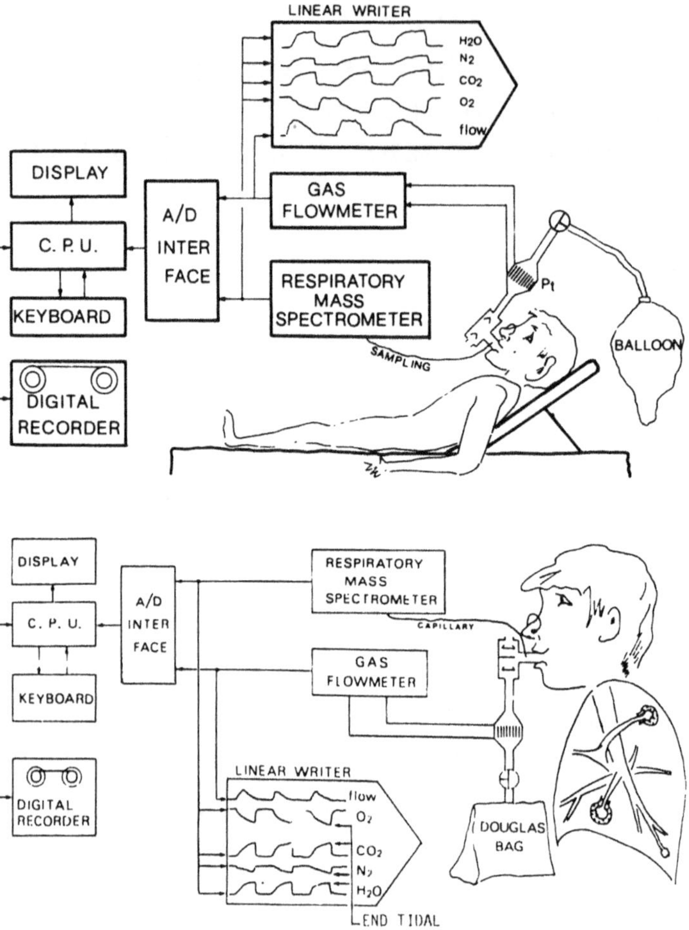

Fig. 1. Scheme of the experimental set up. Semi-recumbent position in critical patients; sitting position in other patients to maintain the physiological distribution of ventilation and perfusion

recumbent position, wore a nose-clip and breathed through a mouthpiece into a Hans-Rudolph valve (34 ml dead space) connected to a pneumotachograph (Fleisch no. 3) for flow and volume measurements. The expired gas was collected in a Douglas bag for 5 min, and at the same time, breath by breath, the expiratory gas concentrations were analyzed by a mass spectrometer (Varian M_3). During the final minute a sample of arterial blood was collected from the radial artery. The blood gas analysis was performed immediately by the standard electrode method (IL 1302). Signals from the mass spectrometer (MS) and flowmeter were fed to a computer (HP 1000) through an AD interface; the sampling rate for each signal was 100 Hz.

The steady state was achieved after a few minutes of adaptation; the operator was able to check the pattern of the signals both on the polygraph recorder and on the computer terminal. The description of the computer program is reported elsewhere Giannella et al. (1981), but is here summarized.

Computer Program

Calibrations of flow and volume were performed by a standard syringe (1 liter in volume), and MS was calibrated by using a water-vapor-saturated known mixture of gases (CO_2, O_2, and N_2). Calibrations are performed before and after the test to correct the possible shift of MS signals. Concentrations of collected gas (in the Douglas bag) are measured by the MS, and blood gas data are entered via the keyboard terminal.

The program provides the identification of

1. the expiratory flow signal and
2. the beginning of the water vapor signal.

The water vapor signal is the fastest among the expiratory gases and it is used to align in time all the MS gas concentrations with the flow. The following parameters are then computed breath by breath:

1. End-tidal fractions (FET) and pressures (PET) of O_2, CO_2, N_2, and H_2O
2. Mean fractions ($\overline{FE}$) and pressures ($\overline{PE}$) of O_2, Co_2, N_2, and H_2O derived from the computation of the area of the concentration-time tidal expirograms
3. Mean respiratory exchange ratio (MRQ) from $\overline{FECO_2}/\overline{FEO_2}$
4. Instantaneous respiratory exchange ratio (IRQ)
5. End-tidal respiratory exchange ratio (ETRQ)
6. Mean fractions, mean pressures, and respiratory quotient from the analysis of the expired gas collected in the Douglas bag, in order to check the results of the mean fractions and the MRQ computed during the breath-by-breath analysis.

Alveolar pressures and AaD for O_2 and CO_2 were computed by the following methods:

1. End-tidal (ETO_2, $ETCO_2$).
2. Bohr equation (BEO_2, $BECO_2$), using the equations

$$PACO_2 = VT \cdot (PECO_2/VT\text{-}VDanat) \tag{1}$$

where VT is the tidal volume and VDanat is the anatomical dead space [the VDanat was computed from the prediction equation of Hart et al. (1963)] and

$$PAO_2 = PIO_2 - PACO_2 \cdot (FIO_2 - FIO_2/MRQ) \tag{2}$$

where $PACO_2$ is derived using Eq. (1).

3. Application of Rahn's definition of mean alveolar gas (RDO_2, $RDCO_2$). In each single breath the algorithm provides the identification of the equality between MRQ and IRQ, considering the MRQ computed in the single breath, and the pattern of IRQ during the same breath. The point of the equality between MRQ and IRQ is considered for the alveolar pressure values of O_2 and CO_2.
4. The ideal alveolar O_2 was computed considering the ideal alveolar air equation ($IPAO_2$):

$$PAO_2 = PIO_2 - PACO_2.(FIO_2 - FIO_2/MRQ) \tag{3}$$

The scheme of the algorithms for the determination of the alveolar pressures by these methods in each single breath is shown in Fig. 2.

The program provides also the computation of different dead space measurements:

1. Physiological dead space, using Enghoff's equation:

$$VD/VT\% = (PaCO_2 - PECO_2)\, PaCO_2 \tag{4}$$

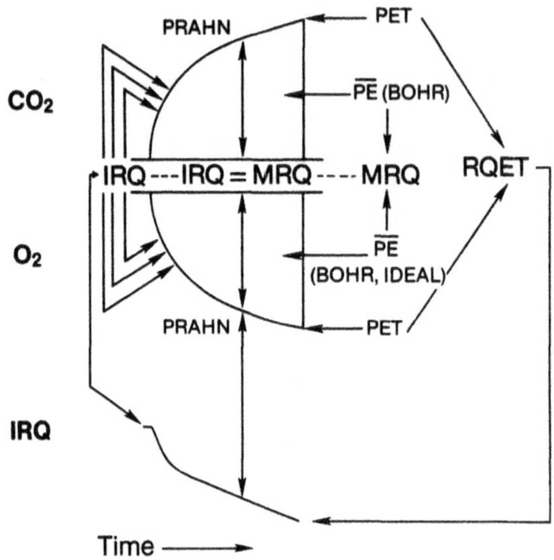

Fig. 2. Scheme of computer algorithms in each single breath. IRQ = instantaneous respiratory exchange ratio: MRQ = mean respiratory exchange ratio; PE = mean pressures; PET = end-tidal pressures; RQET = end-tidal respiratory exchange ratio; PRahn = location in O_2 and CO_2 expirograms of alveolar pressures according to Rahn's definition (where IRQ = MRQ)

2. Alveolar dead space: a) VD alv (Eng)/VT%, subtracting the anatomical dead space measured by the predictions of Hart et al. (1963) in Enghoff equation; b) using the well-ventilated but unperfused index proposed by Severinghaus and Stupfel (1957):

$$\text{VDalv (SE)/VT\%} = aADCO_2/PaCO_2 \tag{5}$$

c) using the correction for the effect of the reinspiration of anatomical space gas proposed by Robin et al. (1960):

$$\text{VDalv(Ro)/VT\%} = aADCO_2/(aADCO_2 + PECO_2) \tag{6}$$

$ETCO_2$ difference was used for the determination of a, b, and c alveolar dead space.

The validation of the computer program is reported elsewhere (Giannella et al. 1981)

This technique has been routinely used since 1982 in our laboratory in patients with various pulmonary diseases and recently has been used in critical patients [PE and acute respiratory distress syndrome (ARDS)].

Results

Results of the application of this technique in patients with severe COLD and acute PE are reported separately.

Cold patients

Sixteen patients (mean age 58.9 ± 9.5 years) were studied. Most were affected by both chronic bronchitis and emphysema. The diagnosis was assessed by clinical history, physical examination, chest radiography, spirometry, and arterial blood gas analysis. Values of PAO_2 ranged from 34 to 60 mmHg and those of $PACO_2$ from 32 to 72 mmHg; mean value of FEV_1 as percent of predicted was 38 ± 23.9.

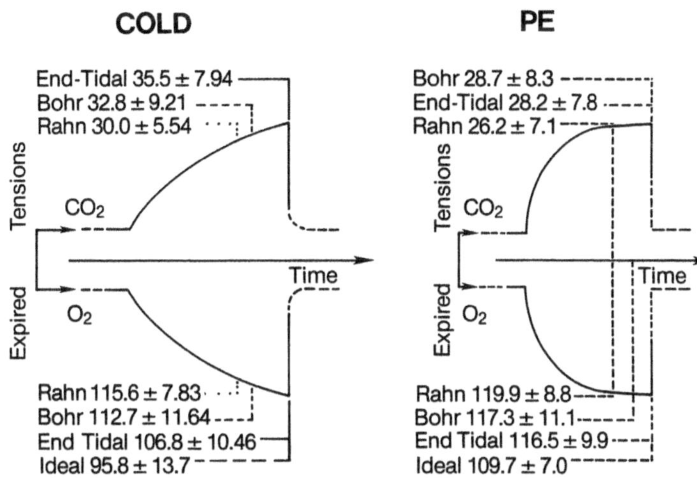

Fig. 3. Location of mean alveolar pressure values by different methods in the tidal expirograms of COLD and PE patients. The shape of O_2 and CO_2 expirograms is representative of the patterns observed in the patients of the two diseases

Gas exchange parameters were determined with patients in a sitting position. The points where the alveolar pressures are located by each method in the O_2 and CO_2 expirograms are represented in Fig. 3; mean values and standard deviation for each method are also reported. Rahn alveolar pressures occur before BE and ET determinations in each tidal expirogram during steady-state breathing. This result indicates the possibility of finding the point where IRQ = MRQ before the end of the expiration. Comparison of the methods (by paired t test) showed that ET O_2 and CO_2 were significantly different from BE and RD. BE and RD were not significantly different. $IPAO_2$ resulted always in the lowest value and was significantly different from the other methods. The same trend and statistical difference were observed for AaD.

Regression analysis of VD/VT% and $aADCO_2$ derived by each method are shown in Table 1. A significant correlation was always found ($p < .001$). However, the slope is somewhat steeper (and thus the correlation coefficient higher) for the ET $aADCO_2$.

PE Patients

Fifteen patients (eight men and seven women, mean age 58 ± 16 years) were studied during the acute episode of PE and at different time intervals after the anticoagulant therapy (Giannella et al. 1982), Diagnostic perfusion lung scan was performed in three projections using albumin macroaggregates labeled with ^{131}I and injected in a sitting position to maintain the physiological base-to-apex perfusion gradient. Measurement of gas exchange parameters was performed in a semi-recumbent position because of the severity of the patient's condition during the acute episode.

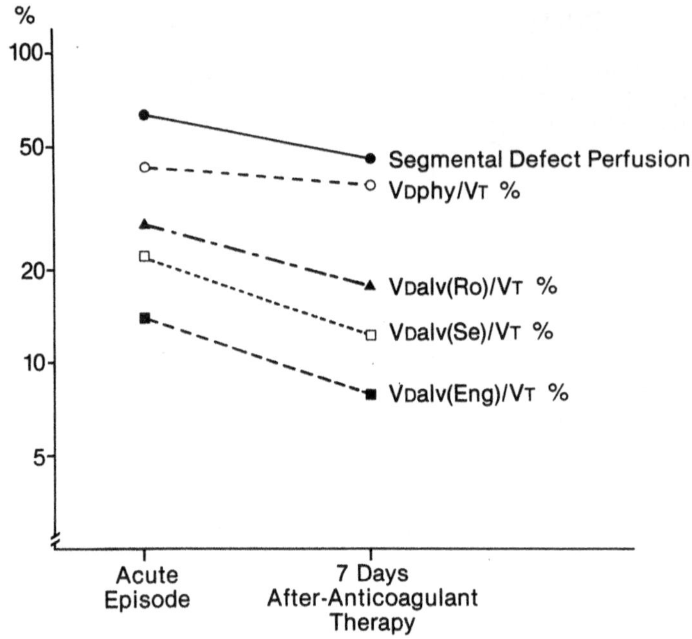

Fig. 4. Relationships between dead space measurements, physiologic (VDphy/VT%) and alveolar (by different methods), and perfusion defects (expressed in percent) measured by the number of unperfused segments at the perfusion lung scan. Relationships are shown in the acute condition and after anticoagulant therapy

Figure 3 shows the points where the alveolar presssures and their mean values and SD by each method are located in the O_2 and CO_2 tidal expirograms. Also in these patients, it was possible to find equality between IRQ and MRQ before the end of the expiration during steady-state breathing. Values of alveolar pressures by all methods were similar, with the exception of $IPAO_2$.

The relationships between different dead space measurements (alveolar and physiological) and the perfusion lung scan defects during the acute episode and after 1 week of therapy are shown in Fig. 4. The number of lung segments without perfusion was used as an approximate index of perfusion impairment (Giannella et al. 1982), and expressed in percent. VDphy/VT% was the closer value to the percent of perfusion defects: however, alveolar dead space measurements were consistently lower than the perfusion impairment. VDalv (Ro)/VT%, was the higher alveolar dead space, both in the acute episode and after 7 days of therapy.

Discussion

The application of this automated technique showed the possibility of measuring alveolar gas pressures by Rahn's definition in each single breath in both groups of patients. This result is different from that of Luft et al. (1979), who were able to find the equality of MRQ and IRQ during steady-state breathing in only 55% of their patients. This difference may be explained by the use of different methodologies. Essentially, our computerized breath-by-breath technique provides an accurate estimate analysis of IRQ in each single breath during the whole period of the test. Luft et al. (1979) measured alveolar gas by Rahn's definition using the Bargeton (1967) technique in a few breaths at the end of the test. Therefore, the accurate IRQ analysis and the computation of MRQ in each single breath (by O_2 and CO_2 mean fractions) permits the breath-by-breath determination of alveolar gas by Rahn's definition. In addition, MRQ computed in each single breath was not significantly different from the respiratory quotient measured by analysis of expiratory gas concentration of mixed expired gas collected in a Douglas bag (Giannella et al. 1981).

Alveolar pressures showed a different pattern in the two groups of patients, except for PAO_2 derived from the ideal alveolar air equation. In fact, $IPAO_2$ was the lowest value and significantly different from the other values in both diseases. This result is explained by the assumption that alveolar CO_2 is equal to arterial CO_2 in the ideal alveolar air equation. Therefore the dead space component, which may be important in COLD, is not evaluated, resulting in incorrect measurement of alveolar O_2 and consequently of AaD.

ET alveolar pressures and AaD were significantly different (by paired t test) from BE and RD in COLD patients. ET values of gas concentrations represent the lung units at low $\dot{V}A/Q$ (West et al. 1957 a, b), especially in patients with COLD, where the extreme asynchronous emptying of the lung units produces the sampling of low VA/Q units. RD alveolar pressures also provide the evaluation of the contribution of high $\dot{V}A/Q$ units because of the location before the ET point. Therefore, RD allows a more precise determination of the alveolar gas because the contribution of high $\dot{V}A/Q$ units (dead space effect) is considered. This component is important in COLD patients as demonstrated by Wagner et al. (1977) using the multiple inert gas technique.

BE and RD values were very similar in COLD patients; however, BE determinations are dependent or the measurement of the anatomical dead space. Our automated technique does not provide direct measurement of the anatomical dead space, because of the difficulty of its determination during steady breathing, especially in COLD patients. Prediction equations (Hart et al. 1963) were used to derive this parameter. Nevertheless, the use of a prediction equation is always questionable, especially for a small volume which strongly influences $PACO_2$ and consequently PAO_2. Therefore we think RD measurement of alveolar gas and AaD better characterize patients with COLD.

Alveolar pressure and AaD by the different methods were similar in PE, except for ideal O_2 determination (Fig. 3). The different pattern from COLD patients is explained by the presence of different shapes of O_2 and CO_2 tracings. In fact, a plateau is present in the final part of the expirograms in PE patients, therefore the allocation of RD alveolar pressures before the ET point does not cause important differences. On the contrary, the presence of a steeper slope in the final part of the O_2 and CO_2 expirograms in COLD patients causes the differences between ET and RD measurements.

Table 1. Correlation between VD/VT% and the three different $aADCO_2$ in COLD patients

Y	vs	X	Methods	Regression	r	P	n
VD/VT%		$aADCO_2$	RD	y = 39.27 + .69 x	.79	<.00001	16
VD/VT%		$aADCO_2$	BE	y = 41.38 + .67 x	.77	<.00002	16
VD/VT%		$aADCO_2$	ET	y = 38.25 + 1.13 x	.84	<.00001	16

RD = Rahn's definition; BE = Bohr equation; ET = End Tidal

The relationships between VD/VT% and $aADCO_2$ in COLD patients were always significant (Table 1); however, VD/VT% is influenced by changes in the tidal volume and does not take account of the dilution of respiratory gases in the physiological dead space (Ross and Farhi 1960), and this may be important in COLD.

The wasted ventilation is better assessed by the measurement of $aADCO_2$, which directly represents the efficiency of the ventilation instead of the VD/VT% value. The good correlations between VD/VT% and $aADCO_2$ (all methods) show that VD/VT% is a satisfactory indirect determination of dead space effect, but must not be considered the reference for the accuracy of $aADCO_2$ measurements (Luft et al. 1979; Nunn and Hill 1960; Pappius et al. 1975).

The analysis of the relationships between different dead space measurements and perfusion defects during the evolution of the disease in PE patients showed that alveolar dead space values were always lower than the estimate (%) of perfusion defects, evaluated by the number of unperfused segments. Air shift from the embolized lung areas has been demonstrated in animal models (Dantzker et al. 1978; Levy and Simmons 1975). In humans this component is not demonstrated. Nevertheless, regional lung ventilation studies by radioisotope techniques show the presence of ventilation in the unperfused area, and this finding is considered a standard diagnostic criterion (Moser et al. 1971). Therefore the lack of correlation between dead space measurements and the unperfused lung zones may be explained by other mechanisms, such as incomplete vessel occlusion (Giannella et al. 1972). VDalv (Ro) was the highest value of the alveolar dead space, pointing out the importance of correction for the reinspiration of anatomical dead space gases.

In conclusion, this paper has summarized some results of the application of this automated technique in different diseases. In particular, this method has been useful on studying some physiopathological mechanisms in COLD and PE. Nevertheless, the technique is very simple and reliable for day-by-day evaluation of gas exchange in pulmonary and critical patients.

Acknowledgements. This study was supported by the Italian Research Council, Special Project on Preventive Medicine, Subproject on Chronic Obstructive Lung Disease, 81-00392.83. Antonio Giannella Neto was a visiting researcher from COPPE/UFRJ (Brazil) with a fellowship from CNP_q.

References

Rahn H (1949) A concept of mean alveolar air and the ventilation-blood flow relationships during pulmonary gas exchange. Am J Physiol 158: 21–30

Giannella A, Fornai E, Paoletti P, Pisani P, Marchesi C, Giuntini C (1981) Computer evaluation of respiratory gases parameters and alveolar to arterial differences in clinical and research pulmonary medicine. In: Proc Internat Conf Computers in Critical Care and Pulmonary Medicine, Norwalk, June

Hart MC, Orzalesi MM, Cook CD (1963) Relation between anatomic respiratory dead space and body size and lung volume. J Appl Physiol 18: 519–522

Severinghaus JW and Stupfel M (1957) Alveolar dead space as an index of distribution of blood flow in pulmonary capillaries. J Appl Physiol 10: 335–348

Robin ED, Forkner CE, Bromberg PA, Croteau JR, Travis DM (1960) Alveolar gas exchange in pulmonary embolism. N Engl J Med 262: 283–287

Giannella A, Fornai E, Paoletti P, Prediletto R, Fazzi P, Di Ricco G, Marini C, Perissinotto A, Giuntini C (1982) Control of ventilation and gas exchange in massive pulmonary embolism with severe hypoxia. Bull Eur Physiopathol Respir 18 (4): 127–138

Luft UC, Leoppky JA, Mostyn EM (1979) Mean alveolar gases and alveolar-arterial gradients in pulmonary patients. J Appl Physiol 46: 534–540

Bargeton D (1967) Analysis of capnigram and oxygram in man. Bull Physio-pathol Respir 3: 503–526

West JB, Fowler KT, Hugh-Jones P, O'Donnel T (1957a) Measurement of the ventilation-perfusion ratio inequality in the lung by the analysis of a single expirate. Clin Sci 16: 529–547

West JB, Fowler KT, Hugh-Jones P, O'Donnel T (1957b) Measurement of the inequality of ventilation and perfusion in the lung by analysis of a single expirate. Clin Sci 16: 549–565

Wagner PD, Dantzker DR, Dueck R, Clausen JL, West JB (1977) Ventilation-perfusion inequality in chronic pulmonary disease. J Clin Invest 59: 203–206

Ross BB, Farhi LE (1960) Dead-space ventilation as a determinant in the ventilation-perfusion concept. J Appl Physiol 15: 363–371

Nunn JF, Hill DW (1960) Respiratory dead space and arterial to end-tidal CO_2 difference in anesthetized man. J Appl Physiol 15: 383–389

Poppius H, Korhonen O, Viljanen AA, Kreus KE (1975) Arterial to end-tidal CO_2 difference in respiratory disease. Scand J Respir Dis 56: 254–256

Dantzker DR, Wagner PD, Tornabene VW, Alazraki ND, West JB (1978) Gas exchange after thromboembolization in dogs. Circ Res 42: 92–103

Levy SE, Simmons DH (1975) Mechanisms of arterial hypoxemia following pulmonary thromboembolism in dogs. J Appl Physiol 39: 41–46

Moser KM, Guisan M, Cuomo A (1971) Differentiation of pulmonary vascular from parenchymal diseases by ventilation-perfusion scintigraphy. Ann Int Med 75: 597–605

Computers in Experimental Pathophysiological Research

R. Schosser, H.-P. Engel, and K. Messmer

Introduction

Although they have been available for more than a decade, only a few monitoring and biosignal processing systems have been installed in research laboratories and clinical departments. This is due not only to the investment expediture, but depends mainly on costs and time to adapt the systems to the particular environment in which they are to be used.

This situation can not be clearly understood without understanding the history of their development. Three issues have to be considered when evaluating "first generation" systems:

1. Memory and disc capacities were expensive at that time and therefore the software was structured primarily to save space.
2. Software was not "engineered" but "programmed," since scientifically based concepts (e. g., structured programming) and appropriate tools (e. g., languages supporting structured programming) were not yet common knowledge.
3. The software was not programmed with general applicability and portability in mind, but was first produced to satisfy specific local requirements.

The result was large "bulky" programs. If, therefore, the software had to be modified, it required great effort to make even minor changes. As a consequence, the software did not usually benefit from these manipulations; quite the opposite, its structure became more complex instead. Even the software available,today has not improved substantially, since most of it evolved from the "first generation" systems.

Although clinical experience and relevance have been reviewed recently (Osswald et al. 1984), *general* concepts and methods of software engineering for biosignal processing and monitoring systems have not been described in the literature. This illustrates how little attention has been paid to the design of biomedical software. On the other hand, it has been realized, that lack of flexibility is one of the major obstacles preventing a more widespread propagation of these systems into different biomedical environments (Swoboda and Polonius 1983).

Environment

The environment can be defined as the sum of all organisational and operational characteristics of a given application which affect software and/or hardware realization of a biosignal monitoring or processing system. Environmental characteristics may be, for example, the analog instrumentation, input and/or output formats, data processing algorithms, and even methods or parameters to be used. The programs are usually designed to satisfy exactly the requirements of a particular application, preferably in the situation in which it has been developed; hence, this software is "tailored" to its environment. If an attempt is made to transfer the software (supposing hardware compatibility) to another evironment with different organisational and operational characteristics, it will not fit. To solve this problem, two alternatives have been tried in the past:

Modification of the Environment. This means a decisive disruption of the organisation and operation of a complex unit such as a research laboratory or an ICU. Therefore it is often not feasible and, if feasible, it is not to be recommended, since the result is usually a low user acceptance of the system.

Modification of the Existing Software. This is an expensive and time-consuming procedure with sucess being doubtful. Despite this fact, software modifications have been performed many times on the same system to adapt it to different environments. Most of the systems which are at present in use emerged this way.

In the research laboratory, unlike routine applications, a different environment is created each time the experimental set-up changes. Therefore the problem of software "portability" from one environment to another is not solely encountered between different units but, even more importantly, within the same unit. It is evident that a study on hemorrhagic shock requires different methods to be applied and different parameters to be measured than a study on artificial ventilation. It is obvious that neither the environment can be adopted to the software, nor the software be modified each time the experimental set-up changes. This dilemma was the reason why we excluded existing systems and started to design a new versatile system by applying modern concepts of software technology.

Method Base Systems (MBS)

The basis of the new software concept is a so-called method base system. Generally, an MBS is a software system which provides the user with programs or entire program systems to solve the problems of a particular application and has two salient features (Dittrich et al. 1979):

1. The system must be easily adaptible to different environments.
2. The handling of the system does not require a detailed background in data processing.

The literature on MBS is rare, widespread, and difficult of access, because it is predominantly related to particular projects and products (Dittrich et al. 1979). Existing MBS are confined to industrial management, public and medical administration, engineering and statistics in social sciences. As far as we know, real-time applications like biosignal processing and monitoring systems have not been realized with MBS.

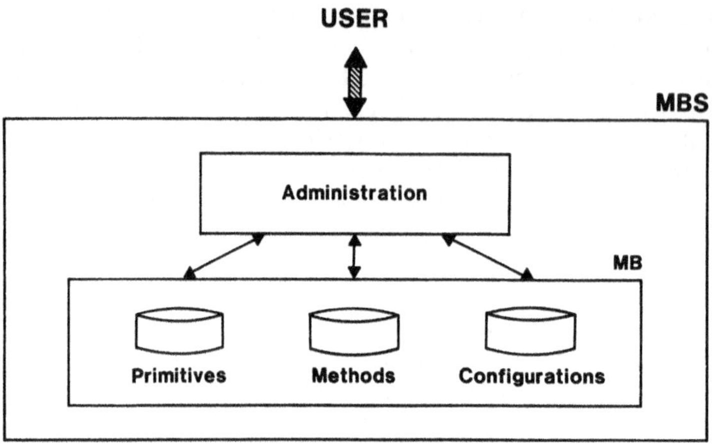

Fig. 1. Components of the MBS

MBS for Biosignal Processing Applications

The MBS concept that we developed, consists of the "method base" (MB), and "administrative" system, and a "run-time" system. The constituents are described in the following sections.

Method Base

The MB comprises three types of components: primitives, methods, and configurations (Fig. 1).

Primitives

Primitives are modules which perform elementary functions. The *structure* of a primitive is uniformly the same (Fig. 2). It consists of an input "connector," the "body" and an output "connector." The connectors have one or several data channels and one or several control channels, which could be described as connector "pins." The connectors are the interfaces to other primitives. The body contains the algorithm to perform the elementary function.

Likewise, the *function* is also the same for all primitives. Together with the control information, the data from the preceeding primitive is entered through the input connector, it is then processed in the actual primitive, and finally both data and control are transferred to the succeeding primitive through the output connector.

The function of primitives is explained in Fig. 3 showing five possible examples:

1. The first primitive serves signal input by digitizing analog signals, e. g., and ECG. By means of variable parameter settings (sampling rate, gain etc.), the *same primitive* may be used for *different signals*. These primitives are attributed "parametrized."
2. A digital filter primitive may be used to reduce signal noise; thus signal quality can be improved. Since the digital filters are parametrized, the same primitive may be applied to different filtering problems, e. g., in the frequency domain.

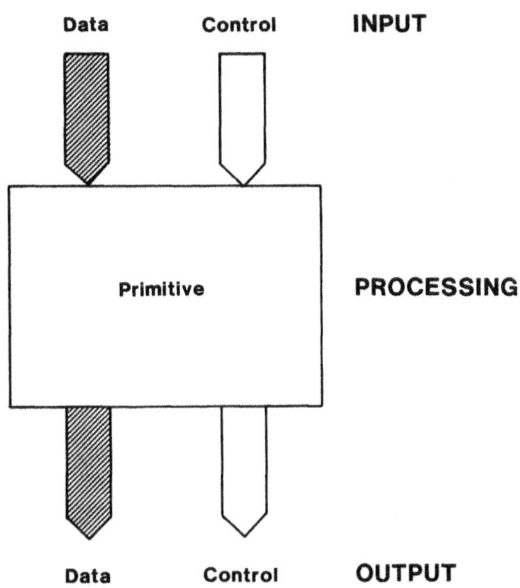

Fig. 2. Structure of a primitive

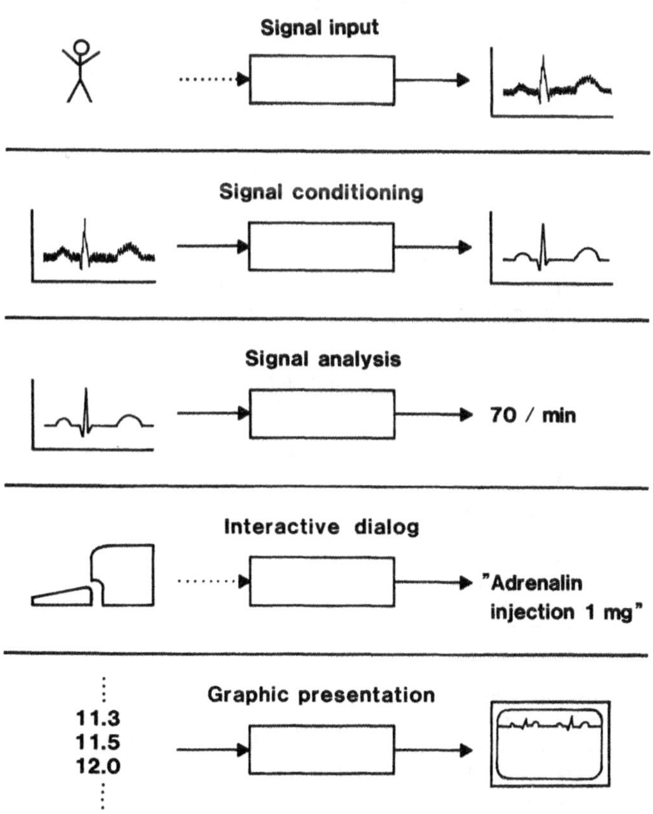

Fig. 3. Examples of primitives

3. With signal processing primitives the signals can be analysed and additional parameters may be derived, e.g., the heart rate from the ECG.
4. With a different type of primitive the interactive dialogue between user and computer can be realized by primitives, e.g., to enter a comment.
5. The graphic presentation of data, e.g., an ECG curve, can also be carried out by primitives.

In general, any process which may be expressed as algorithm with data and control I/O can also be realized as a primitive. However, since primitives perform only elementary functions, they do not usually provide a complete and meaningful method for a given application. Therefore several primitives have to be linked together to form a more complex type of component, the so-called methods.

Methods

A method generally consists of two or more compatible primitives which are linked together in a meaningful manner. A method is complete in itself. Data and control input is transferred directly to the first primitive, and returned from the last primitive within a method.

Figure 4 shows, as a well known example, the method used to obtain the average heart rate from an ECG curve as it can be realized with our system. The signal is entered into the system using a parametrized primitive for data acquisition. The digitized signal is then filtered by another parametrized primitive to improve signal quality. Processing of the ECG curve is carried out by three primitives for detecting the R-peaks, measuring the RR-intervals and computing the reciprocal value. Finally a parametrized primitive performs averaging over any desired time constant.

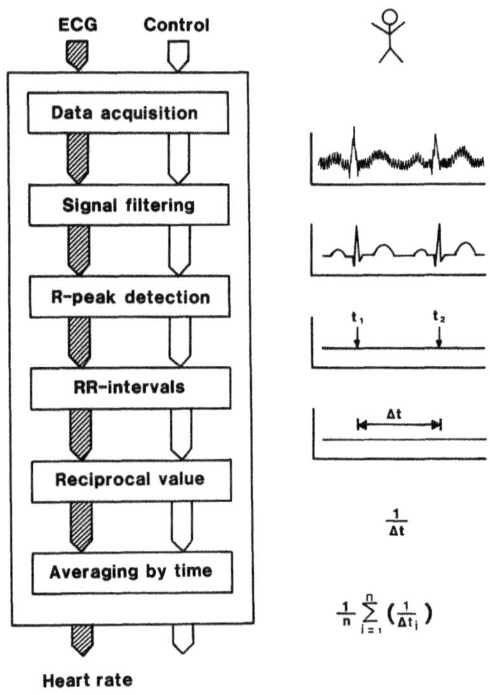

Fig. 4. Structure and example of a method

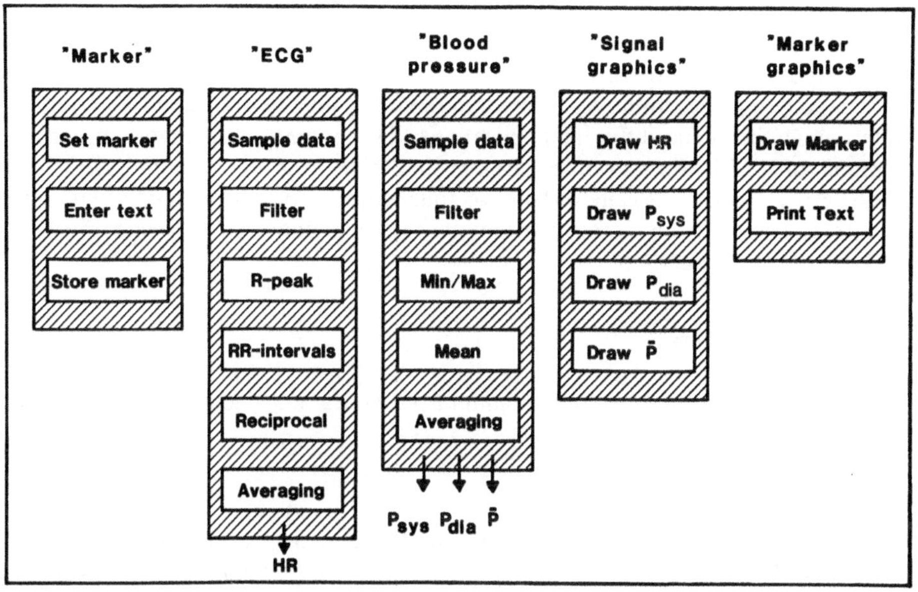

Fig. 5. Structure and example of a configuration

In general, it is possible to construct any method that can be composed of a given set of primitives with compatible data and control channels. The methods may have any level of complexity.

Configurations

One single method, however, is not enough to perform an experiment in the research laboratory or to monitor the vital functions of a patient in the ICU. Several methods have to be combined to form a so-called configuration.

As an example, Fig. 5 shows a simple hemodynamic experiment. This configuration is built from five methods as follows:

1. The method MARKER supports the setting of an event flag together with a text comment to identify the event.
2. The methods ECG and BLOOD PRESSURE are used to enter the ECG and the aortic pressure curve into the computer. After filtering, the signals are analyzed and the average heart rate as well as systolic, diastolic and mean arterial pressures are derived.
3. With the methods SIGNAL GRAPHICS and MARKER GRAPHICS the heart rate and the pressures are displayed on a video monitor along with the markers and comments.

Within the methods BLOOD PRESSURE and ECG, three primitives, namely SAMPLE DATA, FILTER and AVERAGING are identical. Although they are identical, they do not perform exactly the same task since the ECG is digitized with a rate of 250 sampless-, while the arterial pressure curve is digitized only with a rate of

100 sampless-. Therefore, the parameter "sampling rate" is variable, and the actual value is transferred to the primitive via one of the data channels which is characteristic for parametrized primitives.

As a consequence primitives, once programmed, may be re-used in a variety of different methods for different applications. This is one of the most important features of MBS. Furthermore, as can be seen from the method SIGNAL GRAPHICS, which basically consists of four identical primitives named DRAW, primitives may also be re-fused within the same method. In this case the only difference is the input data.

Administrative System

The MBS does not work without an administrative frame, which is described in the next section.

Builder

When the MBS is used for the first time, the MB contains nothing but a library of primitives. With an interactive utility program, named "builder", primitives are selected from the library and linked to appropriate methods. In the next step, the methods may be combined into arbitrary configurations which meet exactly the requirements of the actual environment. Once they are created, both methods and configurations can be stored in libraries for further use.

This generation process may be repeated at any time for both methods and configurations. The libraries may be updated by adding or deleting components. This allows optimal flexibility in "unstable" environments like research laboratories, where the actual environment changes frequently.

Although a configuration has been generated, it is not yet ready to be executed, since the libraries of methods and configurations contain only *descriptions* of the components. Therefore, the logical descriptions have to be translated to a correlate, which can be operated by the computer. This is achieved by a second utility program, the so-called "loader."

Loader

The loader is a stand-alone program which requires no input but the name of a user-specified configuration. The loader then looks up the description of this configuration, reads the referenced method descriptions and finally resolves the primitives that are components of the methods. With this information the loader builds up a configuration image containing all the controll and data information necessary to run the configuration. Finally the configuration image is loaded into a specific memory partition, the "common data and control area."

Run-time System

After the image has been loaded, the configuration is ready to be executed (Fig. 6). Once the system is started, control is transferred to the "execution supervisor" which

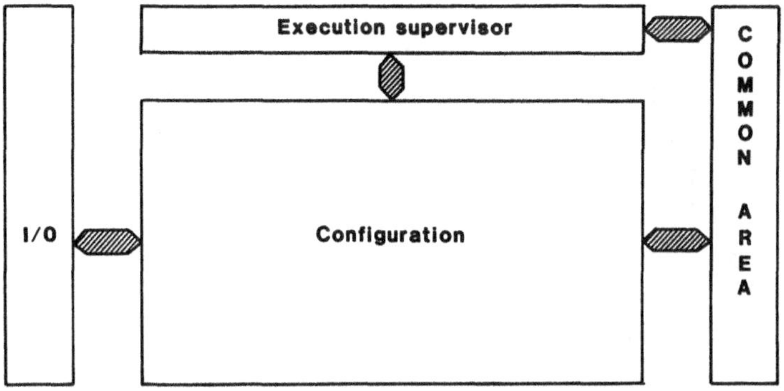

Fig. 6.
Run time system

coordinates all activities within the configuration. At run-time, the configuration physically consists of a number of tasks, each corresponding to one primitive. The execution supervisor starts and synchronizes the tasks, and provides them with control information. Task-to-task and task-to-supervisor communication is performed via the common data and control area. Task-to-peripherals communication, e.g., signal input or graphic output is passed through system I/O directives.

Hardware

The minimal configuration to run this software is a computer with a single-processor structure using a multitasking operating system. Recently, however, computer systems became available which offer multiprocessor capabilities and this is illustrated in Fig. 7.

The system we use at present consists of a master processor and up to 15 co-processors which are connected via the bus. A co-processor is basically a single-board computer which can be referenced as "device" in a similar way as, for example a disc or a terminal. After a program has been located, the co-processor works "parallel" to the master processor. Here it becomes evident to what extent this hardware architecture supports the MBS software concept and thereby increases performance. As an example, those methods could be loaded into a co-processor which require high computational power, like the EEG analysis using a FFT. For a clinical application, one co-processor could be used for each ICU patient, which would allow us to process the data of 15 patients in parallel.

In this hardware architecture the master processor itself becomes a supervisor which coordinates the co-processors and transfers control and data between the components of the system. This structure is very similiar to the run-time system, where the execution supervisor coordinates the methods within a configuration.

Conclusion

Real-time applications of MBS have not been reported so far. However, the MBS as conceptual framework for a new type of biosignal processing software provides the

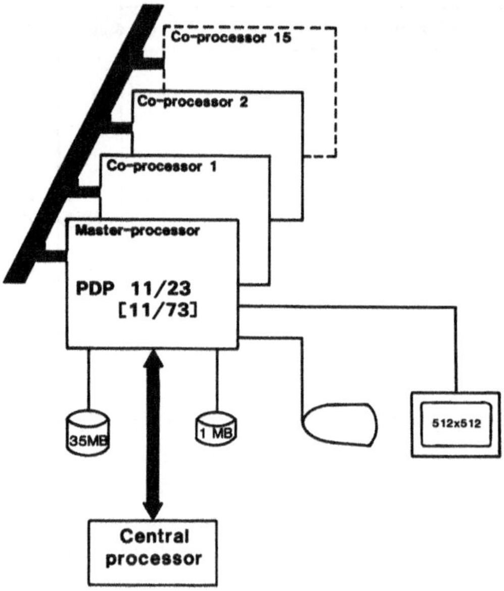

Fig. 7. Hardware structure

user with a very versatile and flexible "interface" to the environment. Therefore, the computer system can be adapted easily to different evironments without software modifications.

Adding new methods or operational characteristics to the system is easy since only a few primitives have to be programmed, this is simple, thanks to their well defined structure and new methods and configurations can then be readily generated. The software structure, however, never has to be changed, which is probably the greatest advantage of this concept.

Finally, this system should help to decrease both costs and the time needed to adapt the application system to different environments, to increase user acceptance and, last but not least, to spread the use of biosignal processing and monitoring systems in research laboratories and ICUs.

Acknowledgements. The authors gratefully acknowledge the support given by the Christine-Jung-Stiftung, University of Heidelberg, and by Ambos GmbH, Munich, FRG.

References

Dittrich KR, Hüber R, Lockemann PC (1979) Methodenbanksysteme: Ein Werkzeug zum Maßschneidern von Anwendersoftware. Inform Spektrum 2: 194–203

Osswald PM, Bender HJ, Hartung HJ, Lutz H (1984) Perspektiven des Computereinsatzes in der Anaesthesie. Anaesthesist 33: 129–133

Swoboda A, Polonius MJ (1983) Kriterien für den Einsatz eines Rechnersystems in der Intensivmedizin. In: Epple E, Frey R, Bleicher W, Apitz J, Schorer R, Faust U (eds) Rechnergestützte Intensivpflege II. Thieme, Stuttgart, pp 209–211 (Intensivmedizin Notfallmedizin Anästhesiologie, vol 44)

Data Bases in Acute Medicine

T. J. Stafford and R. Burney

In chronic medicine, a major direction of computing has been in the field of data bases, with, among other objectives, an ideal of testing hypotheses, seeking patterns. By contrast, computer applications in acute medicine have tended to concentrate on data acquisition, communication, calculation and transformation, control and display, and perhaps some diagnostics.

The unsatisfactory nature of relying on paper records for the management of intensive care data has long been recognized. The logical solution of using a digital computer to capture, store, and display the extremely dense stream of information generated in intensive care found expression throughout the late 1960s and 70s in a number of systems based on minicomputers.

Strictly speaking, this concept has, over the past two decades, proved to be something of a disappointment. Several reasons can be cited: capital cost, support cost, user difficulties, and perhaps preeminently, the lack of a clearly provable benefit, be it time or cost saving. However, the advent of the microprocessor and the consequent fall in computer costs, improvement in network communication, advances in ergonomic design of displays and data entry, increasing sophistication in software development, and above all, increased realism as to what can and cannot be expected from computers in the ICU environment, have in the past 3 or 4 years rekindled hopes for the prospects of ICU systems.

Notwithstanding this, the overall concept has not changed in its main focus of application over these past two decades. Limits to improvement are apparent. For example, the noninterconnectability of peripheral monitoring devices from different manufacturers to any system, centralised or distributed, is a problem which the industry has not faced up to, and probably will not in the conceivable future.

It is probable that any true prospects for computer systems in the near future in acute medicine require a major change in concept. Potentially, ICU data have very many uses:

1. Clinical therapeutics/management (real time)
2. Management reporting
3. Billing/finance
4. Resource utilization
5. Retrospective clinical research
6. Retrospective "expert system" (real time)

To date, both in the "paper systems" and in the existing generation of computer systems, only the first aspect, the real-time clinical management, is catered for. Of course, this is the most immediate, the most pressing, and is fundamental. However, it is somewhat depressing that with such complete data and after such labor in collecting it (up to 20% of nurse ICU time reportedly) its other potential uses (2–6) do not survive its capture: paper records are cabinet stored while computer data are sequestered, tape stored: both are unusable. However, we are now entering another economic climate in the practice of medicine where the efficient management of departments is becoming increasingly important. Planned resource allocation and the accurate cost analysis of medical procedures are vital to the independence of standards of medical practice. For good or ill, economics and medicine are inseparable.

Whereas until recently individual departments could largely ignore costs as long as the organization was not grossly inefficient and could deliver medical care according to internal estimates of good medical practice, this independence is now a thing of the past. Thus, factors 2–5 are starting to become important.

In distinction, factor 6, the real-time "expert" system, the potential of using all of the accumulated data from hundreds of patients as a real time reference, an accumulated "wisdom" and "experience" of the intensive care unit, offers a truly clinical benefit. An example of its use might be a real-time response to the query, "How many long-stay patients on steroids have developed chest infections and please identify them?" The natural follow-up would then be, "How were they treated and what was the outcome?" The clinical benefit would then be, when faced with a patient with that condition, to have instant access to the unit's entire experience, which is almost impossible with multiple statt/split shifts, etc. Again, in no current system can such a facility be offered. Thus, of all the potential uses of automated ICU data, only factor 1 is offered; factors 2–6 are unavailable.

This shortcoming lies in the failure to address the archive component of the system. Again, no commercial computer system has attempted this feature. An explanation for this state of affairs after 17–18 years of computerized ICU patient data management systems is now in order. For all the uses of the patient data other than real-time, therapeutic management (the current focus), it is evident that data base management systems (DBMSs) are the necessary tools.

However, on examining the structure of the stream of data generated in the ICU, one notes that it is characterized by being:

1. Very dense
2. Having a wide range of data types (number, ordered string, free text, etc.)
3. Time asynchronous
4. Potentially open-ended, containing potential areas of data/data types, etc. involving almost any diagnostic/therapeutic procedure in the hospital. Thus, the record can be very highly structured and necessarily sparse, or else unstructured.

Hence, it is evident that full and detailed ICU records are not suitable for DBMS. A logical structure for a system for ICU data management must therefore allow for data reduction of the complete records. Data reduction can be on a daily basis (perhaps the most logical) corresponding to a daily summary, or on discharge of the patient. Such data reduction as entry to a DBMS *can* be the entire system, but this necessarily must be so attenuated (the maximum number of data entries is perhaps 300/400) that many useful clinical (and management) data are inevitably lost.

A more useful approach is to link a DBMS with a structured and attenuated data input set to the complete real-time, time series data generated by the data management system. Acknowledging that these latter data are internally complex and are best analyzed by the clinical viewing them, using the "time-windowing" and other sorting tools which are always part of these data management systems, it is apparent that a usable system results by compartmentalizing an analysis (a) to the DBMS to give unique primary index identifiers, which are then linked by single pointers to (b) the complete and detailed daily record, which can be individually analyzed using the existing data management system tools.

The initial data reduction can be either wholly manual or semiautomatic; some data items and types are suitable for automatic entry, others not. A system as proposed would be interactive, allowing the clinician (nurse/doctor) to enter the data reduction summary set while at the same time being able to view the detailed daily record in order to refresh his/her memory. Thus using the enquiry mode, the user would:

1. Interrogate the DBMS
2. Generate and identify set of patients
3. Using the single pointer, access the complete real-time record for each patient and examine them sequentially

The search possibilities thus must be restricted to the power of the DBMS set. The choice of the most useful data items is therefore crucial, bearing in mind that if the set is too extensive, the data will be poor through fatigue and frustration of the clinician.

The most important question has been left till last. Given the relatively elementary nature of this structure, why have such systems not been implemented? It is likely that the lack of suitable DBMS has been a major drawback. There are today well in excess of 200 commercial DBMS software packages on the market, some of which are suitable for microcomputers. Traditionally, most of these are described in terms of their structure as (a) relational, (b) network, or (c) hierarchical. Currently there is something of a fashion for relational systems as they are supposedly more suitable for development.

A number of these DBMSs have been developed as "medical data bases," and Costar, Clinfo, Misar and Medusa are examples of these. Medusa, being one of the most recently developed, can be taken as, if not typical, then at least representative. Medusa is multibranch hierarchical in structure, and, thereby certainly represents the open-ended loose structure of general medical data. However, both by virtue of this structure and in many other ways, while Medusa is a good systems solution to the generality of medical data, it is in practice unusable by clinicians. It is too complex to use, certainly for a real-time system. Every computer system represents some trade-off between flexibility/completeness and ease of use. If one were to ignore the generality of medical data and restrict consideration to one user, one clinic, and one medical area, it becomes apparent that very much simpler structures of DBMS are entirely suitable.

We have been using a recently developed DBMS, Metabase, which has specifically espoused this concept, and using an extremely simple structure has taken advantage of it to place great emphasis on simplicity and ease of use. Comparison with many of the other medical data bases shows no shortcomings in analytic powers, speed, data storage, etc. Such a type of DBMS is likely to be part of the next generation of patient data management systems.

Computerized Clinical Records in the Neurosurgical ICU with Self-updating of Some Biological Data

R. Urciuoli, M. Knaflitz, G. Balestra, M. A. Arbinolo, M. L. Bellero, R. Bertino, C. Franco, M. Gessa, and A. Guarnaccia

Patients in neurosurgical intensive care units often develop unexpected problems, and the urgency of treatment requires that it is possible to collect and analyze a lot of data concerning vital signs and intracranial events; in some circumstances this information allows one to diagnose intracranial lesions before the patient develops clinical symptoms and suffers adverse consequences. Hence, clinical assessment of these patients involves continuous careful consideration of many physiological variables that must be frequently and efficiently monitored and displayed.

In 1982 we developed at our institute a clinical sheet which proved valuable in following the patients' course. As we have to collect and update a great number of data, this sheet is quite complex; its manual updating is laborious and wastes considerable time. Thus we came to think that a proper computer approach would be able to make clinical form management easier and more efficient and accurate.

Our "Automatic Clinical Form Management" project started in October 1983 and is being carried out in close cooperation by physicians and engineers; as this study is deeply interdisciplinary, we believe this cooperation is essential to achieve good results.

The first step toward our goal was choosing a computer. After a preliminary analysis of the problem, we decided to buy a multiuser system that (a) is able to store much information, (b) is on-line, connected to monitoring instrumentation in order to self-update some biological data, and (e) is able to draw graphics to display in a more effective way trends and histograms. Moreover, our system had to be easily inserted in the monitoring room of the neurological ICU, and we wanted to be able, in future, to increase its configuration and to insert it in a computer network. At present the configuration of the system consists of one MICRO PDP 11/23 by DIGITAL, two video terminal VT100s, one graphic printer LA100; and one A/D converter multiplexer card ADV11-C.

In order to make insertion of data easier, we are now developing a microprocessor-based network consisting of some bedside slave systems controlled by a master that manages the communication between bedside systems and the MICRO PDP 11/23. The criteria followed in developing software are:

- *Reliability:* As the system must run continuously and the whole management of the ICU depends on it, we must avoid a bad analysis.
- *Privacy:* Data must be inserted and updated by authorized users only.
- *Security:* Data must be preserved against damage, i.e., by means of frequent backups.

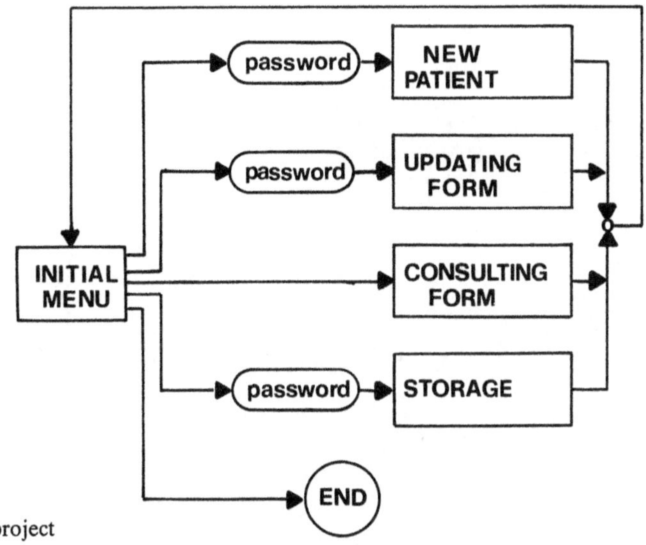

Fig. 1. Block diagram of project

- *Flexibility:* The whole package must be easily transportable to another computer and each part of its structure must be simple to modify.
- *Ease of use:* Our first aim is to create a system that will make physician's and nurses' work easier, and not more difficult.
- *Checking for errors:* In order to avoid as many errors as possible when inserting data, some tests are performed to check the consistency of each input value.

The language used in developing software is FORTRAN 77, and the system runs under the RSX 11-M operative system.

From an functional point of view, the package can be divided into four parts (Fig. 1):

- *New patients:* This procedure allows us to open a new clinical record: general data, recent anamnesis, symptoms, and some notes are inserted.
- *Updating:* Manual and automatic procedures allow the user to insert data concerning neurological examination, water balance, biochemical and diagnostic tests, etc.
- *Consulting:* Data and trends are displayed by means of graphics, histograms, and tables.
- *Storage:* When closing a clinical record, data of interest can be stored in a data base where they are available for future studies.

In order to understand how clinical form management is performed, let us look at Fig. 2. This is the first menu to appear when the user enters the program; through this menu it is possible to select the procedure to be performed: If, for example, the user selects the second item, updating, the menu showed in Fig. 3 appears. By means of this video form he can select the cluster of data that he wants to update, or return to the first menu. If updating of a cluster of data is chosen, this is performed by means of some other forms.

In Fig. 4, for example, we can see the form that allows updating of a part of the neurologic examination, the "side neurological deficit". To update this form, the user only need digit the number corresponding to the answer he chooses from among those

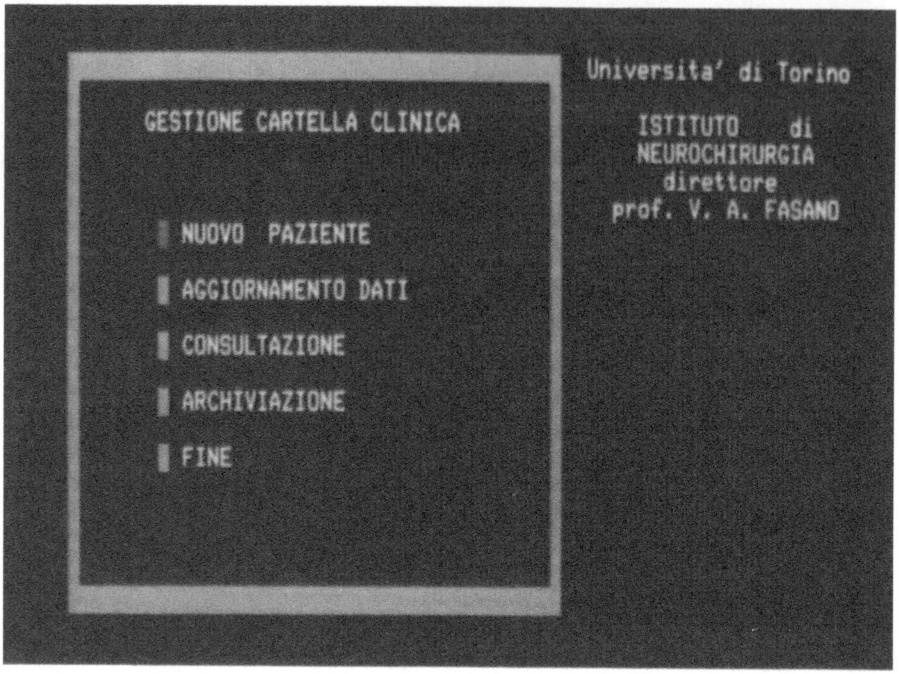

Fig. 2. First menu

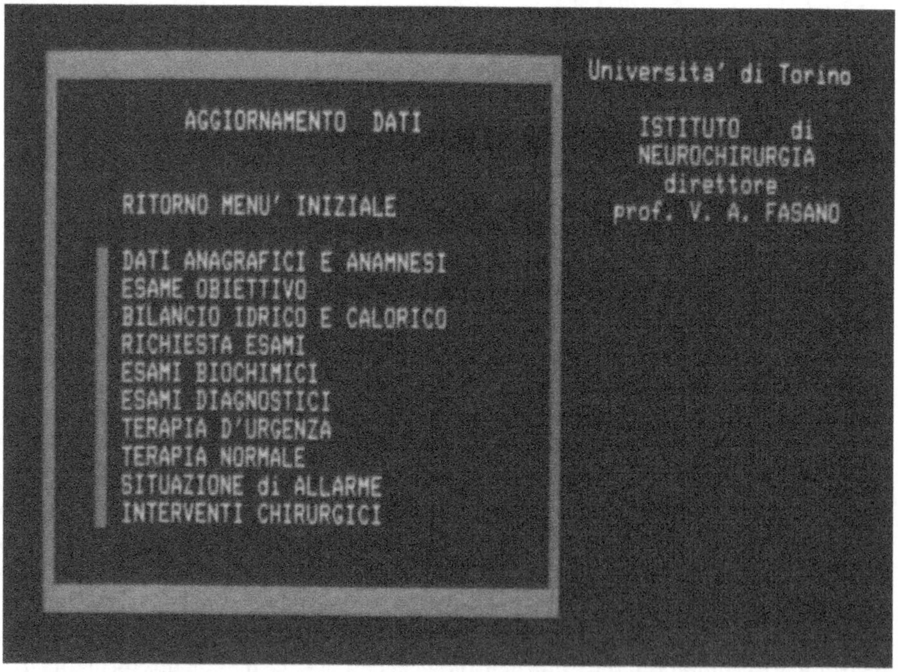

Fig. 3. Second menu

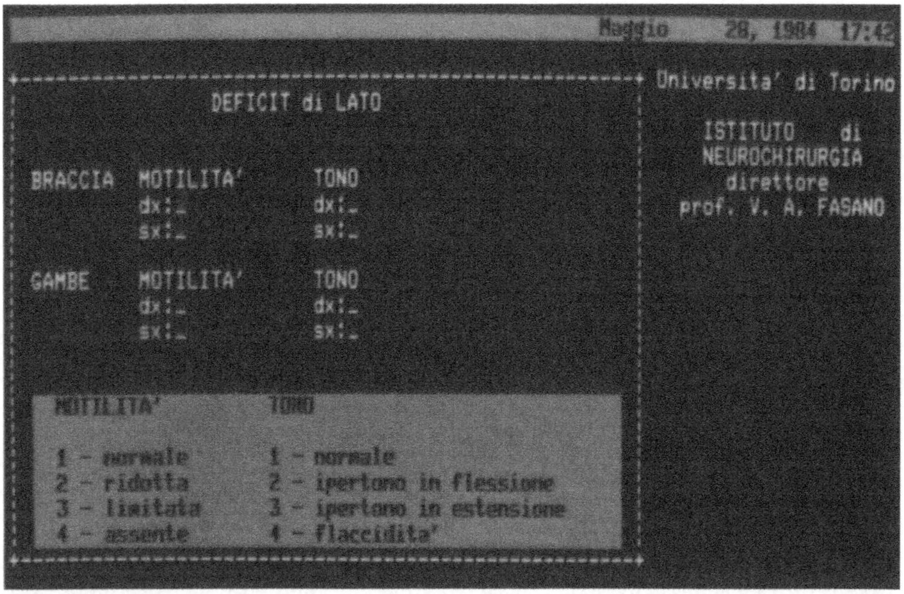

Fig. 4. A videoform

placed in the background area of the form. All these forms should make updating easy, swift, and free of mistakes; put briefly, all the procedures are aimed at optimizing the input from the user's point of view and are structured according to a common scheme.

In order to make it as easy as possible to use the computer, we decided to introduce a training period consisting of two parts: an introduction to computer science and its application on medicine, and training in the use of the package developed.

In future we intend to use data stored in the data base to perform studies involving the identification of exposition factors, the construction of clinical models of interesting pathologies, etc. We are also looking into the construction of expert systems to aid physicians in respect of prognosis and therapy.

Organization and Analysis of Data from Patients with Trauma and Hemorrhage

W. KELLERMANN, K. PETER, U. JENSEN, Y. SUMMA, and D. NEUMEIER

Pathophysiology and Indicative Value of Measurable Parameters

Hemorrhage and trauma cause specific disturbances in physical integrity, which are classed under the general term of shock and whose effects become evident as circulatory shock. Shock may be defined as an acute insufficient nutritive blood flow to vital organs with subsequent hypoxia. This means that the "biological site" of a shock event is not the measurable impairment of macrocirculation, but rather reveals itself in

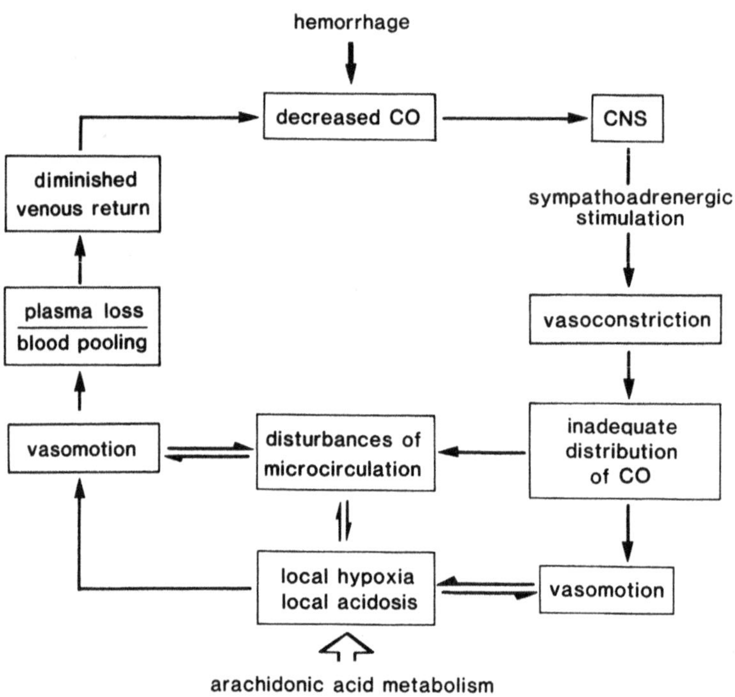

Fig. 1. Pathophysiology of shock. The impairment of macrocirculation is both the cause and the result of microcirculatory alterations. These disturbances in microcirculation result in impairment of cellular functions, in particular a diminished oxidative phosphorylation due to the critically reduced oxygen supply. The effects become apparent, for example, in the metabolism of arachidonic acid and the transport machanisms in the cell membranes, they influence the amount and elimination of metabolites as well as the mobilization of the cascade systems

Table 1. Clinical signs of shock

Cool, humid, pale-cyanotic or marbled skin
Retarded perfusion of nail bed
Restlessness, Clouding of consciousness
Dyspnoe
Tachycardia
Arterial hypotension
Decreased amplitude of blood pressure
Oliguria
Hypoxemia
Metabolic acidosis

microcirculatory alterations such as, for instance, dissociation of capillary blood flow, AV-shunts, changes in capillary permeability and intravascular coagulation disorders, as outlined in Fig. 1 (Schmucker et al.). There are accompanying clinical signs as shown in Table 1 for example.

So far, the spectrum of parameters to be closely observed must include – apart from macrocirculation – the control of gas exchange, blood gases and pH-values as well as the hemogram, coagulation parameters and metabolites (Table 2); therefore the control of the shocked state should ideally include measurement and monitoring of microcirculation, which, however, is not yet possible.

Table 2. Measurement in shock, showing the cardiorespiratory parameters influenced by shock and the corresponding hemogram and blood-gas examinations

Cardiorespiratory parameters		Laboratory examinations
HF	SVI	e.g.
MAP	SWI	Hb
CVP	SVR	Htc
PAP	PVR	Lactate
PCWP		
CO		
$AaDO_2$		Arterial and
$avDO_2$		mixed-venous blood gases
O_2-delivery		
O_2-extraction		
Q_S/Q_T		
V_D/V_T		

Abbreviations used: AV = arteriovenous, PVR = pulmonary vascular resistance, PCWP = pulmonary capillary wedge pressure, $avDO_2$ = arteriocoronary venous O_2 content, $AaDO_2$ = Alveoloarterial O_2-difference, LVSW = left ventricular stroke work, BUN = blood Urea nitrogen, HV = urine output, C_{Kreat} = creatinine content, FE_{Na} = fractional excretion of sodium, HF = hemorrhage factor, MAP = mean arterial pressure, CVP = central venous pressure, PAP = pulmonary arterial pressure, CO = cardiac output, SVI = stroke volume index, SWI = stroke work index, SVR = systemic vascular resistance, PVR = pulmonary vascular resistance

The plots in Fig. 2 are adapted from a study by Shoemaker 1984. They show important parameters of the hypovolemic-hemorrhagic shock. The parameters are plotted against defined time periods, which correspond to the various stages of shock development, i.e., prior to circulatory response, the time when blood pressure reached its minimum, and the recovery phase or late stage of shock, respectively. Shoemaker and his group (Hopkins et al. 1983; Shoemaker et al. 1982) examined more than 100 shock patients (with more than 56000 individual measurements) and determined the variables by which the surviving patients differed from those who died. These prognostic indices for mortality, also investigated by other authors (Augenstein et al. 1976; Siegel et al. 1980), correlated well with the degree of severity of the disease. Apart from the selection of parameters based on pathophysiology, this selective scheme, which is founded on probability criteria, offers another path to rational data acquisition in the case of acutely ill patients. Thus, for instance, traumatic shock patients who survived differed from those who died by a normal pulmonary

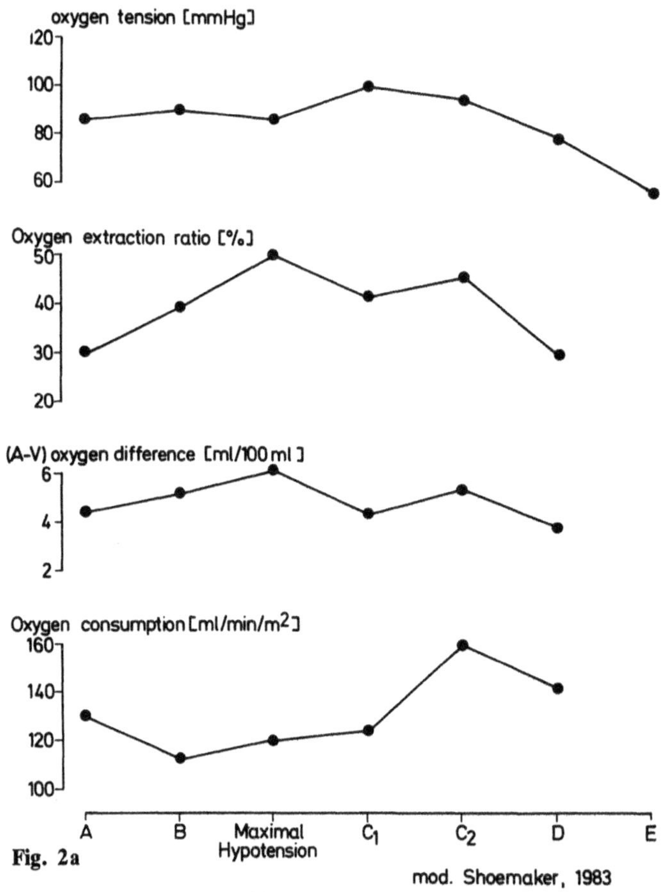

Fig. 2a

Fig. 2a, b. Parameters of hypovolemic-hemorrhagic shock (modified from Shoemaker 1984), plotted against defined time periods: A, prior to circulatory response; B, beginning, point of maximal hypotension; C_1-E, recovery phase. Not only cardiac output and blood pressure, but also oxygen tension, oxygen extraction ratio and oxygen consumption, for instances are affected

vascular resistance (PVR), normal pH-values and stimulation of circulation, while the non-survivors exhibited high PVR and acidosis. The conclusion, that parameters with the most pronounced sensitivity to possible survival ought to be given priority in monitoring, may well be considered as justified. We learn that the measured parameters are as useful for diagnostic purposes as for objectifying therapeutic success and they have a certain limited prognostic value.

Application of Electronic Data Processing for Organization and Analysis of Data

The application of electronic data processing in order to organize and analyze patient data may be classed in three categories, which will be considered in turn: data acquisition and storage; documentation and presentation (tabular or graphic presentation); and analysis and evaluation of data (calculating aids and computer aided decision making).

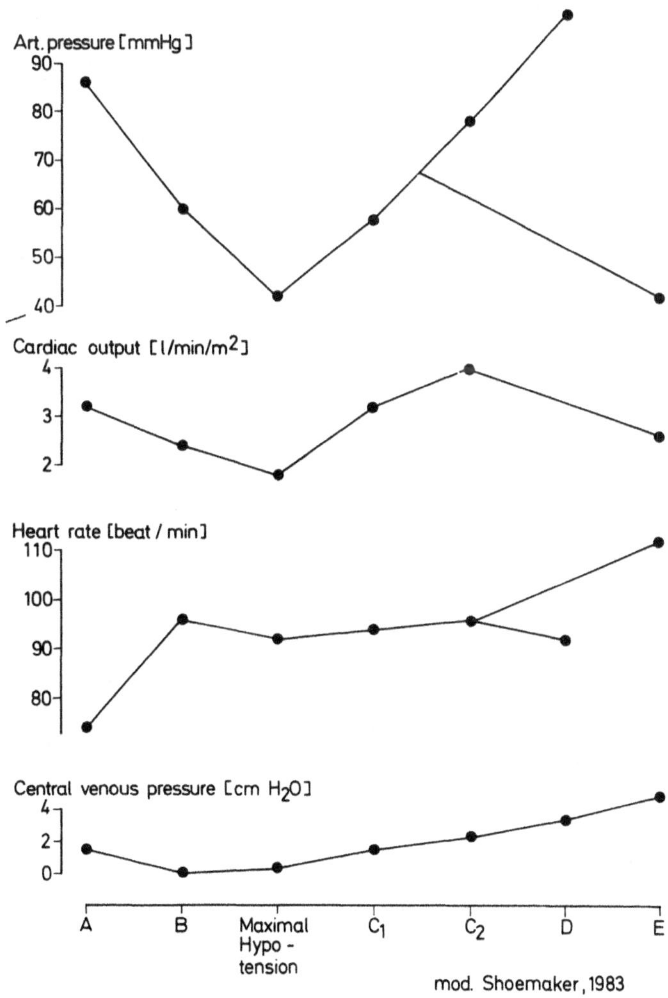

Fig. 2b

Data Acquisition and Storage

Off-line registration of patient data includes, on the lowest level, general descriptive parameters such as name, date of birth, height, weight and so on. Today, the immediate access to this information is a matter of everyday practice in intensive care systems, in x-ray examinations, in laboratories and other institutions. Data transfer between these facilitates routine work; it must be ensured, however, that the rules concerning data protection are strictly observed. In emergency medicine there are stringent requirements with regard not only to speed, but also to reliability of the determinations of laboratory parameters. Since the necessary technical equipment is more and more reduced in size, the practice of direct measurement and processing of the patient's emergency parameters by means of microprocessors is becoming increasingly common in medicine. The measurement of blood gases, largely automated today, may serve as an example of these bedside analysis procedures.

Apart from such methods, in our institution a central laboratory has proved to be efficient (Neumeier and Knedel). This laboratory is interfaced with the laboratory data processing center (Primulabsystem) and linked to the intensive care unit and the operating room by a special tubular post system for fast transport of the blood samples.

In 1983, a total of 2.6 million examinations were done, 27% as emergency examinations (Fig. 3). We note that efficiency criteria for the acquisition of laboratory data include times for transport and analysis as well as control of the data obtained with regard to quality and plausibility. Dependent on the degree of priority desired, vital laboratory parameters, such as those shown in Fig. 4, are available within minutes.

The control of those values deviating from the preliminary findings is rendered possible by color coding on the laboratory monitor. In addition, it is possible to control the course of up to four variables at the same time on the basis of a diagram (Fig. 5). The values are transmitted by direct line to a printer installed in the intensive

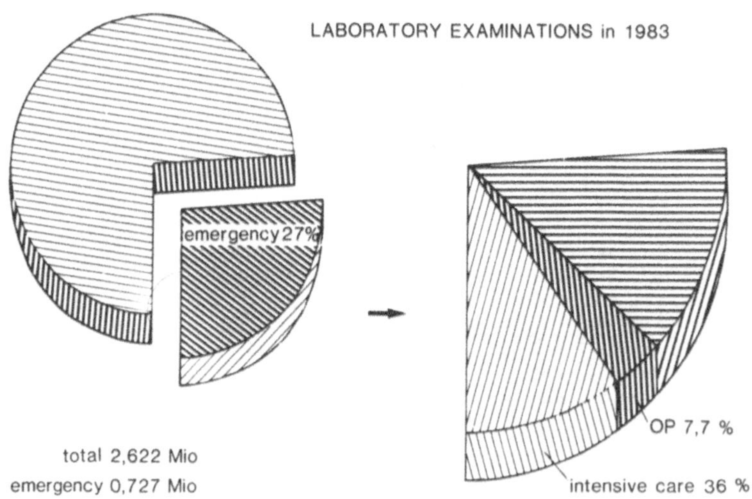

Fig. 3. Scope of emergency examinations in the central laboratory

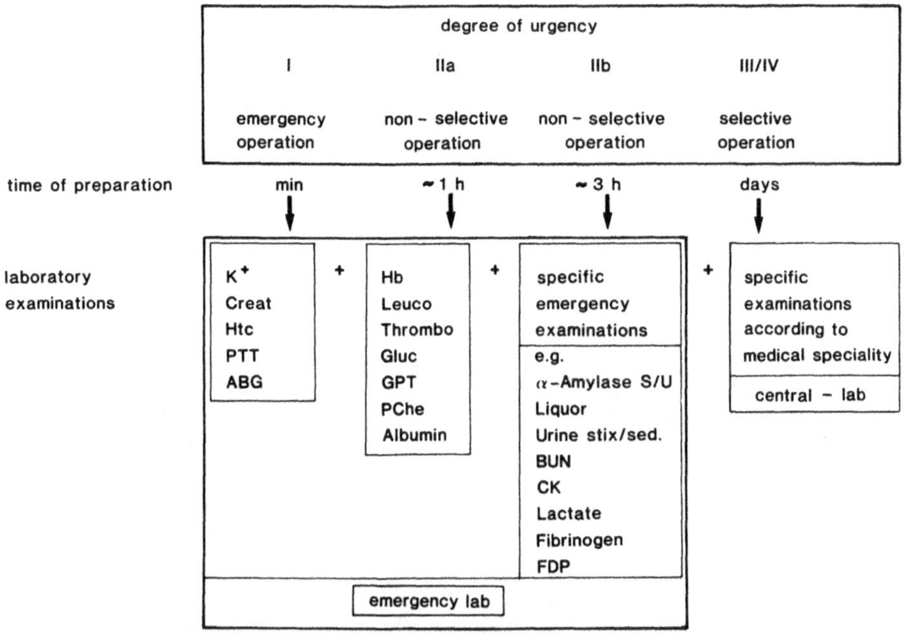

Fig. 4. Laboratory examinations dependent on the degree of urgency. In the case of an emergency, a subset of laboratory parameters is available in minutes. The preparation time increases as more specific laboratory parameters are required

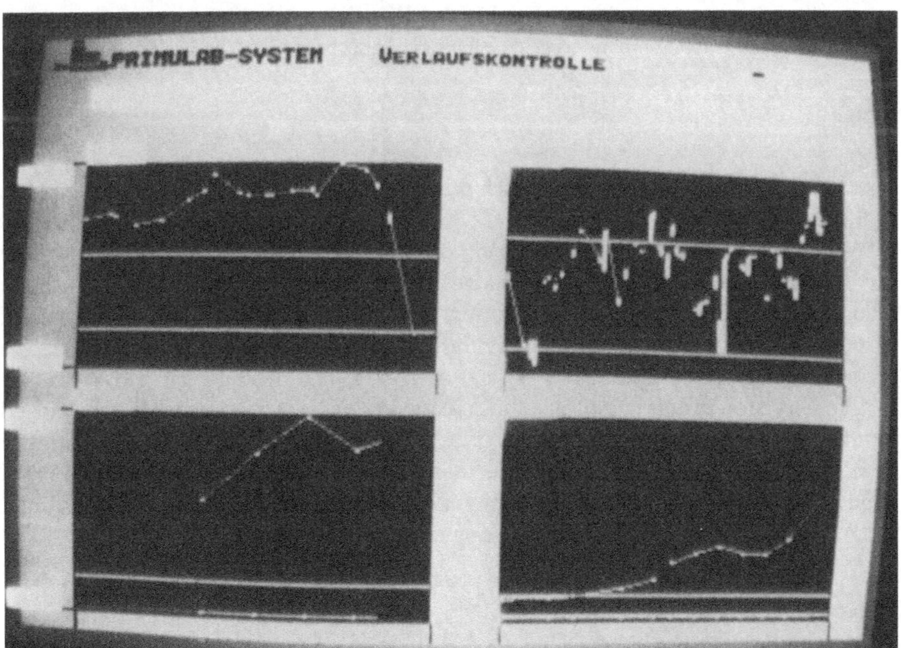

Fig. 5. Primulab system: an example of the simultaneous monitor control of the time course of four laboratory parameters. The (originally colored) picture shows the time course of Na^+ and K^+ *(above)*, BUN and creatinine *(below)*. Emergency examinations are highlighted in different colors

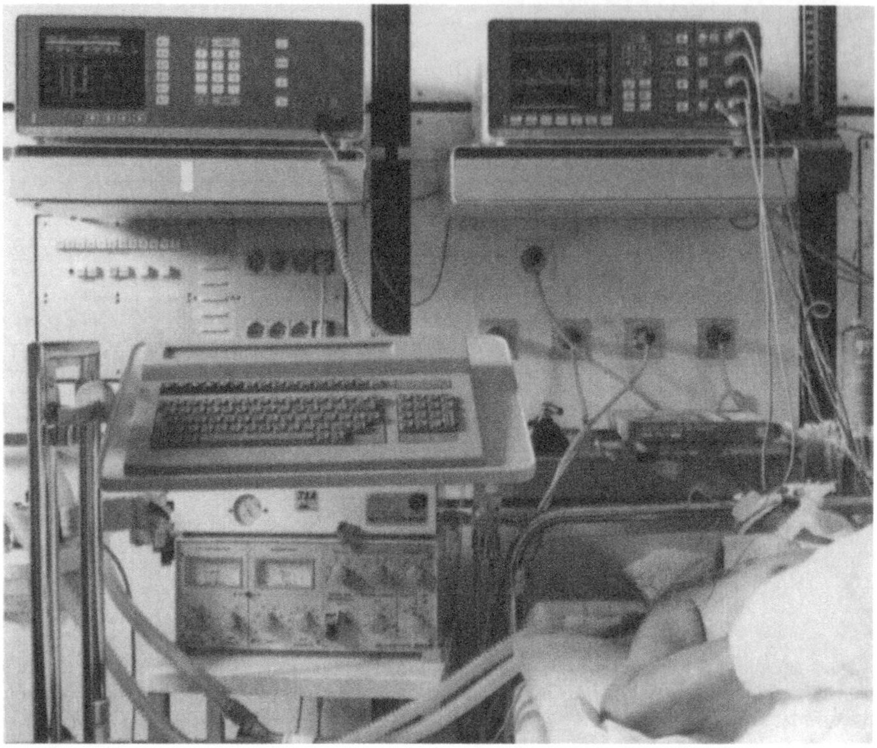

Fig. 6. Modular computer monitoring system for two to six beds (Siemens Sirecust 404 and 425)

care unit. A patient care system, which is equipped accordingly, allows transmission to the bedside monitor.

In addition to the on-line monitoring of cardiocirculatory parameters, so-called intelligent monitors are, moreover, in a position to indicate alarming situations and to recognize artifacts. There are calibrating and adjusting devices, and by means of storage and presentation within previously defined time intervals trends can be recorded (Glaser and Thomas 1975).

A further step in this sector are the so-called patient care systems. Decentralized modular systems, as shown in Fig. 6, offer a high degree of flexibility. By means of such systems it is possible to provide monitoring for one or more "shock beds". Values, which have been measured manually, or comments, may be fed in off-line, reports can be established and computing aids are offered.

Documentation and presentation

An integral part and, as can be seen from the previous remarks on monitoring, an important aspect of electronic data processing is the documentation and presentation of the compiled patient data (Fig. 7). Apart from presentation in the form of tables

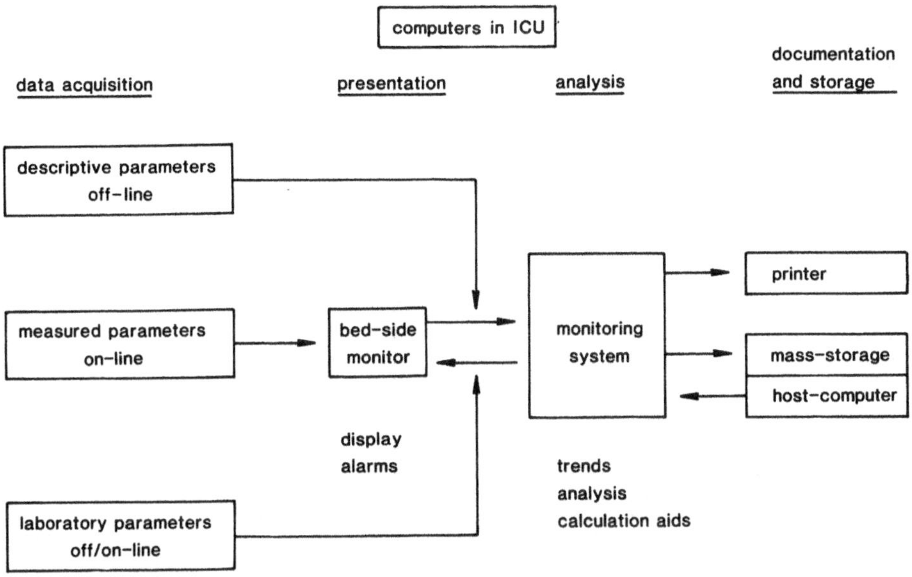

Fig. 7. Computers in ICU. The physical equipment (transducers, monitor, printer) and the corresponding tasks of a computer monitoring system in ICU (data acquisition, presentation, analysis, documentation and storage) are shown

printed on paper at distinct time intervals for documentary purposes, the relevant information is transferred to the viewing screen. Being visualized as diagrams, the data become more comprehensible to the physician. But to a large extent, computer-based trends or computer forecasts are still in a software test stage (Augenstein 1984; Wiener and Weil 1978).

The descriptiveness of diagrams can be made evident by an example. For computing derived cardiorespiratory variables on the basis of a program developed by ourselves, we make use of a desk-top computer. In Fig. 8a and b we show the original printout of the cardiorespiratory parameters of a shock patient, measured at different times. Presentation of such parameters in the form of a diagram, as in Fig. 9, allows more immediate conclusions with regard to time relationships.

Analysis and Evaluation of Data

Following this example, we come to the third catogory, the analysis of the measured data, for which purpose computing aids are primarily employed. In addition to the presentation of data in the form of diagrams, the analysis procedure makes possible a further elucidation of the interdependence of different parameters; thus, for instance, the success of a positive-inotropic therapy or a therapy based on volume replacement can be estimated. For the situation given in the example in the previous section the change of the actual position in the plot of stroke work against PCWP is graphically presented in Fig. 10.

PROGRAMM ZUR ERRECHNUNG VON KARDIOPULMONALEN PARAMETERN
Anaesthesiologische Intensivtherapiestation H2/I2b Klinikum Grosshadern

K
Groesse 170 cm, Gewicht 75 kg, Oberflaeche 1.86 qm, Grundumsatz 1765 kcal/Tag

Messung Nr.	-01-	-02-	-03-	
Datum	13.5.81	14.5.81	14.5.81	
Uhrzeit	17.30	10.00	11.45	h
Dopamin(ug/kg/min)	15.56	55.56	55.56	
Suprarenin(ug/kg/min)	.29	2.22	2.67	
Herzminutenvolumen [l/min]	9.60	8.50	7.80	
Herzfrequenz [Schl./min]	136.00	136.00	128.00	
Mittlerer arterieller Druck [mmHg]	57.00	52.00	57.00	
Mittlerer Pulmonalisdruck [mmHg]	27.00	31.00	30.00	
Zentraler Venendruck [mmHg]	15.00	16.00	15.00	
Wedge-Druck [mmHg]	18.00	18.00	18.00	
Herzindex [l/min/qm]	5.15	4.56	4.19	
Schlagvolumen-I.[ml/1/qm]	37.88	33.54	32.70	
Linksv.Schlagarbeits-I.[gm/qm]	29.36	23.72	25.35	
Rechtsv.Schlagarbeits-I.[gm/qm]	13.91	14.14	13.34	
Periph.Widerstand [dyn*sec/cm^5]	349.56	338.40	430.23	
Pulm.Widerstand [dyn*sec/cm^5]	74.91	122.20	122.92	

Fig. 8a

Groesse 160 cm, Gewicht 70 kg, Oberflaeche 1.73 qm, Grundumsatz 0 kcal/Tag

peep = 5

Messung Nr.	-07-	-08-	-09-	
Datum	17.5.	17.5.	18.5.	
Uhrzeit	15H30	23H	7H00	h
Barometerdruck (mmHg)	716.20	716.00	715.40	
FIO2	.55	.48	.46	
FECO2 (%)	2.90	3.30	3.00	
Atemminutenvolumen (l/min)	18.20	18.20	19.20	
Haemoglobinkonz.(g/100ml)	13.20	13.20	13.30	
Temperatur (oC)	38.10	38.80	38.60	
RQ	.85	.85	.85	
Arterieller PO2 (mmHg)	92.00	101.90	99.00	
Gemess.art. Saettigung (%)	96.80	97.30	97.30	
Arterieller PCO2 (mmHg)	44.10	43.90	43.80	
Arterieller pH	7.41	7.42	7.42	
Gemischtven. PO2 (mmHg)	39.80	39.40	41.90	
Gemischtven. Saettigung (%)	68.50	67.50	67.90	
Gemischtven. PCO2 (mmHg)	52.40	51.80	56.20	
Gemischtven. pH	7.39	7.38	7.38	
Korr. art. PO2 (mmHg)	98.26	112.82	108.55	
Korr. art. PCO2 (mmHg)	46.22	47.40	46.89	
Korr.art. pH	7.39	7.39	7.40	
Errechn. art. Saett. (%)	97.07	97.67	97.53	
Korr. ven. PO2 (mmHg)	43.02	44.75	46.91	
Errechn. ven. Saett. (%)	72.13	70.43	73.77	
Alveol. PO2 (mmHg)	322.55	277.14	263.27	
AaDO2 (mmHg)	224.30	164.32	154.72	
Arteriell. O2-Gehalt (vol%)	17.40	17.52	17.64	
AVDO2 (vol%)	5.17	5.47	5.42	
Intrapulm. R-L-Shunt (%)	19.01	14.24	13.85	
HZV, Fick' Prinzip (l/min)	12.01	12.92	12.50	
Totraumventilation	.58	.54	.57	
'Ratio'	2.28	1.46	1.43	
PO'50' (mmHg)	28.68	28.51	29.98	
O2-Verbrauch (ml/min/qm)	238.75	257.28	247.28	
O2-Transport (ml/min/qm)	803.89	824.53	804.83	
O2-Ausschoepfung (%)	29.70	31.20	30.72	
RQ (errechnet)	1.29	1.36	1.36	
Errechn. Kalorienbedarf (Kcal/h)	136.16	149.50	143.57	

Fig. 8b

Fig. 8a, b. Examples of tabular printout of cardiorespiratory parameters, given by a desktop computer used in our ICU as a calculating aid in patient monitoring

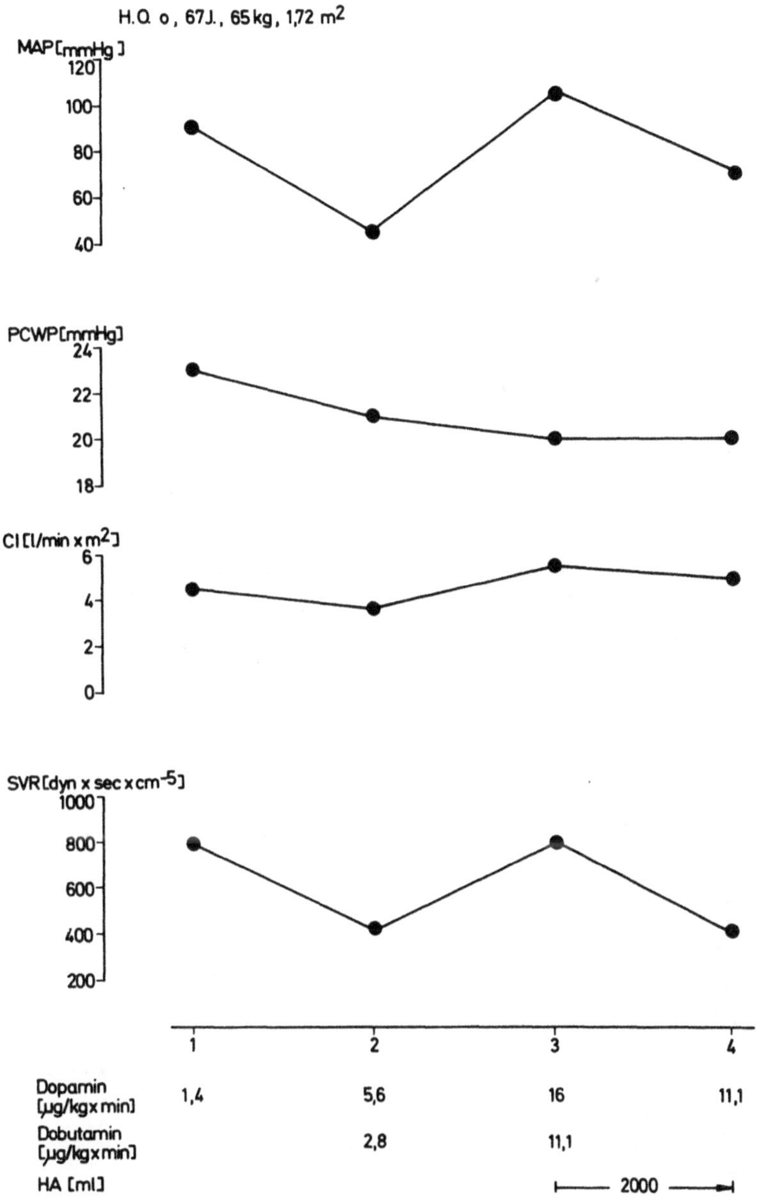

Fig. 9. Graphic presentation of hemodynamic parameters such as those in Fig. 8. Marks 1–4 are time marks representing beginning and recovery of a septic hypovolemic shock

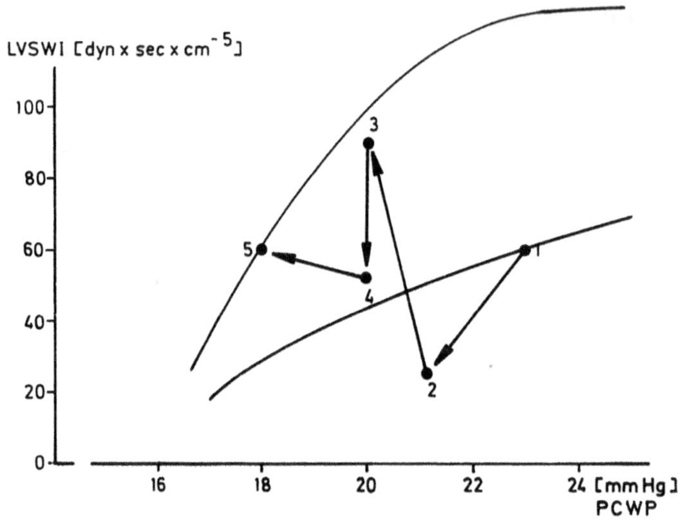

Fig. 10. Plot of stroke work against PCWP from to the measurements shown in Fig. 9. The *arrows* demonstrate the time course of the variations in stroke work against PCWP. The solid curves represent (non-measured) ideal Starling curves for orientation purposes

NN ...., M, 185 CM 102 KG 69 J TKW 50 L OBERFL. 2,26 QM

SAMMELPERIODE: 6.00 H BIS 6.00 H = 1440 MIN
URINVOLUMEN 980 ML = .68 ML/MIN

U OSMOL	302 MOSMOL/KG		
P OSMOL	317 MOSMOL/KG	THEORET. 309, 4 MOSMOL/KG	DELTA 7,6 MOSMOL/KG
U/POSMOL	.93		
C OSMOL	.64 ML/MIN		
Tc H2O	-.05 ML/MIN	EX-OSMOL 296.0 MOSMOL/24 H = 100 %	
U KREAT	15 MG%		
P KREAT	2,70 MG%		
U/PKREAT	5.4		
C KREAT	3,6 ML/MIN	= 3,14 % SOLL (115,95 ML/MIN)	
EX-KREAT	.15 G/24 H	= 7,78 % SOLL (1,89 G/24 H)	
U UREA	540 MG%		
P UREA	228,0 MG%	DELTA P UREA + 32,0 MG%	
U/PUREA	2,5		
C UREA	1,7 ML/MIN	= 47,5 % C KREAT	
EX-UREA	5,29 G/24 H	= 2,47 G H-N (URIN)	88,2 MOSMOL/24 H = 29,8 %
U NA	42,7 MMOL/L		
P NA	137,3 MMOL/L		
EX-NA	41,85 MMOL/24 H		77,4 MSOMOL/24 H = 26,2 %
FRAKT. NA-EXKRETION	5,80 %		
U KA	54,1 MMOL/L		
P KA	4,10 MMOL/L		
EX-KA	53,02 MMOL/24 H		98,1 MOSMOL/24 H = 33,1 %
U GLUC	270		
P GLUC	177 M%		
EX-GLUC	2,65 G/24 H		14,7 MOSMOL/24 H = 5,0 %
KOD	16,0 MM HG	EX-OSMOL REST 17,5 MOSMOL/24 H = 5,9 %	

Fig. 11. Example of a printout of a daily report from the station laboratory concerning renal parameters

Other parameters which were calculated are $avDO_2$, $AaDO_2$, O_2-extraction, O_2-transport capacity, shunt, etc. (Fig. 8 b). Minimizing the computing time makes these values available at the bedside within a reasonably short period of time.

A parameter not to be underestimated when assessing the circulation and volume state of a patient is renal function and this could indicate the necessity for access to a laboratory. For this reason urine controls, on the basis of 24-hour sampling, are carried out in our ICU laboratory by measurement of osmolality, creatinine and urea levels as well as of sodium, potassium, and glucose content of plasma and urine Finsterer et al. 1982. Derived parameters like creatinine clearance, free water clearance, or fractional sodium excretion are calculated by means of a computer. A printout is shown in Fig. 11. The overall progress of an acute oliguric renal failure, as demonstrated in Fig. 12, is made up of such daily reports. This monitoring has proved to be efficient with regard to diagnosis and prevention of disorders in the water-electrolyte balance.

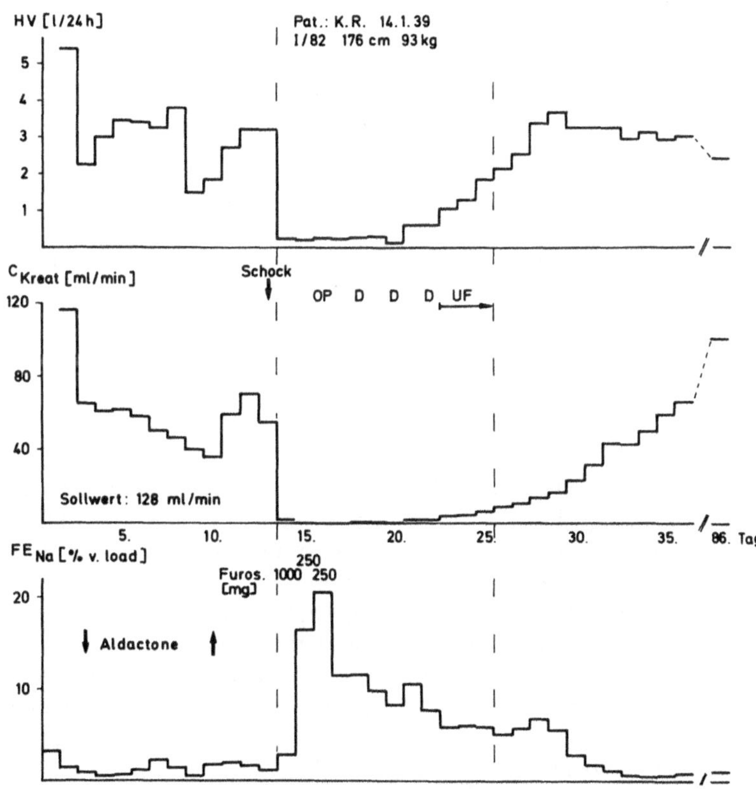

Fig. 12. Time course of a oliguric acute renal failure (ARF), based on daily reports shown in Fig. 11. After a shock event urine output (HV) and creatinine clearance (C_{Kreat}) drop. Simultaneously the fractional excretion of sodium (Fe_{Na}) rises to levels typical for ARF

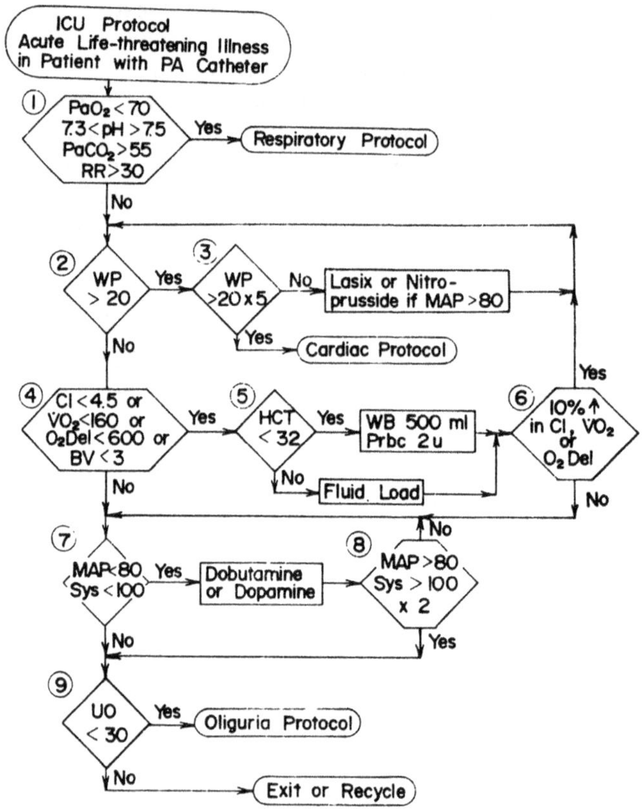

Fig. 13. ICU algorithm (from Hopkins et al. 1983). See text for explanation

A further step in the general development constitutes the "computer-aided decision making". In Fig. 13a so-called ICU algorithm according to Hopkins is shown (Hopkins et al. 1983). On the basis of this algorithm an attempt was made to achieve an optimum volume replacement therapy for a shock patient by means of a stepwise interrogation of the variables, and thus getting suggestions for therapy and aids for decision making. Starting from quantitative data and descriptive variables, such algorithms generally try to form complex parameters with regard to a general status description and determination of the severity of the disease. Such procedures are said to result in a shorter resuscitation time and in a reduction of complications (Hopkins et al. 1983; Shoemaker 1984; Siegel et al. 1980).

There are various possible ways of constructing such algorithms (Augenstein 1984):

1. So-called expert systems or production rules are compilations of rules in the form of packages, which are made up by experts. For example the MYCIN system (Stanford University) makes use of such procedures in the case of sepsis.
2. When drawing up models or simulations a mathematical combination of physiological relations should describe a physiological or pathophysiological sector as closely as possible.

3. In probability analysis the linking up of symptom accumulations according to the Bayes' probability theorem will result in information on diagnosis, prognosis and probably on therapy.
4. Using the method of data-base analysis, an analysis of stored clinical experiences is carried out in order to get information on prognosis and choice of therapy. For this purpose earlier similar cases are selected and linked up with one another and the new data. An example of a general clinical data base system based on this method is ARAMIS at Stanford.

Conclusion

The disadvantage of all these procedures is to be found in the relative inflexibility of electronic data processing. Ensuring a prognosis *quoad vitam* is inconceivable, since the influx of advances in the medical sector is too slow. In addition, clinical decisions will always have to be based on incomplete sets of data. But, despite of some limitations still existing, patients in shock after hemorrhage and trauma need all the technological support modern medicine can offer.

References

Augenstein JS (1984) Use of data-processing systems in clinical decision making. In: Shoemaker WC, Thompson WL, Holbrook PR (eds) Textbook of critical care. Saunders, Philadelphia

Augenstein JS, Civetta JM, Herman FN, Schenkman JH, Shroder MM (1976) Prediction of survival in intensive care patients. Crit Care Med 4: 107

Finsterer U, Kellermann W, Jensen U, Beyer A, Unertl K, Butz A, Ciossek D, Summa Y (1982) Monitoring der Nierenfunktion. In: Organversagen während Intensivtherapie, INA 45. Thieme, Stuttgart

Glaser DH, Thomas LJ (1975) Computer monitoring in patient care. Annu Rev Biophys Bioeng 4: 677

Hopkins JA, Shoemaker WC, Chang P (1983) Results of a clinical trial on the use of an algorithm for resuscitation of surgical emergencies. Crit Care Med 11: 621

Neumeier D, Knedel M (to be published) Technologische Entwicklung in der Labormedizin – Nutzen für die Intensivmedizin. In: 5. Internat. Symposium über aktuelle Probleme der Notfallmedizin, INA. Thieme, Stuttgart

Schmucker P, Peter K, Jensen U, Jesch F (to be published) Schock. Enke, Stuttgart

Shoemaker WC (1984) Pathophysiology and therapy of shock syndromes. In: Shoemaker WC, Thompson WL, Holbrook PR (eds) Textbook of Critical Care. Saunders, Philadelphia

Shoemaker WC, Appel PL, Bland R, Hopkins JA, Chang P (1982) Clinical trial of an algorithm for outcome prediction in acute circulatory failure. Crit Care Med 10: 390

Siegel JH, Cerra FB, Moody EA, Shetye M, Coleman B, Garr L, Shubert M, Keane JS (1980) The effect on survival of critically ill and injured patients of an ICU teaching service organized about a computer-based physiologic CARE system. J Trauma 20: 558

Wiener F, Weil MH (1978) Computer-based monitoring and data management in critical care. Methods Inf Med 17: 252

Computer Assisted ICU Monitoring

T. OYAMA, H. ISHIHARA, A. MATSUKI, M. YAMASHITA, K. ISOZAKI, and T. SUZUKI

It is crucial to monitor critically ill patients continuously and to store all data collected in a readily accessible way. The minicomputer has been used for storing large amounts of data; however, it requires a considerable space in which to locate it and this is not always feasible in the limited space of the ICU. Our ICU is so small that the restricted space must be used for the monitoring system. The microcomputer system (NEC Saneisokki Co. Ltd.) has been developed in our ICU to fulfill the above mentioned aim. The stored data of serial ECG tracing from each patient are also available by using this system.

Six beds are equipped for continuous monitoring. Our system consists of bedside monitor, central monitor, on-line laboratory data system, and respiratory data processing system, as shown in Fig. 1.

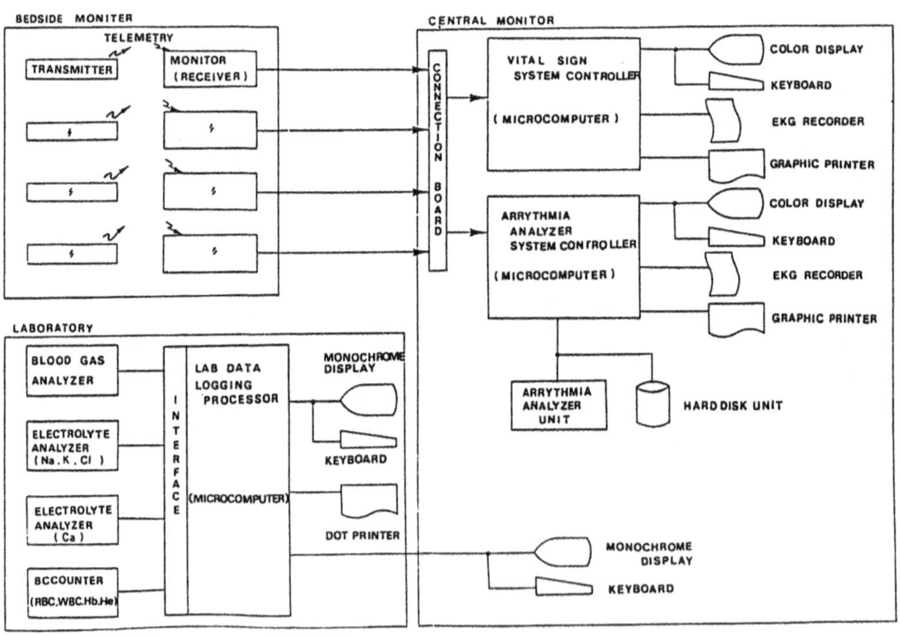

Fig. 1

Bedside Monitor

Display and computer terminals are located at each bedside. A computer terminal connects with the central microcomputer (NEC Saneisokki) which is placed in the separate computer room. Data measured, including arterial blood pressure, pulmonary artery pressure, ECG tracing, and body temperature, are input to the bedside monitor using a compact telemeter (51 × 176 × 180 mm in size) which monitors continuously for 10 days without changing the battery.

Central Monitor

The central monitor consists of the central display of the six bedside monitors, arrhythmia analyzer and display of laboratory data.

Central Display of six Bedside Monitors

On-line measured data from a bedside monitor are displayed on the color screen and are stored in a microcomputer by five minute sampling periods. The information is stored on data-file and is available using digital or graphic methods (Fig. 1).

Arrhythmia Analyzer

A microcomputer system is also adopted to store serial ECG tracing for 24 h for all patients. A hard disc (RAM 19.7 Mbyte) is utilized to store these data. Information for every 24 hour period on arrhythmia is thus available quickly (Figs. 2, 3). Analysis of arrhythmia and warning signals are also generated. The following diagnoses are made by the system:

1. Cardiac standstill, ventricular fibrillation, ventricular tachycardia.
2. Short run, VPC, tachyarrhythmia, bradyarrhythmia.
3. ST segment change, prolonged R-R interval, supraventricular arrhythmia, pace maker failure.
4. Artifact.

Laboratory Data Display

The central monitor is connected to a microcomputer in the laboratory located elsewhere. On-line data from blood gas analysis, electrolytes (Na, K, Cl, Ca), CBC (RBC, WBC, Ht, Hb) are input and stored in the computer. Other data, such as blood levels of glucose and lactate, are also input using the keyboard. Derived respiratory or cardiovascular indices from cardiac output, pulmonary artery wedge pressure and blood gas analysis are calculated and stored in the microcomputer. These indices include: cardiac index (CI), systemic vascular resistance (SVR), pulmonary vascular resistance (PVR), available oxygen, pulmonary shunt, and dead space.

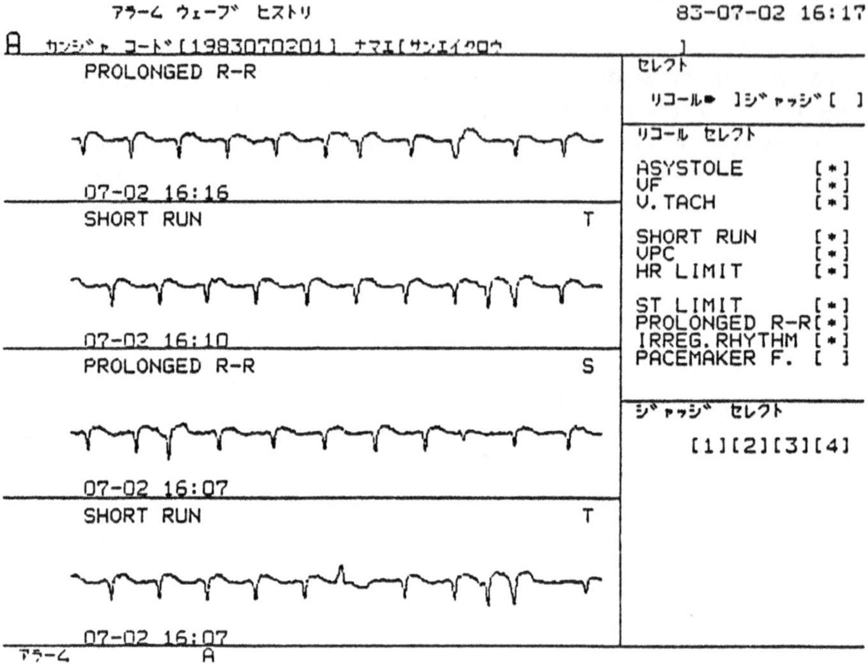

Fig. 2

A カンジャ コード[1983070201] ナマエ[サンエイクロウ]

ヒヅケ	ジコク	EVENT	RESET	ヒヅケ	ジコク	EVENT	RESET
07-02	16:38	PROLONGED R-R	T	07-02	16:20	PROLONGED R-R	S
	16:37	SHORT RUN	T		16:19	SHORT RUN	S
	16:37	ASYSTOLE	T		16:19	SHORT RUN	S
	16:37	PROLONGED R-R	S		16:16	PROLONGED R-R	T
	16:37	HR LIMIT	S		16:10	SHORT RUN	T
	16:37	ASYSTOLE	T		16:07	PROLONGED R-R	S
	16:37	PROLONGED R-R	S		16:07	SHORT RUN	T
	16:37	SHORT RUN	S		16:07	PROLONGED R-R	S
	16:36	SHORT RUN	T		16:05	PROLONGED R-R	S
	16:36	HR LIMIT	T		16:05	SHORT RUN	S
	16:36	ASYSTOLE	T		16:04	SHORT RUN	S
	16:36	PROLONGED R-R	S		16:02	HR LIMIT	S
	16:35	SHORT RUN	T		16:02	ASYSTOLE	T
	16:35	SHORT RUN	S		16:02	PROLONGED R-R	S
	16:33	ASYSTOLE	T		16:01	ASYSTOLE	T
	16:33	PROLONGED R-R	S		16:01	PROLONGED R-R	S
	16:33	SHORT RUN	S		16:01	ASYSTOLE	S
	16:32	ASYSTOLE	T		16:01	PROLONGED R-R	S
	16:32	PROLONGED R-R	S		16:00	SHORT RUN	S
	16:32	SHORT RUN	T		16:00	ASYSTOLE	T
	16:31	SHORT RUN	T		16:00	PROLONGED R-R	S
	16:29	SHORT RUN	T		16:00	VPC	S
	16:27	ASYSTOLE	T		15:58	HR LIMIT	S
	16:27	PROLONGED R-R	S		15:58	ASYSTOLE	S
	16:27	PROLONGED R-R	S		15:58	PROLONGED R-R	S
	16:24	PROLONGED R-R	T		15:57	SHORT RUN	S
	16:21	VPC	T		15:52	PROLONGED R-R	A
	16:21	HR LIMIT	S		15:48	SHORT RUN	S
	16:21	ASYSTOLE	T		15:45	HR LIMIT	S
	16:21	PROLONGED R-R	S		15:45	ASYSTOLE	A
	16:20	HR LIMIT	S		15:45	PROLONGED R-R	S
	16:20	ASYSTOLE	S		15:44	PROLONGED R-R	T

アラーム A

Fig. 3

Respiratory Data Processing

Our system consists of a gas mass spectrometer, a heated wire flowmeter and a 16-bit microcomputer. Oxygen consumption and carbon dioxide production are calculated by the adjoining computer. The system allows us to detect optimal weaning from the respirator, and metabolic requirements in critically ill patients immediately.

Automatic Signal Analysis and Prediction in Intensive Medical Care

A. Swoboda and E. Epple

In many areas of human life, science and technology system modelling has become a powerful tool in understanding system behavior as well as in assessing possible consequences of outside interference with the system under study.

Often the appropriate methods have to be used in an iterative manner, requiring a remarkable amount of skill and judgment (Box and Jenkins 1976). As hardware is becoming smaller and cheaper and more powerful at the same time, micromachines will also be able to handle more sophisticated algorithms. Thus the next thing to do seems to be to study the possibilities of fully automating the algorithms suitable for system identification and modelling.

Under certain assumptions which will be mentioned later, the characteristics of a nondeterministic system may be estimated from the processes the system is generating. The time series of various measurements taken from such a system may then be considered to be one of several in which ways the system is expressing itself in an observable manner. Therefore the parameters describing the process emanating from a system should in some way reflect the characteristics of the generating system. The problem of automating identification and modelling of a system as well as predicting reactions and developments may thus be approached by identifying and modelling the process emanating from it (Endresen and Hill 1977)

The main steps of the procedure proposed, utilizing the identification, modelling, and forecasting capabilities of time series analysis and spectral analysis, would be:

1. To use spectral analysis first in order to locate any existing concentrations of spectral mass and determine the main frequencies.
2. To estimate the process parameters of the stochastic model reproducing the original time series, considering at the same time any seasonal or polynomial components.
3. To associate the process parameters estimated by 2. with the nature or state of the process generating system using external criteria thought to be characteristic for the specific application.
4. Vice versa, to estimate the state of the generating system from the process parameters.
5. To use the latter in forecasting future time series and possibly system state as well.

While items 1, 2, and 5 are mathematical procedures, the other two involve difficult interpretation, depending greatly on the specific application. As a rule this job will have to be done by somebody who is familiar with the system under study.

One of the assumptions mentioned pertains to the stationarity of the stochastic process. At first glance, this might look like a severe handicap. However, this is not the case, since nonstationary time series segments can be handled by suitable differencing. Therefore the behavior of a system may be observed throughout time. Assuming that any outside interference with the system might be expected to show up as a local nonstationarity of the emanating stochastic process, the classification of the generating system should be feasible.

When attempting full automation of process identification and modelling, two main difficulties are met:

1. How can the (mostly iterative) algorithms for identifying and modelling the process be combined in such a way as to perform automatically, once a representative part of the emanating series has been selected?
2. How can such a representative section of the original input series be selected automatically as well?

One can think of a variety of areas, ranging from scientific to industrial applications, where real-time automatic modelling would seem to be of some value for the user.

Two criteria play an important part in process analysis and model fitting: the autocorrelation function (ACF) of the time series and the residual variance of the working series after preliminary fitting. The usual procedure is to look at the first few lags of the ACF, compare them with the single or double bounds of the estimated standard deviation, and then decide on the trend and type of model. Having calculated the selected model's parameters, the residual variance of the working series is estimated. A small residual variance is usually considered to be an indication in favor of the model chosen.

This procedure has been tested on several time series segments representing measurements of vital signs sampled from patients under treatment in a cardiovascular intensive care unit. In the course of this investigation it was found that both variables should be used more as general guidelines than as reliable criteria. In some instances, for example, the variables, minimizing residual variance primarily did not yield the stochastic model reproducing the original input series in a satisfying manner. Nor did looking at the first few lags of the ACF suffice to decide on the trend and model type. The author's experience is that the significance of the single and double standard deviation bounds of the ACF may sometimes be overestimated and that it is indeed the shape of the ACF indicating presence or absence of trend. Subtracting distinct seasonal patterns helps in reducing variance. Therefore preliminary spectral decomposition is an important step in detrending time series.

Starting from these facts, an algorithm is suggested that may be suitable for automatic model selection, taking into account mainly the variance of input data and their frequency distribution. Fig. 1 is an example of arterial systolic pressure sampled at 1-min intervals over a period of 8 h. Beginning in section A the algorithm gathers about 30 data points before starting the cycle. The model found describes the series by a fixed mean value with an additional white noise component. After 45 min a change in the characteristic of incoming data can be observed, suggesting an increasing influence of seasonality.

As may be expected, a high noise level may seriously endanger algorithm efficiency. In the presence of signal noise it may become quite impossible to decide

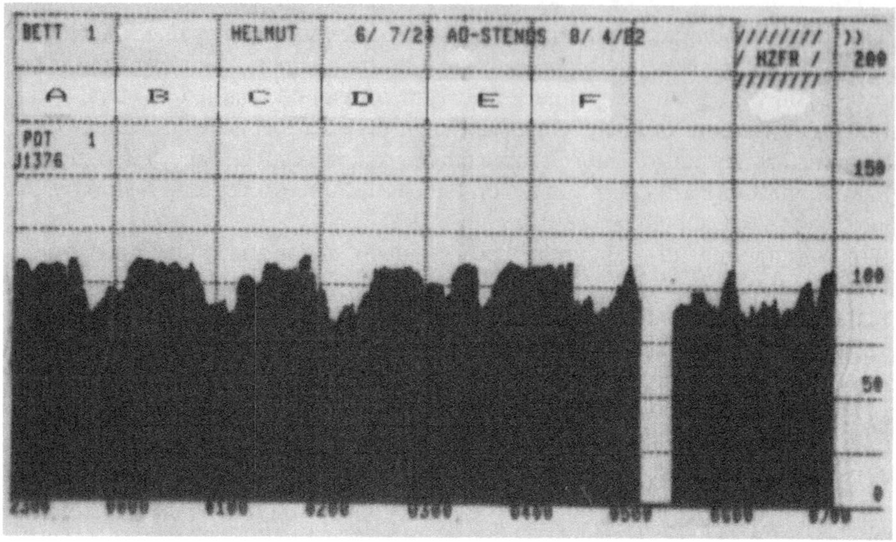

Fig. 1. Systolic arterial pressure

whether detrending should be applied or not. Special care has to be given to detrending as overdoing it may introduce artificial patterns into the working series. On the other hand, existing process patterns may be hidden completely by signal noise as the signal to noise ratio becomes worse.

Using the model (2, 0, 0) * (0, 1, 0) with a period of 70 min model forecast and data actually sampled after prediction are compared in sections B and in the left half of section C. In Fig. 2, * marks the forecast, + stands for sampled data, and U and L give the upper and lower 95% confidence limits of the model forecast. The maximum absolute forecast error is 13.0 and the mean absolute forecast error is 5.9 units.

The process resulting from long-term monitoring of vital signs is slow enough that a full cycle identification – modelling–forecast may be repeated any time new data are available. Another example demonstrating the differences to be observed in the

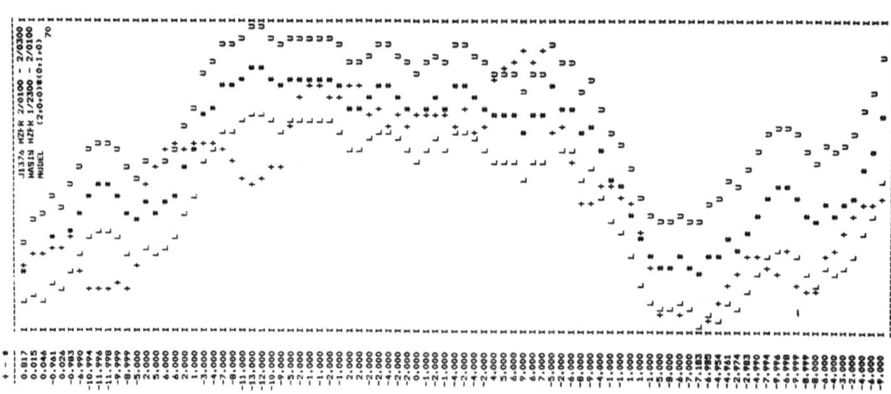

Fig. 2. Model forecast (*), sampled data (+), and forecast error (+ − *)

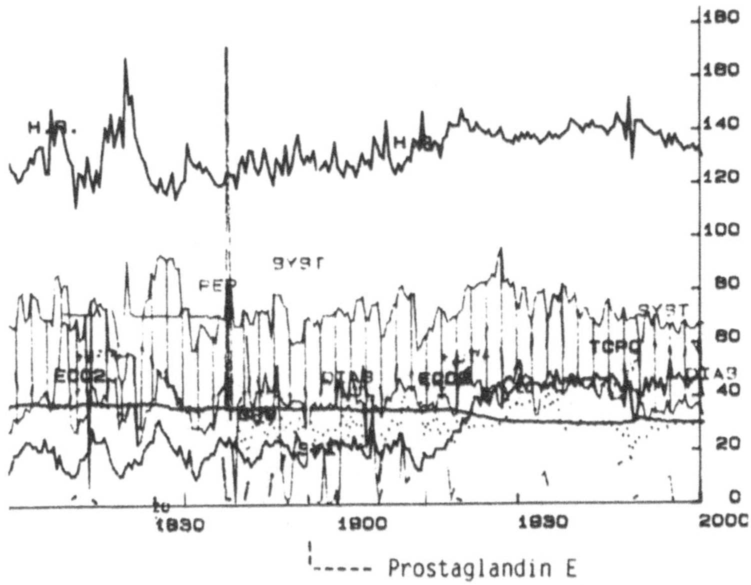

Fig. 3. Hemodynamics of patient suffering from pulmonary atresia. Note the change in the oscillatory component after administration of prostaglandin E at 18:55. (By courtesy of the Division of Peadiatric Cardiology, University of Tübingen)

models fitted to the data are the heart rate (HR) and the oxygen pressure in blood using a transcutaneous probe (TCPO), sampled at a rate of 2 per minute during pulmonary atresia (Fig. 3).

Both series display distinct oscillations, with a common period of about 8.5 min. This can be seen in Fig. 4, which shows the power spectrum estimate of HR and TCPO calculated from a segment of 40 data points (i.e., 20 min). Fig. 5 gives the cross correlation between HR and TCPO, displaying a time lag of about 5 min in the shape of TCPO relative to the shape of HR. Using this information on TCPO a model of the form (1-B**18) *z (t) = (1 + 0.13*B) *a (t) with a mean of 20.0 and a variance of 15.8 can be calculated. The TCPO forecast from this model for the next 20 min and the forecast error are given in Fig. 6.

Now prostaglandin E is administered and the next 20 min (i.e., 40 data points) are studied. Fig. 7 gives the power spectrum of HR and TCPO.

Obviously this spectrum is flat and widespread as compared to the former one, a spectrum considered to be characteristic for data essentially free from seasonal components. Also, the cross correlation between HR and TCPO (Fig. 8) looks quite different from the one before, indicating weak short-term variability as well as a time lag of about 2 min of TCPO shape relative to HR.

Calculation of a stochastic model now yields z (t) = a (t) with a mean of 20.9 and a variance of 8.5. Indeed, this section of the series may well be described by a fixed mean disturbed by white noise. The model forecast is the mean itself.

There remains the problem of how to select basic input data in real time in such a way that the segment chosen may be considered to be truly representative for the state of the process generating system. Obviously, careless selection of input data segments

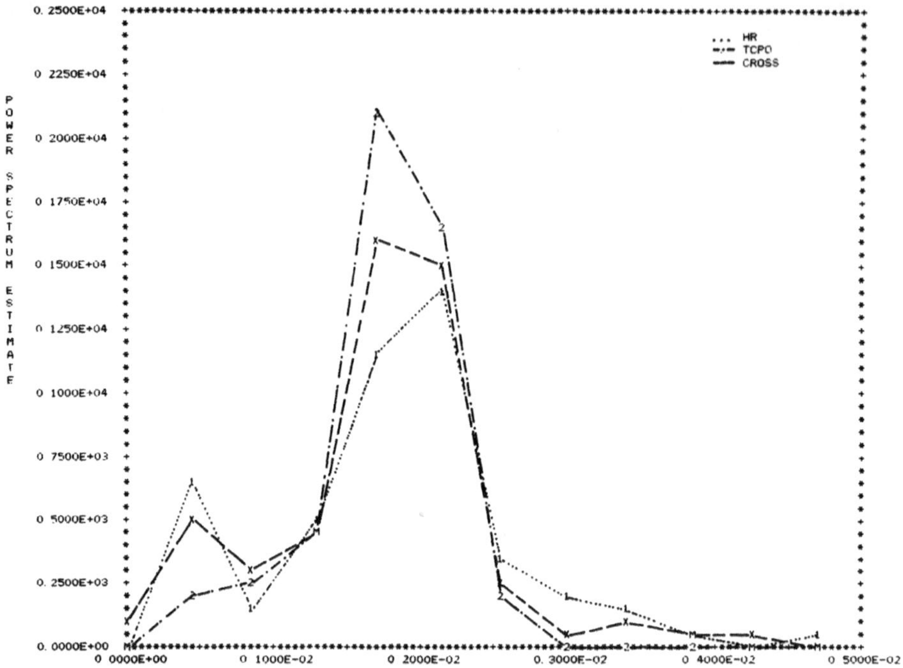

Fig. 4. Power spectrum estimate of HR, TCPO, and cross spectrum during pulmonary atresia

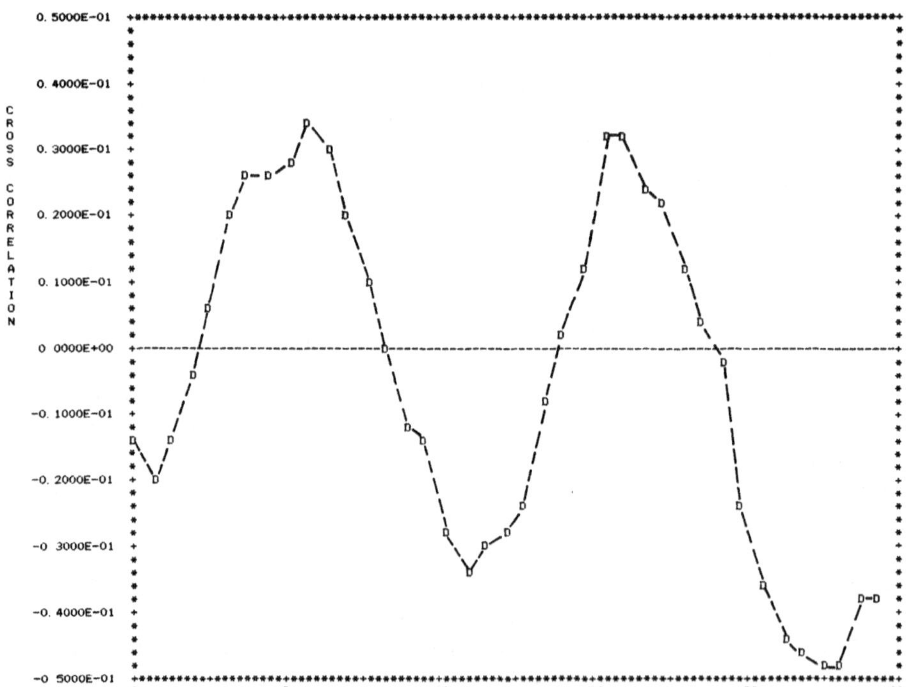

Fig. 5. Cross correlation of HR and TCPO (lag positive)

MODEL FROM: TUEB2 18:32:30-18:52:00 TCPO
* FORECAST FOR 18:52:30-19:12:00 TCPO

+ACTUAL	ERROR
19.200	-4.665
17.600	-3.200
19.200	0.000
16.000	0.000
14.400	-3.200
14.400	0.000
20.800	4.800
20.800	3.200
17.600	0.000
22.400	0.000
22.400	-1.600
20.800	-1.600
19.200	-3.200
24.000	0.000
24.000	0.000
24.000	0.000
20.800	-1.600
24.000	1.600
22.400	-1.465
22.400	1.600
20.800	1.600
25.600	9.600
20.800	3.200
22.400	8.000
19.200	3.700
17.600	0.000
17.600	0.000
27.200	4.800
22.400	-1.600
19.200	-3.200
17.600	-4.800
22.400	-1.600
22.400	-1.600
19.200	-4.800
24.000	1.600
22.400	0.000
25.600	1.735
24.000	3.200
20.800	1.600
20.800	4.800

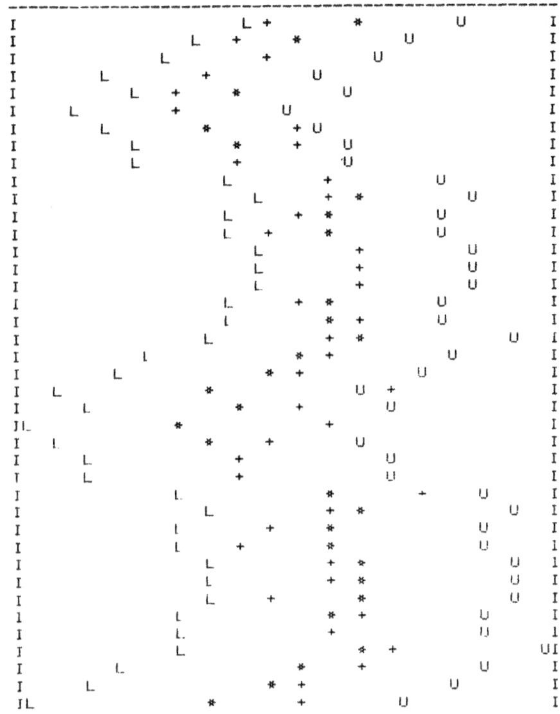

Fig. 6. TCPO model forecast (*), sampled data (+), and forecast error

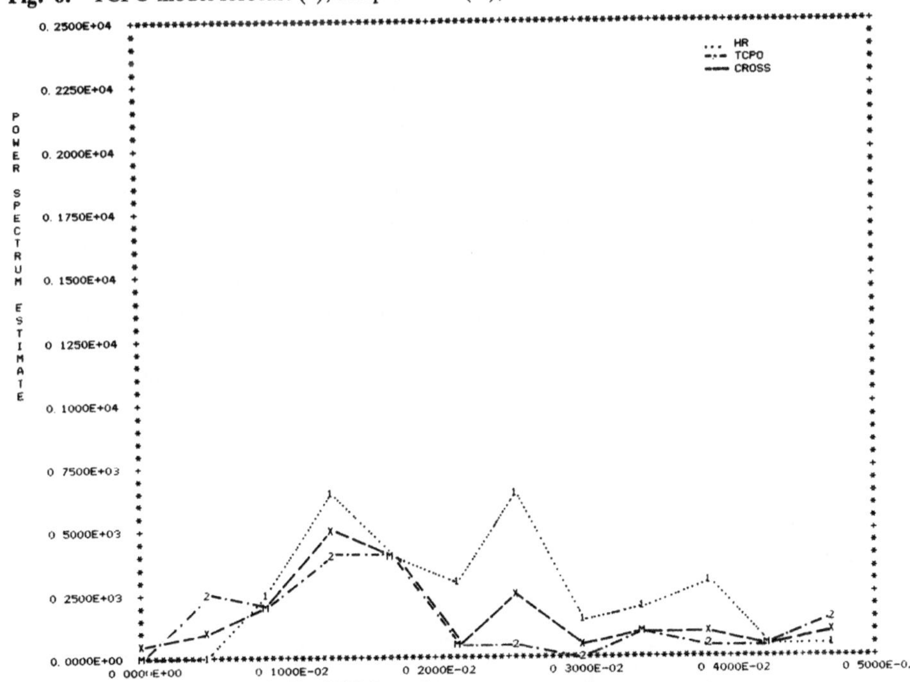

Fig. 7. Power spectrum of HR, TCPO, and cross spectrum after treatment

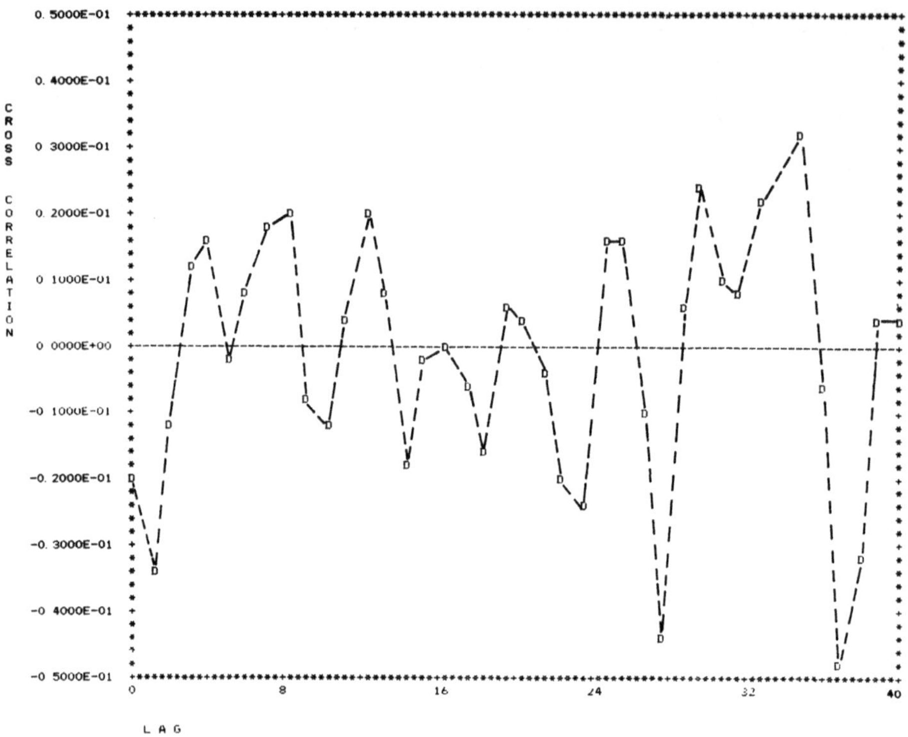

Fig. 8. Cross correlation of HR and TCPO after treatment (lag positive)

may have fatal consequences for the output of the modelling algorithm to follow. This is the time when a priori knowledge of the system becomes of crucial importance. This could contain such items as, for example, already known patterns in the series and their relation to the external system state, bandwidth of reasonable system responses, and system response times, so that suitable filtering may be performed whenever necessary without losing valuable information. As may be expected, an input data selecting algorithm strongly depends on the character of the specific application and should therefore be thought of as being part of the system analysis phase. Indeed, in the authors' opinion one of the most important capabilities such an algorithm should have is to know when to do just nothing and wait for better input data.

References

Box GEP, Jenkins GM (1976) Time Series Analysis. Holden-Day

Endresen J, Hill DW (1977) The present state of trend detection and prediction in patient monitoring. Intens Care Med 3: 15–26

Artifact Processing in a Computerized Intensive Care Unit

W. Bleicher, E. Epple, M. Kopp, and H. Junger

After the installation of our computerized intensive care system, one of our physicians voiced the following opinion: "We have a wonderful system to register data. What we now need is to reduce the huge amount of artifacts which I can see on the computer-generated trend charts."

In Fig. 1, courses of vital parameters are registered which look very likely to have been induced by artifacts. But if one expands the time axis (Fig. 2), one recognizes ordinary behavior of the various) parameters registered, i.e., heart rate, respiration rate, and intracranial pressure. It was proved that the spikes were in fact caused by real physiological changes. This leads us to the question: What is an artifact?

As outlined in Table 1 we can differentiate distortions of physiological signals into three classes. Unfortunately, however, there is no clear distinction between these classes. "Spontanoues changes" and "provocations" are often hard to differentiate

Table 1. Artifact definition

Changes in a physiological signal are
– spontaneous changes, if caused by the patient himself
– provocations, if induced by therapeutical or care measures
– artifacts, if not caused by the signal emitting source

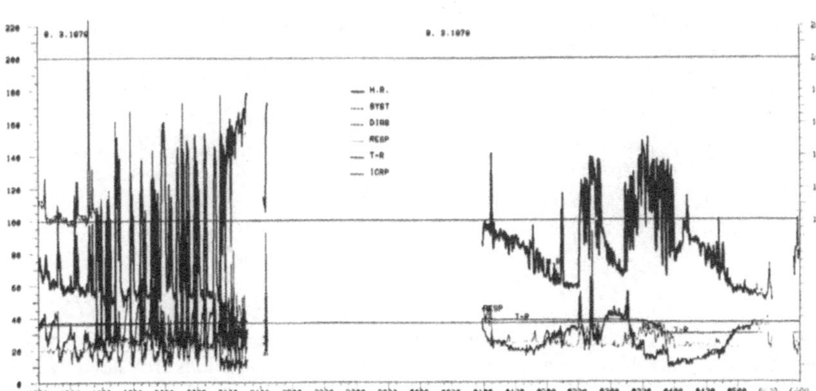

Fig. 1. Patient chart (time span 12 h) with rapidly varying courses in the vital parameters

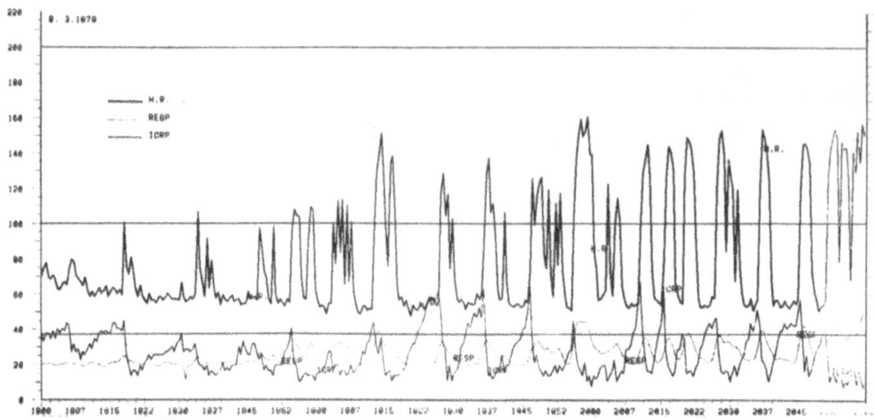

Fig. 2. Expanded view of Fig. 1 (time span 3 h) with only heart rate, respiration rate, and intracranial pressure selected

because the patient-environment interaction is very complex, while in many cases the signal level provides no clear distinction between "provocations" and "artifacts." Let us consider the ECG: Distortions of the signal by loose electrodes or even by muscle tremble are clear artifacts, while distortions caused by extrasystoles can be either spontaneous or the result of a provocation, e. g., drugs. However, some baseline shifts may appear to the monitor like extrasystoles.

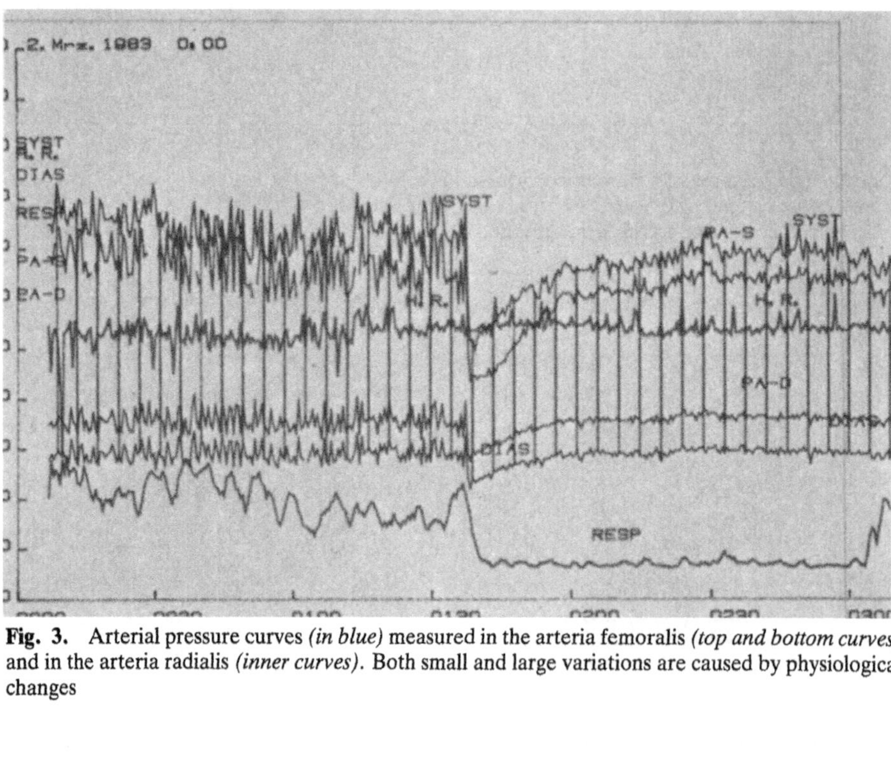

Fig. 3. Arterial pressure curves *(in blue)* measured in the arteria femoralis *(top and bottom curves)* and in the arteria radialis *(inner curves)*. Both small and large variations are caused by physiological changes

In measuring invasive blood pressure, there may be damping effects of the catheter system which produce artifacts, but respiration effects can be either artifactual or real.

When nurses or physicians read values from the digital display of a monitor, they will take an average value of the small variations and consider the large ones to be artifacts. Normally they will wait some seconds and read a new, more stable value. However, as we can see from our trend curves, both small and large variations are in general true physiological events. Fig. 3 illustrates this statement. There the arterial blood pressure has been measured with two different catheters. The top and bottom curves correspond to the systolic and diastolic pressure in the arteria femoralis, while the inner ones have been measured in the arteria radialis. The differences in the absolute values correspond to the physiological difference, but nearly every deviation in one pressure can be seen in the other course, too. What does this mean? We can state that when the same kind of variation appears in two or more independently measured parameters, the variation is very likely to be physiological and not artifactual.

Figure 4 shows this effect with other parameters: Here the same spikes appear in nearly all parameters. Therefore the variations must be physiological. In fact, it was proven that they were caused by a provocation which induced stress.

But let us return to real artifacts. Fig. 5 shows the processing of a physiological signal on its way from the patient to the monitor, together with external influences on the patient. Therapeutic measures (e.g., drug administration, ventilator settings), care measures (e.g., bedding, washing), but also environmental factors like light, noise, room temperature, and interaction with the staff or with visitors influence the physiological state of the patient; we term these external influences "provocations." Apart from the effect of these provocations, the patient regulates his state spontaneously.

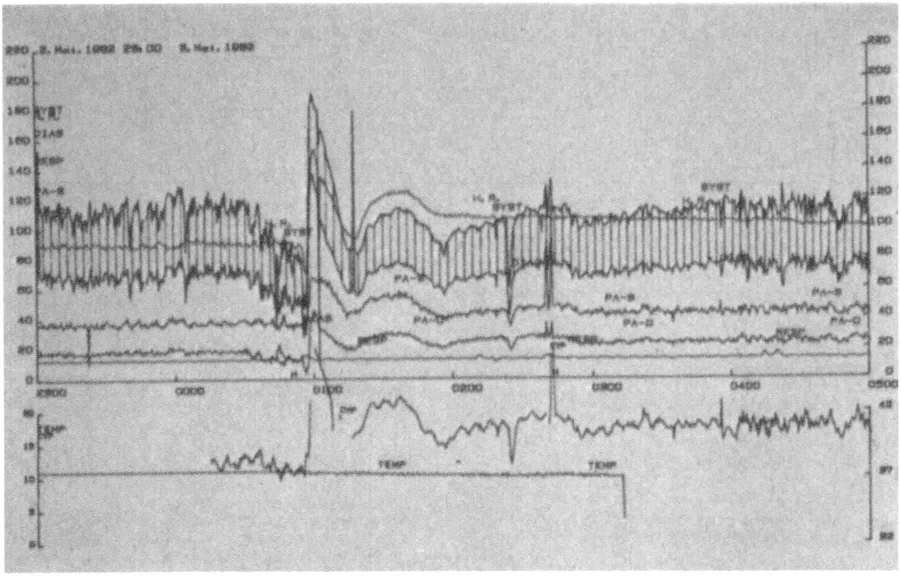

Fig. 4. Coincident variations in different parameters, indicating a physiological change

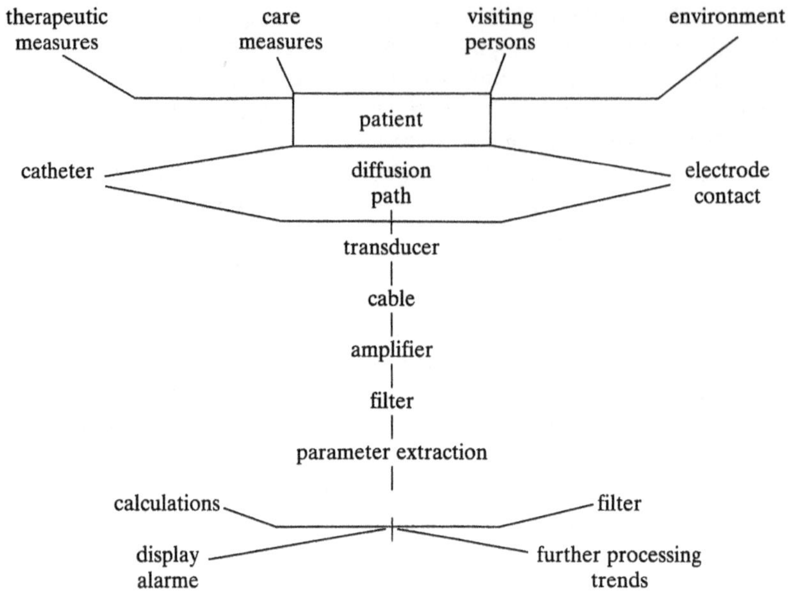

Fig. 5. Signal processing path

The possibility of artifacts begins within the patient himself (e.g., due to muscle tremble in the ECG); they may be induced by catheter, by diffusion or contact problems, or by the transducer. Furthermore, artifacts can occur in cables, in the preprocessing unit, and in the parameter extraction unit. Possibilities of detecting and suppressing artifacts in these steps are dealt with in the literature in great detail. Here we shall concentrate on artifact handling after the parameter extraction in the monitor.

Table 2. Possibilities of artifact suppression and processing

Possibilities of artifact suppression

a) Low pass filtering, short time intervale
b) Low pass filtering, long time intervale
c) Validity check
- upper and lower limite
- changing velocity
- pattern recognition

Possibilities of artifact processing

a) Statue-parameters
- good signal
- noisy signal
- signal not processable
- ...

b) Presentation of parameter courses

Most of the monitors today are equipped with low pass filters, which produce a more or less average value over several seconds. We have asked some manufacturers the reason for these filters. They answered that filtering provides the user with a stable digital number on his monitor and that it reduces artifacts. Both reasons apply to the reading of digital numbers only and are without importance for trend curves.

Figure 7 shows possibilities for artifact suppression after parameter extraction.

- Besides low pass filtering over short time intervals, there are methods for averaging over longer time intervals, but these are meaningless in intensive care because of the short interaction time.
- The checking of data values for validity with upper and lower limits makes sense only when artifact values are clearly distinct from real values.
- The same applies to the comparison of changing speeds: It is clear that no patient can change his core temperature by 3°C in 1 min, but most other parameters can change physiologically from one second to another.
- Similarly, efforts to differentiate artifacts from real values by pattern recognition are only possible in a few well-known cases; much research will have to be done to prove the usefulness of this method.

We have seen that artifact *suppression* after parameter extraction is not feasible at present. The only thing that can be done is to detect and perhaps eliminate artifacts before or during parameter extraction. Nevertheless, it is useful to have a status attribute with every data value which gives information about the quality of the data, e.g.,

- Good signal
- Noisy signal
- Signal not processable
- Loose electrodes

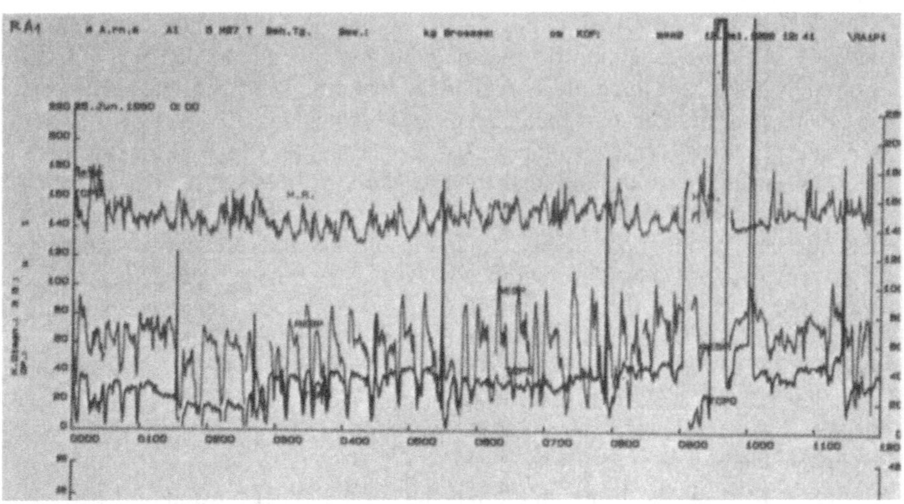

Fig. 6. Artifactual spikes in the transcutaneous PO2 *(bottom curve)* caused by changing the position of the electrode

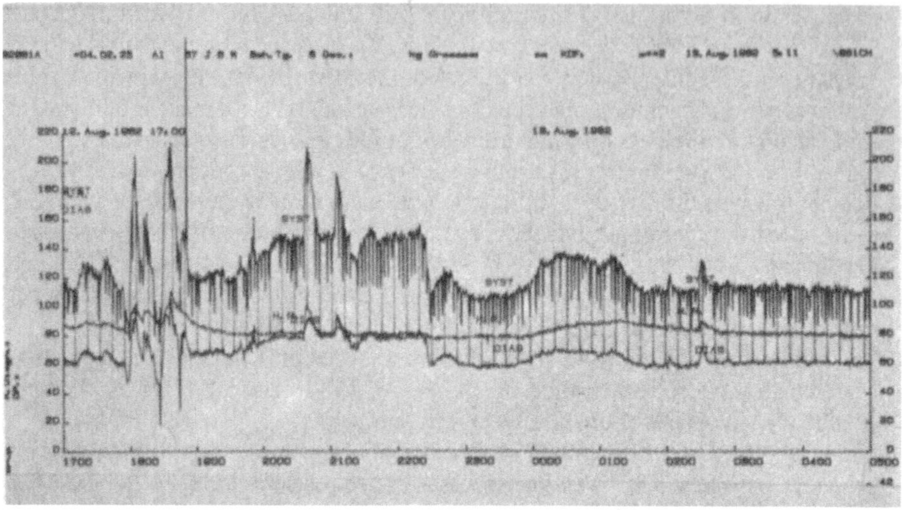

Fig. 7. Intermittent breaks in the systolic arterial pressure *(top curve)* caused by a defective monitor

If there is no possibility of suppressing artifacts, what else can be done to judge the quality of a parameter? We propose a good and detailed *presentation* of the parameter courses, together with their above-mentioned status attributes. Most artifacts produce characteristic trend patterns. For example (Fig. 6), to obtain transcutaneous P02, the position of the electrode must be changed regularly to avoid skin burning. We see the changes induced by this process on the slide. It is possible to suppress these artifactual trends, but we have found that it is better to see them because they give information on the appropriate time of repositioning and the proper functioning of the electrode.

In Figure 7, intermittent spikes can be observed in the systolic blood pressure (SYST). After investigation of the original signal, we found that the spikes were caused by a defective integrated circuit in the monitor. The occurrence of this pattern is now used as an indication that a circuit needs changing.

Some problems, however, still persist. For example, it is well known that most blood pressure curves are influenced by respiration. In Fig. 8 such an effect on the central venous and the arterial blood pressure is registered, the nature of which could be either artifactual or physiological. On the left side, the recorder was running very slowly, on the right side at normal speed. If we register the extracted values not beat-to-beat but only intermittently, we will get values by chance, giving such a picture as is shown in Fig. 9. This tells us something about the overall variability, but not about its periodic behavior nor about its origin. Worse, when the respiration rate and the sampling rate are close to an even multiplication factor, we will get so-called aliasing, which we can see on the right side of Fig. 9. This means that registration of a periodic signal may have a wrong wavelength.

In Fig. 10 this is illustrated in more detail. In the upper portion of the figure, the parameters were registered every 30 s, while the respiration rate was about 15/min, which gives this oscillation in the pressure parameters with a frequency of about 20 per

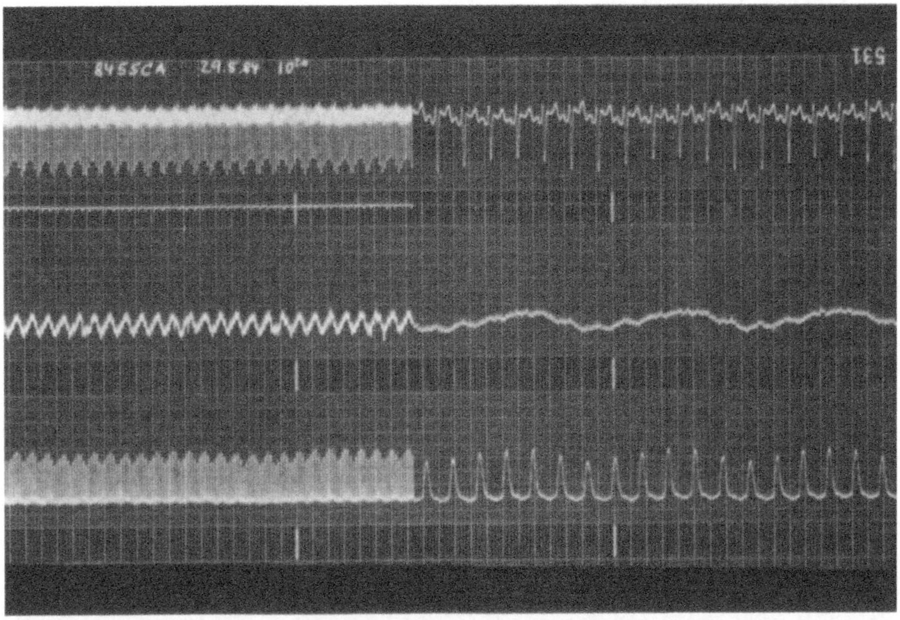

Fig. 8. Recording of ECG, central venous pressure, and arterial pressure at low and medium speed to show the respiration-induced dependency

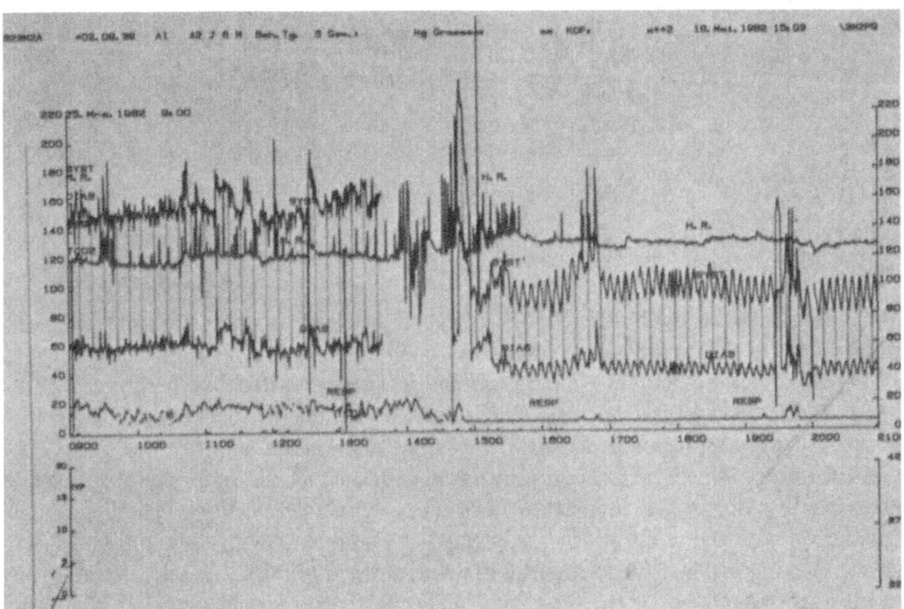

Fig. 9. Alteration in the arterial blood pressure pattern caused by changing from intermittent mandatory ventilation to controlled ventilation: the random variations were followed by an oscillatory behavior

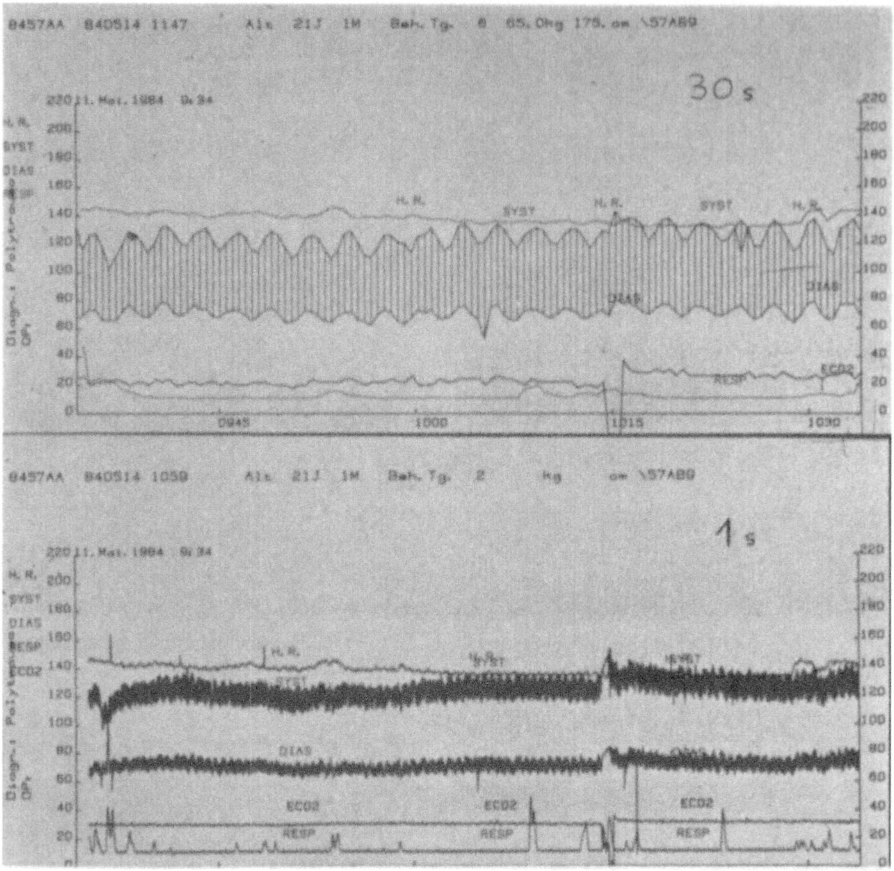

Fig. 10. Effect of the sampling rate on an oscillatory pattern. With a sampling rate of 2/min, the oscillation frequency of 21/hour is caused by an aliasing effect. As indicated with a sampling rate of 1/s, the actual frequency is about 11/min

hour. If one registers every second, one will get a picture like that in the lower portion of Fig. 10. This shows the actual oscillatory behavior.

There are two ways to overcome this difficulty: The first is to choose a sampling rate that is twice the respiration rate, according to Shannon's theorem. This means sampling every second or every 2, which is not economical and in most cases not readable either. However, a short registration with such a high sampling rate is useful for inspecting the actual oscillation rate. The second possibility is to trigger the registration with the respiration, for example to sample only in the end-expiratory phase. This algorithm is implemented in some newer monitors. In our opinion, the actual implementation of this good idea has two major drawbacks: (a) the end-expiratory phase is detected by the changes in the pressure curve itself and not by the respiration wave, if there is one; (b) the triggering is only done in determining venous and pulmonary pressure values, not arterial pressure. With regard to the latter, ordinary low pass filtering is performed to obtain a mean value over the whole respiration period; but as mentioned above, filtering destroys information about variability. To maintain this information, it would be better to register not only one value in the sampling interval, but also a variability measure for this interval, e.g., maximum and minimum value or standard deviation. It should be recognized, however, that good presentation of such an amount of data is very difficult. A lot of ectopic beats or series of artifacts can make a presentation completely unreadable, and it may be that one has to choose between several registration and presentation forms.

References

Blumlein S, Haywood LJ, Harvey G, Murthy VK (1981) Detection of signal associated with noise. Computers in cardiology. IEEE Catalog 81CH1750-9: 339–342

Ellis D (1983) An algorithm for reduction of respiration artifact in pulmonary artery pressure measurement. 34th Annual Meeting of the Pennsylvania Society of Anesthesiologists, May 13, 1983 (Hewlett-Packard P/N 5953-7352)

Gardner R (1983) Artifact detection and elimination in intensive care pressure monitoring systems. In: Epple E (ed) Rechnergestützte Intensivpflege, vol 2. Thieme, Stuttgart

Kraemer M (1975) Ein rechnergestützter EKG-Verstärker für die computer-gestützte Intensivüberwachung Biomed Tech 20:

Rehse E, Kraemer M, Stahl HJ, Mueller K (1977) Zur Behandlung von Störungen bei Biosignalen in der rechnergestützten Schwerkrankenüberwachung. Coping with signal interference in computer-aided monitoring of the critically ill. Biomed Tech 22: 100–105

Wolf M, Bleicher W, Budwig G, Frey R, Fiderer F, Faust U (1983) Möglichkeiten der Artefaktunterdrückung bei Biosignalen In: Epple E (ed) Rechnergestützte Intensivpflege 2. Thieme, Stuttgart

Personal Computers for Gas Exchange Measurements in the ICU

G. Wiesspeiner, S. Schuy, H. Metzler, and W. List

Introduction

Fast and exact measurement and uncomplicated noninvasive monitoring of respiratory and metabolic parameters in the ICU still makes some requests. Only continuous breath by breath analysis for all inpiratory and expiratory cycles assures clear physically based results without assumptions. But this technique of measurement makes great demands on sensors and can only be realized with the help of sophisticated computer real time processing.

Recent microcomputers make available considerable processing capabilities at low prices, but they usually require a lot of additional hard- and software to fit the desired application. In our case an own number base had to be defined and special interrupt-structures had to be developed to run the continuous breath-to-breath analysis. Furthermore, machine and higher programming languages had to be selected carefully.

The demands placed on a computer system for online gas exchange measurement based on continuous breath by breath analysis and the problems that arise from use of a personal computer are described here on the basis of 6 years experience.

Methods of Gas Exchange Measurement

In principle, gas exchange can be measured in four different ways.

In a *closed system* (Fig. 1) like "Crogh's spirometer" (Pichotka 1970) with CO_2 washout, oxygen uptake can be measured directly by the decrease in the initial volume. A computer has no advantage in this case.

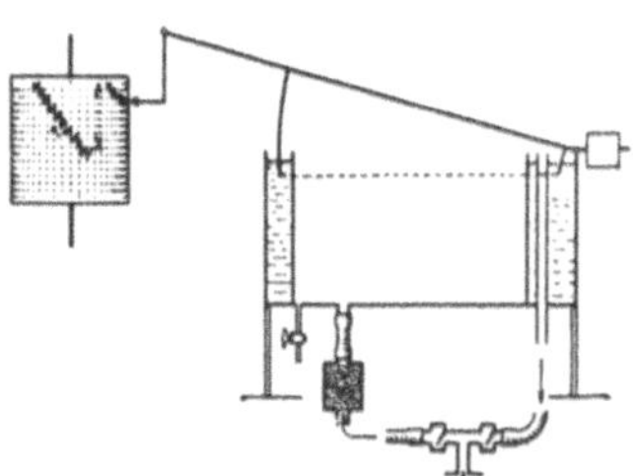

Measurement	:	Volume
Time	:	Minutes
Processing	:	$V_{O2} = V_{Start} - V_{end}$
Computer	:	not necessary

Fig. 1. Example of a closed system

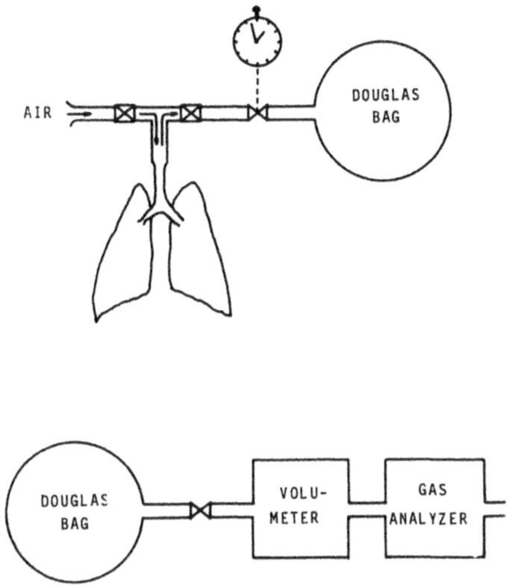

DOUGLAS BAG

Measurement	:	Volume & Gas fraction
Time	:	Minutes
Processing	:	$V_E = V$
		$V_{O2} = V \cdot (F_{IO2} - F_{EO2})$
		$V_{CO2} = V \cdot F_{ECO2}$
Computer	:	Calculator

Fig. 2. Use of a Douglas bag

By using a *Douglas bag* (Fig. 2), expired gases are collected over a given period. In a second step these gases are released through a volumeter to a gasanalyzer. To calculate O_2 uptake and CO_2 production, only a few simple mathematical expressions must be calculated after the procedure of about 10 min duration. Any low cost calculator is sufficient for this computation.

The most common method of measuring gas exchange is the use of *mixing chambers* (Fig. 3); inspiratory and expiratory gas flow is continuously measured by (an integrating) flowmeter and gas analyzer (e.g., Beckmann: Metabolic Measurement Cart.). If inspiratory gases other than air are used, the exact composition must be known or must also be measured in an additional inpiratory mixing chamber (e.g., Engström: Metabolic Computer). Because of the slow changing input variables, results must be calculated at intervals of several seconds. Any simple home computer or personal computer would satisfy the requirements for processing capabilities and speed. Programs may be written in BASIC.

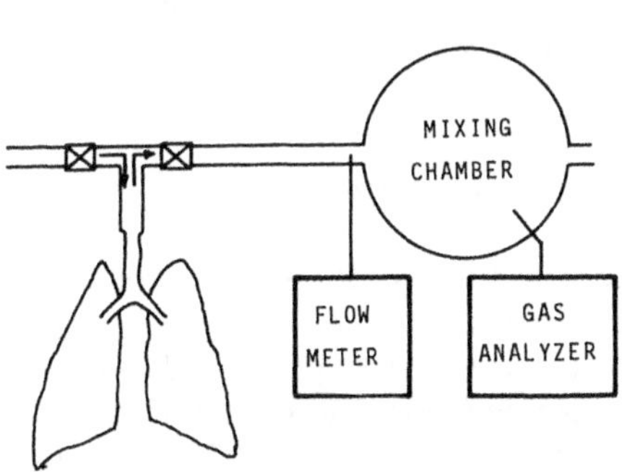

MIXING CHAMBER

Measurement	:	Flow & Gas fractions
Time	:	Seconds
Processing	:	$V_E = \int \dot{V}\, dt$
		$V_{O2} = V_E \cdot (F_{IO2} - F_{EO2})$
		$V_{CO2} = V_E \cdot F_{ECO2}$
Computer	:	Microcomputer
Language	:	Basic

Fig. 3. Use of a mixing chamber

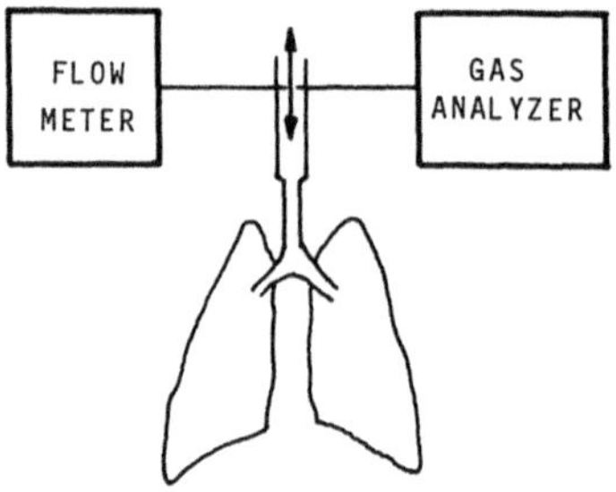

BREATH BY BREATH

Measurement	:	Flow & Gas fractions
Time	:	20 milliseconds
Processing	:	$V_T = \int \dot{V}\, dt$
		$V_{O2} = \int \dot{V}_I \cdot F_{IO2}\, dt - \int \dot{V}_E \cdot F_{EO2}\, dt$
		$V_{CO2} = \int \dot{V}_E \cdot F_{ECO2}\, dt$
Computer	:	Real Time Processor
Language	:	Assembler, Fortran, Pascal, ..

Fig. 4. Breath by breath analysis

As already mentioned, continuous *breath by breath* analysis (Fig. 4) for all inspiratory and expiratory cycles assures clear, physically based results without assumptions but places great demands on transducers and processing capabilities (Swanson et al. 1981; Fletcher et al.; Mitchell 1979). Transducers must display a fast response to the rapidly changing and bidirectional input variables; this is achieved, for example, by the mass spectrometer for gas analysis or the balanced thermistor aneometer (own development) for flow measurement.

At least every 20 ms signals must be sampled and evaluated to partial volumes by the integration of flow value multiplied by gas concentration, separately for each gas component as well as for inspiration and expiration. It is evident that only a fast, real time processing computer can do this job.

Personal Computers

Formerly used analog computers failed with problems like drift, pattern recognition, and decision making. Mainframes or minicomputers are unhandy or too cost-intensive for real time signal processing in an ICU.

Modern personal computers offer remarkable processing capabilities (16 bit word, 128 k RAM, mathematical coprocessor, etc. However, personal computers usually require a lot of additional hard- and software to fit the desired application.

Personal Computer Preparation for Gas Exchange Measurement

In 1978 we started to develop a gas exchange measuring system based on continuous and online breath by breath analysis with the help of a personal computer (Fig. 5). At that time we chose Commodore's PET 2001 because it was a complete single unit with a complete workstation (consisting of a microcomputer, keyboard, video display, and data recorder) and we already had some years of experience on the MCS 6502 central microprocessor.

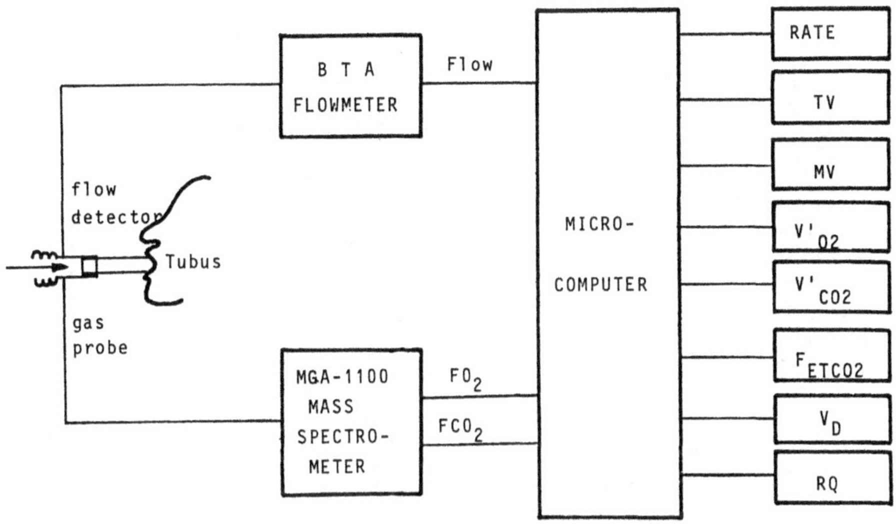

Fig. 5. Gas exchange measuring system based on continuous, online breath by breath analysis, developed with the aid of a personal computer

Hardware Extension (Fig. 6)

For interfacing the mass spectrometer and the flowmeter to the PC, a preamplifier and 16-channel ADC (analog-digital-converter) card was developed. For memory extension and digital I/O (input/output) interface (pen recorder control, alarms) the BMT multiprocessor (Wiesspeiner et al. 1977) is used. A 6-channel trend recorder (Gould) is interfaced by the appropriate digital to analog converter card (own development). These cards are powered by an additional power supply.

To keep the single-unit feature, all additional hardware is built into the original personal computer housing.

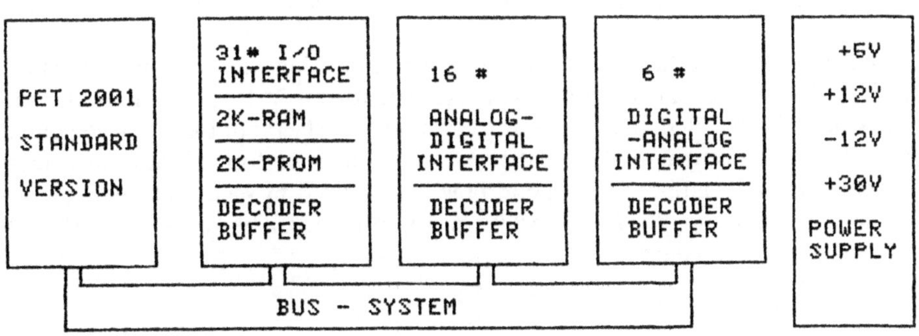

Fig. 6. Hardware-configuration

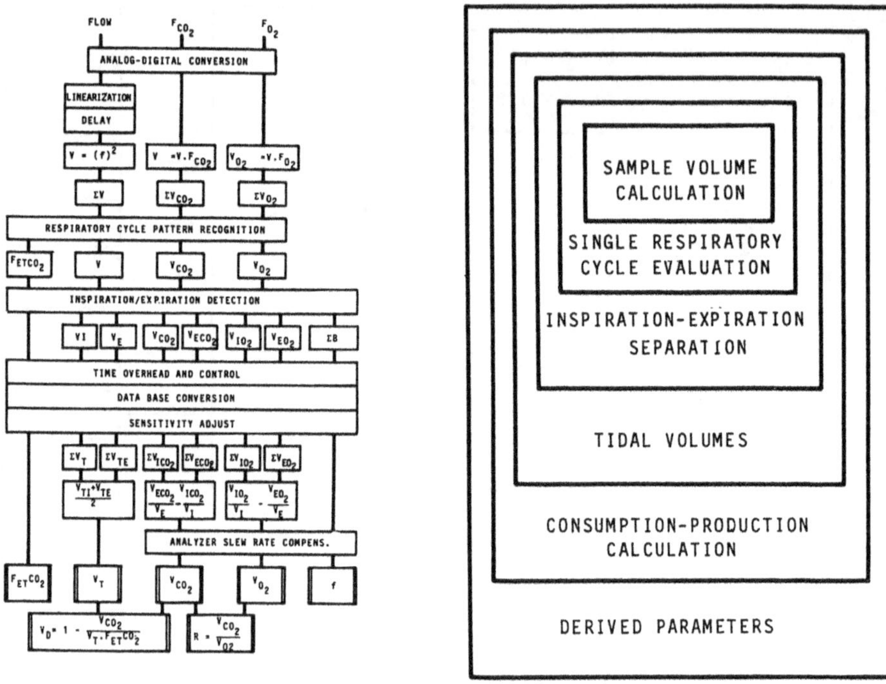

Fig. 7. Software-analysis

Software Extension

The formulas in Fig. 4 only represent a small proportion of the necessary computations, and ignore pattern recognition and program control. More detail is given in the simplified calculation tree in Fig. 7, which should demonstrate that interrupt structures and programming language must be selected carefully to achieve processing and results online.

Inner kernel (Fig. 7) and first overlay are called up every 20 ms, while the two next overlays are needed at the end of every single breath (1–3). Results for output only have to be calculated on request. In our case this automatic update occurs every minute.

It should be noted that about 80% of program functions are written in ASSEMBLER. For even faster execution a data base for mathematical expressions developed by us had to be installed; this speeds up calculations by a factor of 100–1000 compared with BASIC. Only final results and data presentation are performed with convenient-to-write BASIC routines. If program flow is organized in such a manner, even a personal computer supplied with an 8-bit microprocessor can be told to run the breath by breath analysis online.

Problems with Personal Computers

Although personal computers offer the complete hardware to support sophisticated software, from the practical point of view a lot of problems arise with the application of personal computers for real time signal processing. Insufficient *information* hinders selection of the right device. Nowadays personal computers are no longer sold by specially trained personnel but along with various other equipment in computer shops or even in supermarkets.

Insufficient *documentation:* In the beginning we did not even receive an user's manual, not to mention a technical description. This state of affairs has now changed, but available hard- and software documentation cannot be compared with professional computer systems. In most cases it is too shallow for the implementation of specialized hard- and software functions.

Only a few *interfaces* for medical use are on the market. You must be prepared to develop your own.

Most operating systems of personal computers are *real time* interrupt driven and will not support further real time interrupts of user programs. Take care that there is no interference with disk operations or memory refresh cycles.

Software: Many different personal computers use the same microprocessor and support the same operating system. Nevertheless, software is not directly exchangeable because of different utility systems and I/O configurations. Where can one obtain error-free software? It must be considered that the cost of reliable software will be about five to ten times the hardware cost if written by software professionals and much more if written by computer freaks.

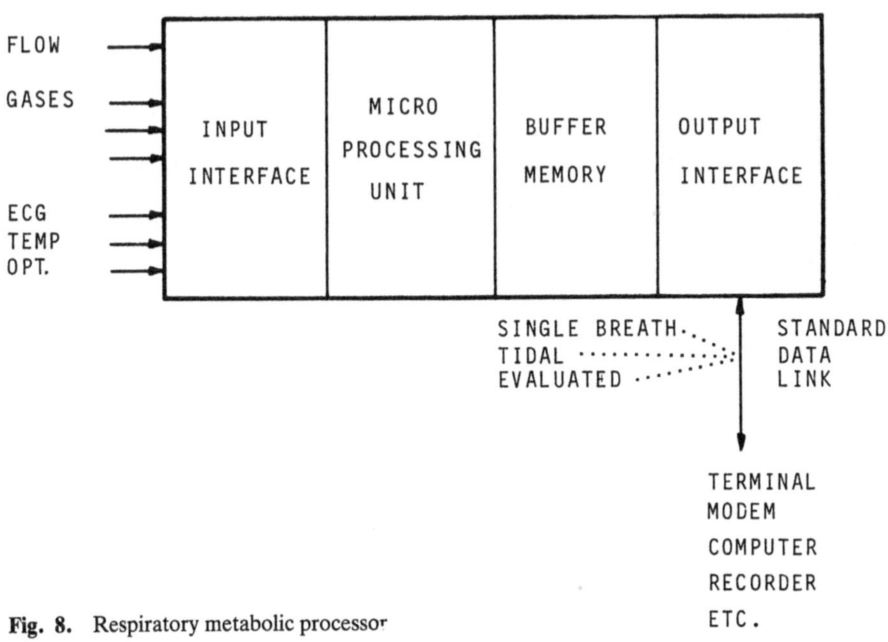

Fig. 8. Respiratory metabolic processor

Very often *service* is a disregarded matter. For clinical use machines must be available at any time. For mainframe computers or clinical equipment that is self evident. That will not be true for a personal computer, because this is a low-cost device with sometimes self-built interfaces and a self-written or modified software.

Conclusion

Taking into account the advantages and disadvantages of personal computers for gas exchange measurements and in order to make continuous breath by breath analysis (Wiesspeiner 1983) available for common use in the ICU, we intend to reorganize our system into two independent parts (Fig. 8):

1. Respiratory and metabolic preprocessor: A dedicated interface between any mass spectrometer, temperature and ECG monitor with an integrated BTA flowmeter on the one side, and a standard data link on the other. The built-in microcomputer should perform over the whole time critical processing and buffer the single breath, tidal, and evaluated data in memory for further computation by external devices (standard link).
2. Optional (personal) computer for investigation, presentation, or documentation of results prepared by the respiratory metabolic preprocessor.

References

Fletcher R, Werner O, Nordström L, Jonson B, Sources of error and their correction in the measurement of carbon dioxyde elimination using the Siemens-Elema CO_2 analyzer. Br J Anaesth 55: 177–185

Mitchell RR (1979) Incorporating the gas analyzer response time in gas exchange computations. J Appl Physiol 47: 1118–1122

Pichotka J (1970) Der Stoffwechsel der Organismen. In: Keidel WD (ed) Kurzgefaßtes Lehrbuch der Physiologie, Thieme, Stuttgart, pp 154–155

Swanson GD, Sodal IE, Reeves JT (1981) Sensitivity of breath to breath gas exchange measurements to expiratory flow errors. IEEE Trans Biomed Eng 28: (11): 749–754

Wießpeiner G (1983) Mikrocomputersystem zur Messung respiratorischer und metabolischer Parameter. Dissertation an der TU Graz, Dezember 1983

Wießpeiner G, Grübler R, Schuy S (1977) Modulares hierarchisches Multiprozessorsystem mit gemeinsamem Arbeitsspeicher. Tagungsberichte der Informationstagung Mikroelektronik, Wien 1977, pp 176–179

Integration of a New Computer HP 9816S in the Pulmonary Calculator System HP 47804S. Advantages of Using the Screen for Graphic Presentation of Flow-Volume Curves

K. ERDMANN and J.-P. JANTZEN

Since March 1979 we have performed 3000 pulmonary function testings in the Department of Anesthesiology, University of Mainz Medical School, using the Hewlett Packard Pulmonary Calculator System HP 47804S. This computer-supported system includes three pneumotachographs in combination with gas analyzers for nitrogen, carbon monoxide, and helium (Fig. 1) (Voigt et al. 1975). The device measures forced expiratory flow patterns, static lung volumes (by open spirometry or nitrogen washout), ventilatory disturbances, and carbon monoxide diffusing capacity.

An HP 9825A desk computer calculates the results from the digitized measurements. All volumes are automatically corrected for BTPS conditions. Messages are displayed by a 32-character LED, enabling the operator to run the test procedure by question-and-answer sequences. After being displayed in part, the results are printed by a modified HP 9871A impact printer which is equipped to be used as a graphic printer as well.

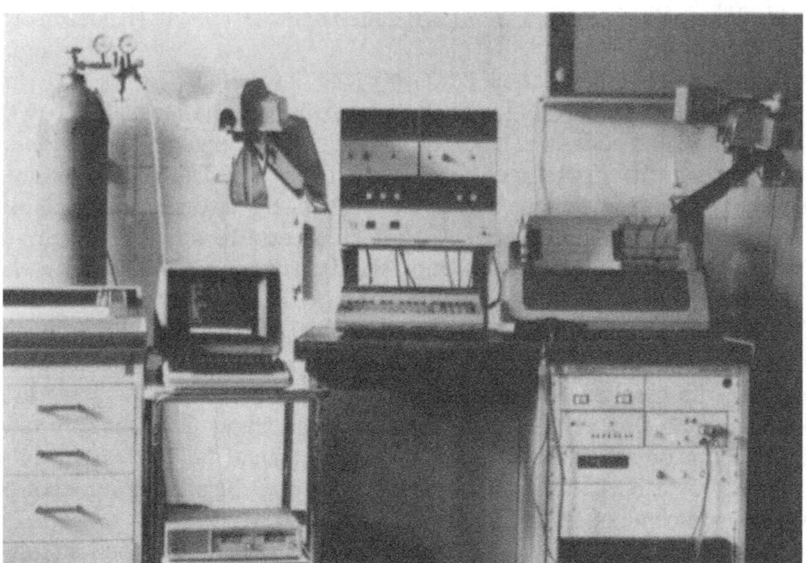

Fig. 1. Pulmonary Calculator System HP 47804S modified by integration of HP 9816S and HP 7225B

indicator for the patient's cooperation

shape of the curve is effort dependent

reproducibility in consecutive tests

detailed and precise information

characteristic patterns in various diseases

obstruction of large and peripheral airways

graphic presentation - fast interpretation

easy and fast performance - clinical relevance

Fig. 2. Value of flow-volume curves

Among these tests the results of the expiratory forced vital capacity maneuver, including the flow-volume curve, are of great clinical relevance (Hyatt 1965; Hyatt et al. 1958). Obstructive and/or restrictive lung diseases can be verified and differentiated. In addition, the reproducibility of the flow-volume curves is a good indicator of the patient's ability to cooperate (Fig. 2).

From this test several parameters are measured or calculated. The most relevant parameters include FEV_1, FVC, FEV_1/FVC, $FEF_{25\text{-}75}$, peak flow rate, and the flow-volume curve (Hyatt 1965, Knudson et al. 1976; Konietzko 1983; Morris et al. 1975). Additional parameters (like FVC, FEF 0.2–1.2, FEF 75–85, MEF 50, and MEF 75) yield additional information for interpretation of the test results (Knudson et al. 1976; Morris et al. 1975).

Careful analysis of abnormal patterns in the flow-volume curves, including information about FVC, FEV 1, and peak flow rate in combination with history, physical examination, and additional laboratory tests, gives detailed and precise information about the underlying pulmonary disease and its severity. This makes measurement of the FVC or the flow-volume curves the most widely used physiological test for the detection of pulmonary disease. Analyzing consecutive flow-volume curves allows assessment of the patient's cooperation and thereby the reliability of the whole test.

Flow volume curves, FEV_1, FEV_1/FVC, and $FEF_{25\text{-}75}$ are valuable in determining the patient's perioperative risk (Konietzko 1983). This is of special importance in poor-risk patients (e.g., geriatric patients, patients in poor general condition, or patients with cerebral disorders), especially when they are undergoing thoracic or upper abdominal surgery. Therefore the results of pulmonary testing are valuable for the decision on whether a surgical procedure should be carried out as planned, modified, or cancelled. Furthermore, they provide helpful information as to the probable outcome of an operation.

The testing requires the patient's cooperation. Cooperation is poor in children and the persons mentioned above. A facilitated testing procedure may solve the problem

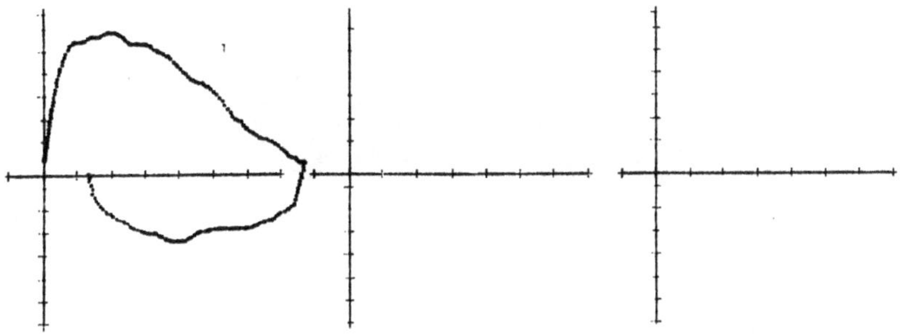

Fig. 3. Printed flow-volume curve – tall adult

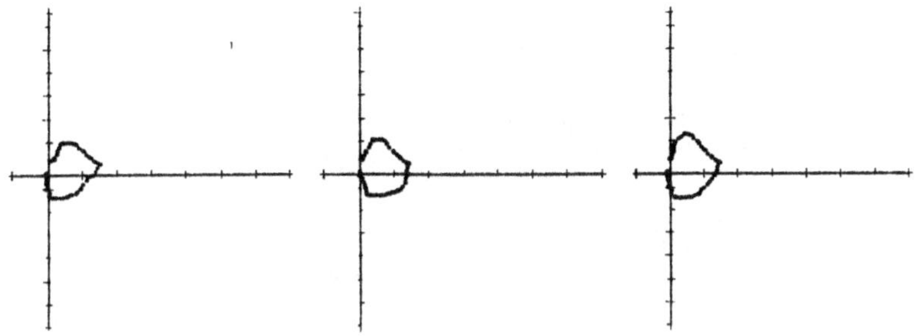

Fig. 4. Printed flow-volume curve – child, 7 years of age

for the patient and the examiner as well. The limitations of the HP 47804S are set by the lack of a screen. Thus the results have to be printed, which is a time-consuming and paper-wasting procedure. The results cannot be seen for acceptance or abolishment of the test before being printed. Besides, the tests can be repeated only 3 to 6 times. While in tall adults the printed curves give good information, the results in small children are rather poor (Figs. 3, 4).

We solved the problem by integrating the HP 9816S desktop computer into the system (Fig. 5). This computer belongs to the HP Series 200 family, which are based on the MC 68000, a 16-bit Motorola microprocessor with 32-bit internal architecture and an 8 MHz clock rate. A 9-inch CRT with a resolution of 400 dots horizontal ×300 dots vertical is integrated. The RAM storage capacity of 512 K bytes provides easy handling of programs and data. An additional HP 7225B plotter gives high-quality plots of the flow-volume curves if wanted (cf. Fig. 1).

The program was transferred from an HP 9885M flexible disk drive to the HP 9825A and via an HP-IB bus to the HP 9816S, then to an HP 9121D flexible disk drive. The screen facilitates software changes and thus test modifications. The program is written in HPL 2.0 and modified to fit our needs. A menu technique is used instead of the special function keys of the old version to guide the operator through the test procedure. Fig. 6 shows a small boy in the test position. His standard flow-volume curve gives poor information.

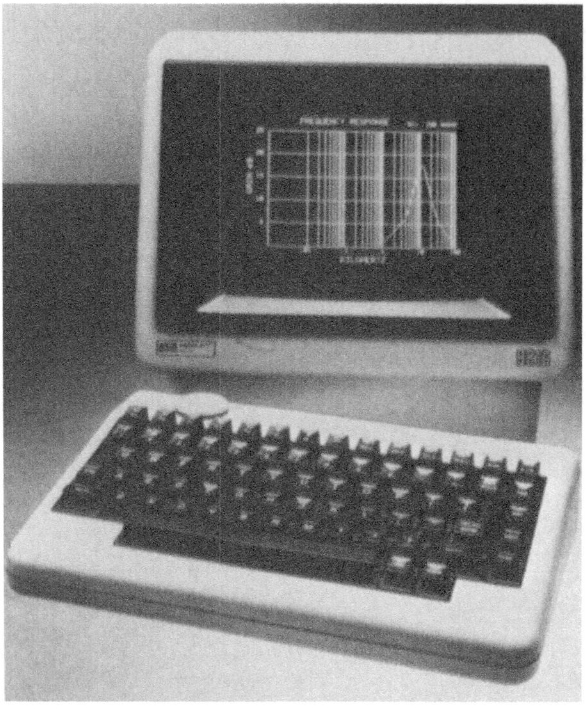

Fig. 5. HP 9816S desktop computer

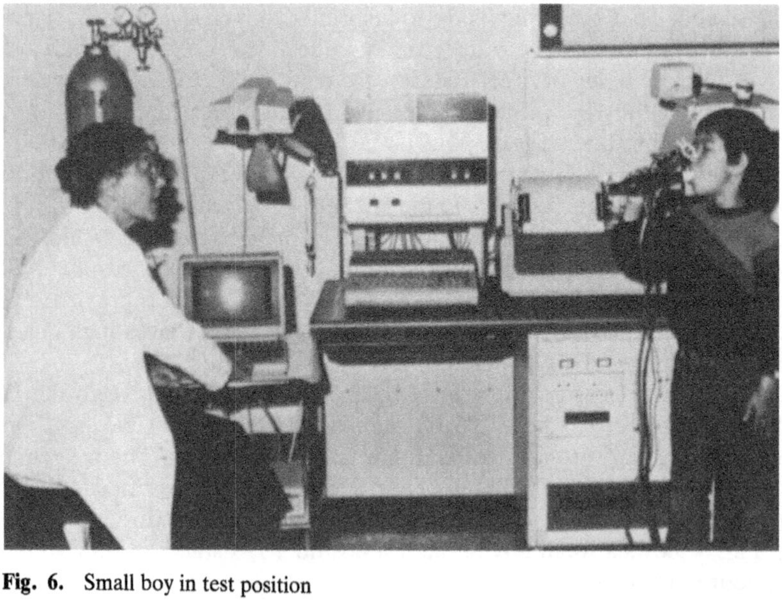

Fig. 6. Small boy in test position

The default values are 7 l for the maximal volume and 12 l/s for the maximal flow rate. By reduction of these values the flow-volume curves are enlarged for volumes of 3 l and 1.5 l, as shown in Figs. 7–9. Through this enlargement the curves give detailed information even in children or in patients with excessive restrictive lung disease. The FVC of some adult male patients exceeds 7 l. By incrementing the maximal volume to 10 l, the flow-volume curve is reduced in size and thus fully visible on the screen. Failed trials can be abolished easily and rapidly, while accepted trials are printed and

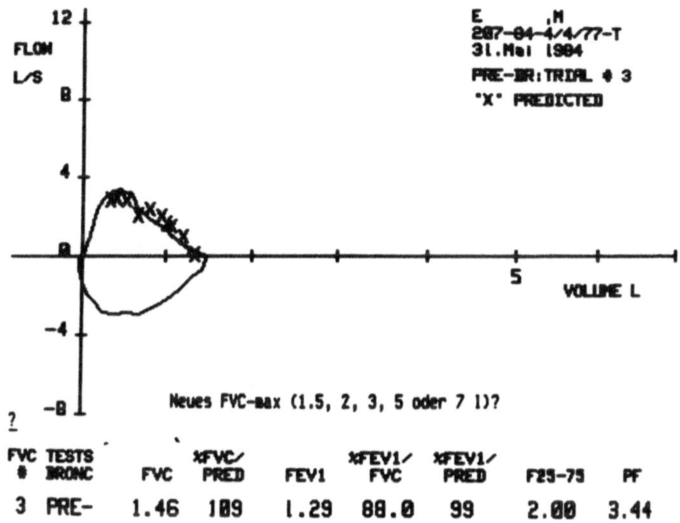

Fig. 7. Flow-volume curve on screen (small child)

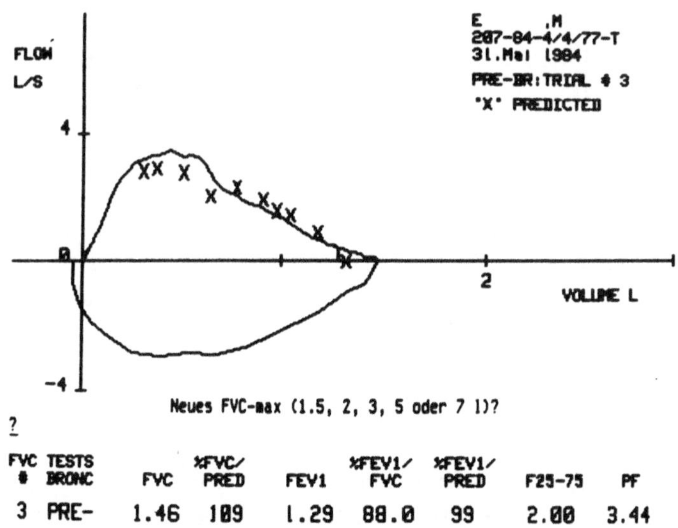

Fig. 8. Enlargement of curve on screen (cf. Fig. 7)

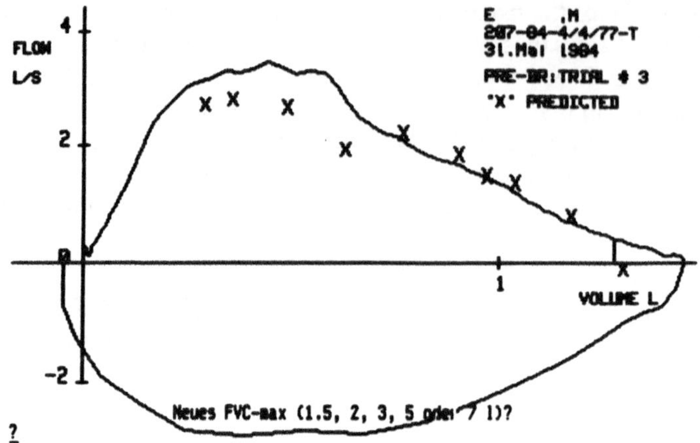

FVC TESTS # BRONC	FVC	%FVC/ PRED	FEV1	%FEV1/ FVC	%FEV1/ PRED	F25-75	PF
3 PRE-	1.46	109	1.29	88.0	99	2.00	3.44

Fig. 9. Maximal enlargement of curve on screen (cf. Fig. 7)

stored for later documentation in a pulmonary function report. The flow-volume curves can be plotted and enlarged in the same manner, providing better information (Figs. 10, 11).

This new system enables us to examine patients with poor cooperation, such as children aged 5 years of age or less, geriatric patients, and patients in a poor general condition or with cerebral disorders (Fig. 12).

By this modification of equipment and test procedures, pulmonary function testing became easier, faster, and applicable even to patients who have not previously been easily accessible.

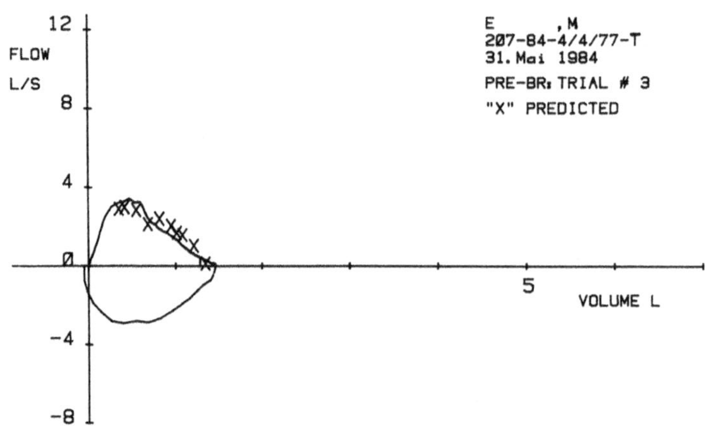

FVC TESTS # BRONC	FVC	%FVC/ PRED	FEV1	%FEV1/ FVC	%FEV1/ PRED	F25-75	PF
3 PRE-	1.46	109	1.29	88.0	99	2.00	3.44

Fig. 10. Plotted flow-volume curve (cf. Fig. 7)

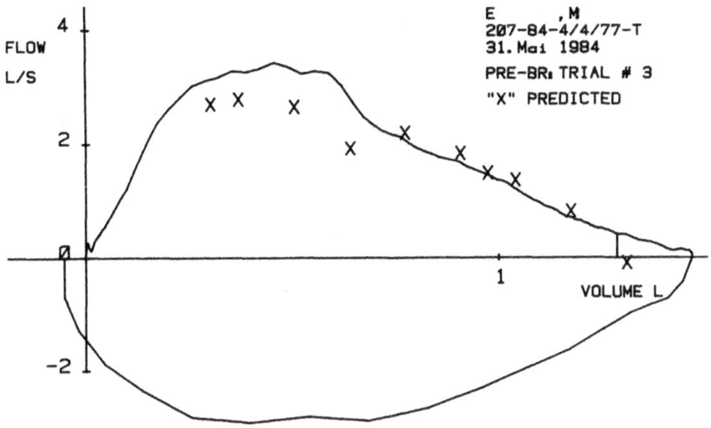

FVC TESTS #	BRONC	FVC	%FVC/ PRED	FEV1	%FEV1/ FVC	%FEV1/ PRED	F25-75	PF
3	PRE-	1.46	109	1.29	88.0	99	2.00	3.44

Fig. 11. Enlarged plotted flow-volume curve (cf. Fig. 7)

testing of patients with poor cooperation

small children (less than 5 years old)

geriatric patients - poor general condition

excessive restrictive lung diseases

detailed information by curve-enlargement

test - software modifications easier

time and cost saving

Fig. 12. Advantages of the new system

References

Hyatt RE (1965) Dynamic lung volumes. In: Fenn WO, Rahn H (eds). Handbook of physiology. Section 3. Respiration. vol 2. American Physiological Society, Washington DC, pp 1381–1397

Hyatt RE, Schilder DP, Fry DL (1958) Relationship between maximum expiratory flow and degree of lung inflation. J Appl Physiol 13 (3): 331–336

Knudson RJ, Slatin RC, Lebowitz MD, Burrows B (1976) The maximal expiratory flow-volume curve. Normal standards, variability, and effect of age. Am Rev Respir Dis 113: 587–600

Konietzko N (1983) Deutsche Gesellschaft für Pneumologie und Tuberkulose. Empfehlungen zur präoperativen Lungenfunktionsdiagnostik. Prax Klin Pneumol 37: 1199–1201

Morris JF, Koski A, Breese JD (1975) Normal values and evaluation of forced end-expiratory flow. Am Rev Respir Dis 111: 755–762

Voigt E, Braun U, Schorer R (1975) Ein neues Gerät zur Lungenfunktionsdiagnostik. Anaesthesist 24: 276–281

Measurement of Oxygen Uptake with a New Method

H. Metzler, G. Wiesspeiner, and W.F. List

Most systems now available for continuous assessment of oxygen uptake and CO_2 production are based on methods that include sampling from a mixing chamber. In 1983 at the 2nd International Symposium "Computers in Anesthesia and Intensive Care" in Rotterdam we presented a new system (Wiesspeiner and Metzler 1983). In contrast to other systems, flow and gas concentration are calculated from a single sensor close to the airway and not by sampling of the mixed expired volume.

Components of the System (Fig. 1)

1. The single proximal sensor unit for flow and gas concentrations is positioned directly on the endotracheal tube or face mask. It measures inspiratory and expiratory variables at the same point simultaneously and is synchronized. Flow is measured by balanced thermistor anemometry (BTA), gas concentration by mass spectrometry (Perkin Elmer MGA 1100 AB).

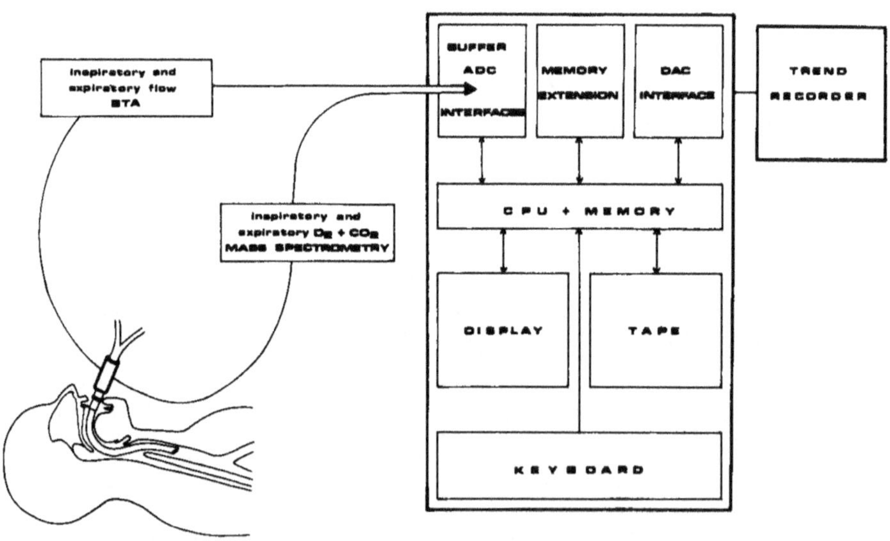

Fig. 1. Block diagram of the system

2. PET 2001 Commodore Microcomputer. The flow data are interval stored and are synchronized to the delayed data of gas concentration adapted to the length of capillary. Delay time is 300 ms, the sampling rate of the computer 60 Hz.

If flow and gas concentrations are measured in the airway dynamically, thermistor anemometry is unable to detect and separate the two phases of a respiratory cycle – inspiration and expiration – because of a constant positive flow signal. The second problem is to recognize the beginning and the end of the inspiratory and expiratory phase exactly. These two steps are managed by a special computer program based on a breath to breath respiratory pattern analysis. The flow curve is divided into three parts by thresholds. The beginning of a respiratory phase is determined by the absolute minimum after crossing threshold 2 and before crossing threshold 1. In the same way the end of a respiratory phase is determined by the absolute flow minimum after the point of the highest flow and crossing threshold 2 (Fig. 2). Separation of the inspiratory and expiratory phase is obtained by CO_2 analysis (Fig. 3).

From the input data the following variables may be measured or calculated:

f	breathing rate
V_T	tidal volume
$\dot{V}_E$	minute ventilation
$\dot{V}_{02}$	oxygen uptake
$\dot{V}_{CO2}$	carbon dioxide production
RQ	respiratory ratio
FIO_2	inspiratory oxygen fraction
$F_E'CO_2$	end-expiratory CO_2
F_ECO_2	mixed expiratory CO_2

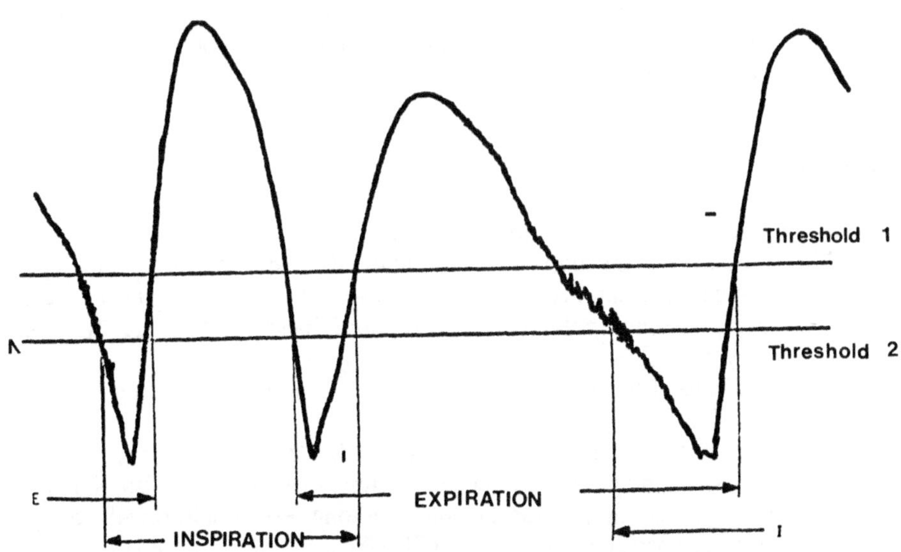

Fig. 2. Recognition of the beginning and end of inspiration and expiration

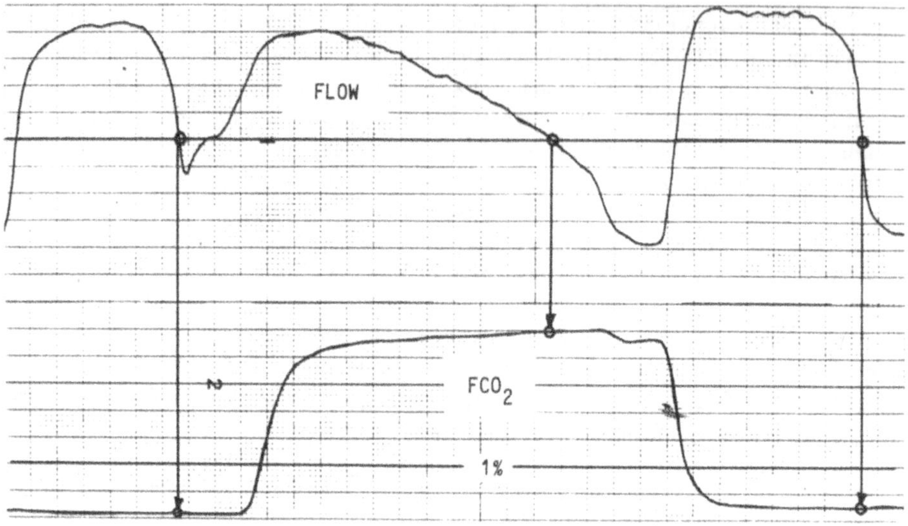

Fig. 3. Separation of inspiration and expiration

Advantages of the System

1. Placing the sensor near the airway reduces errors of compressible volume and ineffective separation of inspiratory and expiratory gas (Braus and Turner 1983; Fletcher et al. 1983).
2. Measuring the two variables flow and gas concentration at the same point, errors of calibration and linearity are reduced (Fletcher et al. 1983; Henderson et al. 1983; Norlander 1983).
3. The system is applicable to different modes of ventilation and ventilatory pattern.
4. Mass spectrometry provides accuracy also with a high FiO_2. Breath to breath analysis eliminates errors of rapidly changing FiO_2 with unstable oxygen blenders (Westenskow et al. 1984).

Problems

1. Every system which measures flow or gas concentration close to the airway has problems resulting from interference by humidity, expectoration, mucus, and excessive coughing, Humidity may block the capillary to the mass spectrometer, and foreign particles may pollute the high vacuum. These problems are effectively eliminated by inlet filters.
2. The damage caused to the heated BTA wires by excessive coughing is still an unsolved problem.

Based on breath to breath analysis, the system is especially designed for rapid registration of oxygen uptake and derived parameters. In addition it is also well suited as a long-term trend analysis monitor. For short- or long-term monitoring the computer is used to select a special program in the ICU which combines oxygen uptake with other relevant hemodynamic, metabolic, or respiratory parameters.

Conclusion

The developed system realizes the concept of computer-based respiratory pattern analysis. It contributes to the current trend of establishing systems for measuring oxygen uptake with high accuracy, applicable to the clinical routine in the ICU.

References

Braun U, Turner E (1983) Problems of indirect calorimetry for nutritional assessment in critically ill patients. ESPEN, Brüssel

Fletcher R, Werner O, Nordström L, Jonson B (1983) Sources of error and their correction in the measurement of carbon dioxide elimination using the Siemens-Elema CO_2 Analyzer. Br J Anaesth 55, 2: 177–85

Henderson AM, Mosse CA, Forrester PC, Halsall D, Armstrong RF (1983) A system for the continuous measurement of oxygen uptake and carbon dioxide output in artificially ventilated patients. Br J Anesth 55, 8: 791–800

Norlander O (1983) Monitoring of artificial ventilation. 4th Int. Symp.: Die maschinelle Beatmung gestern – heute – morgen. Münster

Westenskow DR, Cutler CA, Wallace WD (1984) Instrumentation for monitoring gas exchange and metabolic rate in critically ill patients. Crit Care Med 12, 3: 183–187

Wießpeiner G, Metzler H (1983) Microcomputer system for online gas exchange measurements based on a continuous breath to breath analysis. Second Int. Symp. on Computing in anesthesia and intensive care

A Microcomputerassisted System for the Monitoring of Cardiorespiratory Variables in the Critically Ill

K. Hankeln and H. Michelsen

Physiologic monitoring techniques have given detailed functional insight into circulatory and respiratory systems. In addition, they have provided the scientific basis as well as the clinical impetus for the development of modern critical care medicine. Continuous measurements of the pressure values in in the systemic and pulmonary circulations are now standard features of monitoring systems for critically ill patients. The pulmonary arterial catheter with measurements of cardiac output by the thermodilution technique provides a clinically applicable method of collecting mixed venous blood and evaluate cardiovascular function at discrete intervals.

The usefulness of monitoring these variables has been demonstrated in shock from accidental trauma, in surgical operations, and in myocardial infarction. The adquisition of cardiorespiratory data has led to the introduction and evaluation of new methods of treatment. However, to utilize all the diagnostic and monitoring measurements that are available today necessitates a lengthy period of time for calculations. During acute therapy the attending physician often does not have the time needed for these calculations. In most cases, calculations can only be carried out at a later date and are only available for retrospective analysis. However, with on-line, real-time monitoring it is possible to make rapid clinical decisions based on physiologic data to "tritrate" therapy.

To achieve this goal, a microcomputer-assisted monitoring system has been developed and clinically evaluated in our ICU since 1978 in order to realize bedside real-time calculations of the important cardiorespiratory variables (Schipulle 1983).

Processing of the measured values was carried out every 7.5 min by this system. The units used were a Hellige Servomed System, a Datascope 502 CO_2 analyzer, a Beckman OM 11 O_2 analyzer, and a computer-driven gas-mixing and -collecting system linked to the CBM 8032 computer with two disk drives and a printer. The system was completed by an interface system of our own design to accept the incoming signals from the monitoring units. A graphics monitor completed the system to provide continuous 24-h trends for the most important cardiopulmonary data. The complete setup is schematized in Fig. 1.

The pulmonary artery wedge pressure was measured by the computer at least four times daily, to assess the effects of changes in status or therapy; extra measurements were carried out at shorter intervals. Arterial and mixed venous blood gas analyses were entered manually into the computer via the keyboard to calculate the dependent parameters. Also input at the beginning of each study were the patients body weight and height, to determine body surface area.

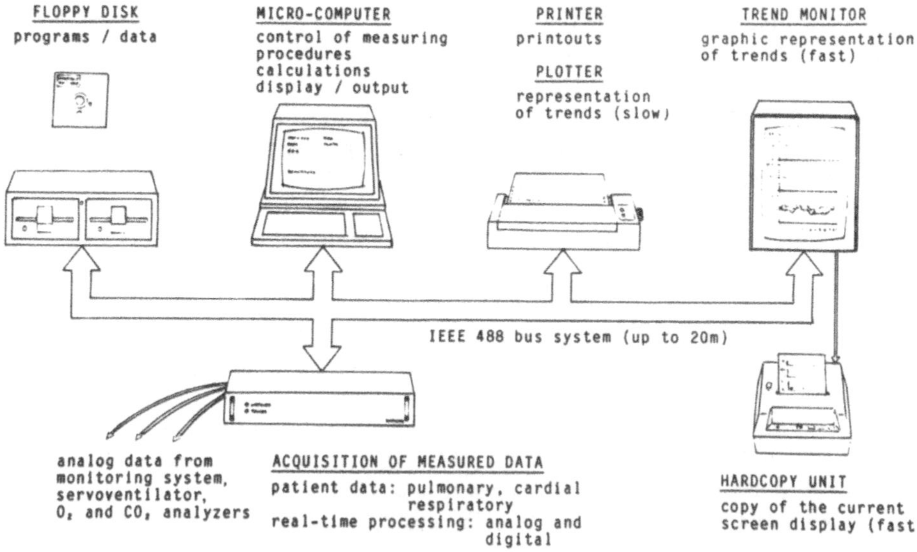

Fig. 1. Microcomputerized monitoring setup

The cardiac output was calculated by the computer according to the Fick principle. In order to determine the oxygen consumption, the computer controlled collections of gas specimens from the inspiratory and expiratory air via a solenoid valve. From these measurements a large number of cardiorespiratory variables were calculated real-time. The computer was programmed to collect all the values automatically at 7.5-min intervals and store them on a floppy disk. At the same time, via a CRT-type graphics monitor 24-h trends for the following parameters were generated; systolic and diastolic arterial pressure, pulmonary artery pressure, central venous pressure, heart rate, cardiac output, cardiac index, pulmonary diastolic pressure, left and right ventricular stroke work index, pulmonary vascular resistance index, systemic vascular resistance index, central and periperal temperature difference, inspiratory and expiratory airway resistance, and total compliance.

The trends gained in this way were also stored on the floppy disk and could be output on a video display unit. The variables calculated in the 7.5-min cycle could also be printed out at the time of measurement or in blocks of 2 h for evaluation.

Discussion

Therapy of critically ill patients, particularly patients in shock, requires monitoring of a large number of measured and derived cardiorespiratory variables. The importance of these variables in critical care has been frequently emphasized.

Our computerized data-acquisition system was designed to process the most important measured and derived cardiorespiratory variables at the bedside as continuously as possible and in on-line operation.

The continuous display of pressures obtained from standard monitoring is now routine. However, cardiac output, which can be determined by the thermodilution method, may only be obtained at repeated intervals to provide a "snapshot" or series of snapshots. However, continuous monitoring of this important parameter is not possible by this method. In the proposed monitoring system, cardiac output could be additionally determined by the Fickmethod where $\dot{V}O_2$ and AV difference in O_2 concentration are the major measured variables.

The continuous monitoring of oxygen consumption has proved to be a valuable mesure of the circulatory status. An important feature of the shock condition is a reduction of blood flow to the peripheral tissues that results in a reduction and or maldistribution of blood flow to the peripheral tissues (Shoemaker 1979).

Reduced $\dot{V}O_2$ was reported to be the common physiologic denominator of shock of various etiologies (Bland et al. 1978). Turner and coworkers (1982) advocate continuous monitoring of $\dot{V}O_2$ for assessing cardiovascular function and for early recognition of hypovolemia in patients following cardiac surgery. Noe and associates (1980) have shown that acute changes in $\dot{V}O_2$ indicate serious disorders of the circulatory and pulmonary function during anesthesia. Because of these and other reports, monitoring of $\dot{V}O_2$ was incorporated in the proposed system.

In critical circulatory conditions we found reduced cardiac output regularly linked with reduction in $\dot{V}O_2$; moreover, both variables rose as circulatory conditions improved (Fig. 2).

Furthermore, the system was helpful in "titrating" therapy in individual drug interventions.

The collected data can also be processed statistically by the same system. For this purpose a statistical package was developed allowing comparative studies in different therapeutic regimens.

One result of the frequent measurements and the large number of measured and calculated variables is a flood of data. It requires considerable effort for the clinician to follow large numbers of independently changing variables. For practical purpose, the system was developed to solve these problems in steps:

First, it is possible to see a list of all the current values via the screen monitor or a hard-copy printout.

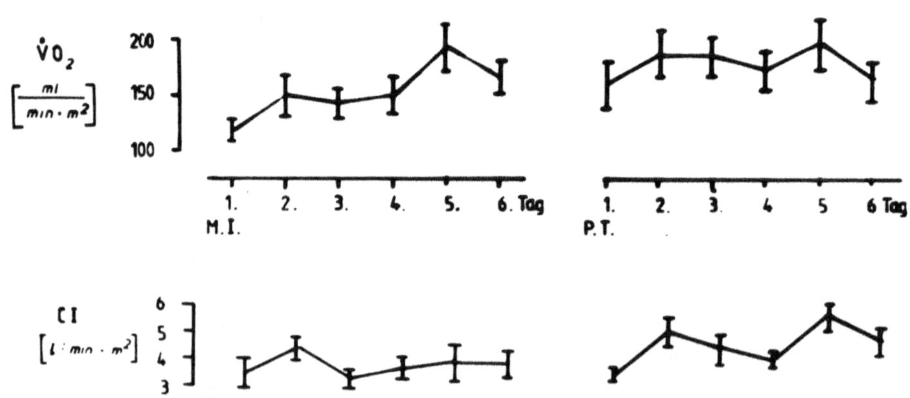

Fig. 2. Changes in $\dot{V}O_2$ and cardiac index (CI) during the first 6 days of treatment

Second, to facilitate an overview and evaluation of the individual data, these lists also show optimal reference values on a white background. These latter values were proposed as therapeutic goals on the basis if extensive investigations of cardiorespiratory data of postoperative shock and trauma patients.

Third, data compression is carried out by means of graphic representation of the trends of the important parameters over time. Graphs from previous days are available to be called up at any time and are printed out as a hard copy as documentation over the course of treatment. These trend graphs visually display the effects of each therapeutic intervention. In our experience, this leads to a better understanding of hemodynamic interrelationships and results in a more consistent and purposeful therapeutic approach.

References

Bland R, Shoemaker WC, Shabot MM (1978) Physiologic monitoring goals for the critically ill patient. Surg Gynecol Obstet 147: 833–841

Noe FE, Whitty AJ, Davies KR, Wickham BL (1980) Noninvasive measurement of pulmonary gas exchange during general anesthesia. Anaesth Analg, 59: 263–269

Schipulle M (1983) Praktische Anwendung eines mikrocomputerunterstützten Überwachungssystems zur Erfassung und Verarbeitung kardiorespiratorischer Parameter auf der Intensivstation. Dissertation, Medizinische Hochschule Hannover, pp 24–28

Shoemaker WC (1979) Pathophysiologie und Therapie von Schockzuständen. In: Berk JL, Sampliner JE, Artz JS, Vincour B (eds) Handbuch der Intensivmedizin. Karger, Basel, pp 198–227

Turner E, Braun U, Leitz KH, Hilfiker O (1982) Überwachung der Sauerstoffaufnahme bei koronarchirurgischen Eingriffen. Anaesthesist 31: 280–286

Selective Lung Ventilation

H-J. Hartung, P. M. Osswald, and H. J. Bender

Introduction

Separate investigation of gas flows in the right and left lung, i. e. bronchospirometry, was conducted by Jacobaeus (Jacobaeus et al. 1932) in 1932 within the framework of spirometric studies. In 1949 Carlens (1949) developed a double-lumen catheter which was relatively simple to manipulate and was subsequently adopted more as an anesthetic appliance in lung surgery than for diagnostic purposes. Carlens and Björg (Björg and Carlens 1950) were thereby able to prevent contamination of the dependent and the healthy lung by the contralateral lung. A few years later, Jenkins (Jenkins and Clarke 1958) and Newman et al. (1961) claimed obligatory application of such tubes in lung surgery. Selective lung, ventilation (SLV) offered advantages not only in anesthesiology, but also in surgery; for example, less motion in the area of operation, more extensive control. The technique has only been adopted in intensive care treatment in the past decade (Trew et al. 1976), and with developments in the variety of instruments employed has become a method for highly differentiated ventilation which can often be successful where conventional ventilation has failed. Technical prerequisites, monitoring, clinical studies, and practical experiences are presented in the following.

Endobronchial Intubation

A number of tubes have been developed for endobronchial intubation. The Carlens catheter and the Robertshaw tube are suitable for separate intubation and subsequent ventilation, but these tubes often cannot meet the requirements for safe application, which are as follows:

1. Easy insertion and minimal risk of injury. Injuries of a serious nature have been described in particular with the Carlens catheter, whose hook rides on the carina (Schaps et al. 1978; Faure 1976).
2. Physiological acceptability of the tube material, especially the cuffs. The latter have to be designed as low-pressure systems.
3. Low resistance values, with lumina as wide as possible to facilitate suction and possible use of a bronchoscope and to enable spontaneous breathing.
4. Disposability, for reasons of hygiene.

A partial solution to these problems was only possible after further development of the Robertshaw tube (Broncocath), a double-lumen tube modified according to Robertshaw and manufactured from thermolabile PVC material (Reinhold and Heller 1982). The left main bronchus is intubated, with inflation of a bronchial and a tracheal low-pressure cuff. This tube has relatively wide lumina, with the result that the resistance is about 50% lower than in traditional tubes of comparable size on the Charrière scale, thus making bronchofibroscopy possible. Use of the low-pressure cuffs diminishes the risk of pressure ulcers of the mucosa and permits long-term intubation.

Since the tube is preshaped at two places – at the tracheobronchial and pharyngolaryngeal transitions – there are usually no problems in intubation. The tip of the tube points to the left and hence slides into the left main bronchus. Correct positioning is therefore possible without a hook, and is objectified by alternating ventilation of the two lungs with auscultation and by chest X-ray.

Shapiro et al. (1981) recommends insertion with the aid of a bronchofibroscope and describes a reduction in faulty placing of tubes.

Critical importance attaches to secure fixation of the endobronchial tube, since on deflation of the bronchial cuffs there is a tendency for the tube to be pushed out of the bronchus (Rafferty et al. 1980). This problem can be exacerbated by copious secretion from the mucosa or by respiratory movements. The location of the tube must be checked very carefully after each suction and each change in position of the patient.

Because of increased difficulties in suction, the ventilating gas has to be optimally moist in order to prevent crusting of secretion. Experiences with endobronchial intubation have been reported on, for example by Read et al. (1977). In the case of all their patients it was possible to effect an endobronchial intubation, but a primary complete isolation of right and left lung could only be attained in 75%. A separation of gas flows in a further 10% was achieved after repeated repositioning. In our own studies it has so far always been possible to arrive at a correct position and function.

Ventilation Methods

Various methods for ventilation have been presented, based in the main on three principles: (a) ventilation with one ventilator and two breathing circuits, (b) ventilation with two ventilators synchronously, or (c) ventilation with two ventilators asynchronously for both lungs. SLV with one ventilator requires two breathing circuits in parallel (Gallagher et al. 1980).

The system described enables synchronous separate ventilation of the lungs. Tidal volumes and PEEP may be regulated individually for each lung. In addition, intermittent or continuous mandatory ventilation may be applied. A higher flexibility has been attained with this system than with the techniques Rivara et al. (1979) and Powner et al. (1977) have published. Powner et al. (1977), Cavanilles et al. (1979) and Rivara et al. (1979) describe much simpler breathing circuits, the tidal volumes for each lung being regulated by elevation of the flow resistance. PEEP may, however, also be applied, in which case the tidal volumes are pressure-dependent, and no longer constant on sudden changes in compliance.

Carlon et al. (1978a), on the other hand, used two synchronized ventilators (Bennett MA/1). Synchronization was effected with a home-made timer linked via a relay to the manual breath switch on each ventilator. This guarantees the integrity of both ventilators, so that tidal volumes, PEEP, flow rates, FiO_2, etc. remain selectively adjustable.

In contrast, Labrousse et al. (1979) and our team (Weller et al. 1982; Osswald et al. 1983; Hartung et al. 1982) employ electronically controlled servoventilators (Siemens-Elema, Sweden). The control elements for the ventilation rate are linked in hierarchy, so that one respirator is dependent on the other with respect to the rate. Master and slave are defined, the rate or the pulse to trigger an inspiration is given by the respiratory frequency switch of the master. All other functions of the two ventilators are maintained, so that tidal volumes, PEEP, inspiration/expiration (I/E) ratio and, FiO_2 remain individually controllable, as in the system used by Carlon et al. (1978a). The linkage is reversible at any time; the respirators remain fully functional.

Hillman and Barber (1980) used two nonsynchronized respirators and attained a still higher flexibility with these, since the respiratory frequency may be selected separately for each lung. One advantage of this technique is that the labor of synchronization, with the attendant risk of error, can be avoided. It could be a disadvantage that the adaptation of the patient to asynchronous ventilation might be made more difficult if heavy sedation or relaxation is not induced (Hillman and Barber 1980). There is of course a cost disadvantage in comparison with the single-respirator system.

It is impossible to decide which philosophy is the best on the basis of experience to date. In principle, SLV may be performed with all the systems presented. Attention should be paid to a readily apparent arrangement of the systems which precludes confusion. The usual safety appliances for each respirator should be available selectively for each lung.

Monitoring and the Use of Microprocessors

Little has so far been published on systematic implementation of and necessity for a selective monitoring. There are four aspects to be borne in mind here: (a) selective monitoring of the mechanical parameters of both lungs, (b) inspiratory and expiratory gas concentrations, (c) selective monitorings of the perfusion of both lungs, and, (d) hemodynamics.

Selective monitoring of mechanical ventilation parameters includes the parameters usually measured noninvasively in ventilation patients, such as respiratory pressures (peak pressure, pause pressure, endexpiratory pressure), and respiratory volumes (tidal volumes, minute volumes), and rated. In addition, the compliance and resistance of both lungs should be calculated and monitored in order to detect mechanical changes and disorders.

An extended monitoring of lung mechanics is possible through preparation of pressure volume, pressure flow, and CO_2 concentration volume diagrams (Prakash et al.) (1982). Mechanical disorders in the breathing system may be clearly differentiated in this manner. Parameters of lung function such as functional residual capacity or diffusion capacity are, on the other hand, very laborious to monitor.

The inspired and expired gases are relatively simple to monitor, and in the first instance, small and simple devices are adequate for clinical requirements. For scientifically exact analyses, recourse has to be made to an expensive mass spectrometer. In basic monitoring the inspired FiO_2 and the expired CO_2 concentrations are measured. Extended monitoring includes the O_2 uptake and output and the CO_2 production Suter (1983).

Selective monitoring and observation of the course of perfusion in both lungs may be effected by both invasive and noninvasive methods. Thus the relative perfusion situations may be ascertained by separate determination of the CO_2 minute production in the right and left lungs, (Osswald et al. (1983)). Flow measurements by flouroscopy or with radioactive xenon are more laborious (Carlon et al. 1978b; Oliveira et al. 1981). Exact absolute figures are obtainable by thermodilution, using two Swan-Ganz catheters which should be placed in the left and right pulmonary arteries.

In the case of this kind of differentiated therapy, monitoring of the hemodynamics will have to be extensive and invasive in order to permit an effective and controlled application of selective ventilation. Continuous direct measurement of pressure in the systemic and pulmonary circulations, together with determination of the cardiac output, represents the standard. The arterial lines – both the systemic and the pulmonary – enable blood-gas analyses to be obtained from these circulations. In this manner it is possible, in conjunction with the remaining hemodynamic parameters, to obtain and represent an exact profile of the patient, objectify positive and negative changes through alterations in ventilation, and assess the quality of the SLV.

Technical advances, miniaturization, and microprocessors permit comprehensive representation and automatic calculation of this large number of parameters. Representation of the course of measurements facilitates prompt assessment of developments in the course of the condition and the therapy. In addition, relationships and interactions can be detected more easily and quickly (Osswald et al. 1981).

A simple system for calculation of mechanical ventilation parameters meeting clinical needs is provided by, e.g., the lung calculation units from Siemens-Elema, Sweden. These compact units enable digital representation of the respiratory pressures, complicance, and resistance. Changes in the latter parameters are detected without delay. Ventilation parameters such as effective and ineffective tidal volumes or dead-space ventilation are similarly to be monitored with this system. The lung calculation units, moreover, enable assessments of the relative perfusion in the two lungs by determination of the CO_2 tidal and minute productions (Olsson et al. 1980). It is thereby possible to monitor both lungs simultaneously. Trends may be represented graphically or numerically through appropriate microprocessor systems (Bender 1981) in parallel for the left and right lungs.

Automated presentation of pressure-volume or pressure-flow diagrams (Prakash et al. 1982) and computer-aided evaluation of such diagrams, permit differentiated statements on the respiratory system or the function of the lungs (Suter 1983). Computer-aided calculation of the complicated physiological parameters derived and representation of their course enable differentiated consideration and assessment of the physiological profile of the patient (Osswald et al. 1981). Off-line-input yields automatic representation of shunt, $AVDO_2$, $AADO_2$, vascular resistances, and O_2 transport capacity.

It has been possible to give an introduction to microprocessors here, but it is apparent that changes in the respiratory pattern of both lungs and the effects of the former can be monitored and assessed more effectively with the aid of such technology. Routine application of the microprocessors makes considerable demands on personnel and necessitates in-house development of programs.

Experimental Studies in Animals

Various reports validating SLV have been published. Kusayima et al. (1975) have been able to demonstrate the effects of SLV in an experimentally induced fatty acid pulmonary embolism confined to one lung. The embolized lung was ventilated with PEEP, the contralateral lung with ZEEP. The results document the possibility of influencing perfusion by changing the vascular resistance through PEEP. Perfusion of the affected lung was reduced, and the shunt volume diminished to almost normal values.

Pace and Westenskow (Pace et al. 1982) investigated the effects of various tidal volumes after unilateral hydrochloric acid aspiration. In this animal model nonselective ventilation was compared with SLV. The tidal volumes were on the one hand exactly halved, and on the other hand adjusted so that the end-expiratory CO_2 concentrations were the same left and right.

The results make it clear that the most efficient oxygenation and the lowest shunt volume occur when the end-expiratory CO_2 concentrations of both lungs are the same.

Other studies (Benumhof et al. 1979; Mink et al. 1981) have similarly confirmed the effectiveness of SLV after experimental induction of unilateral pneumonia or atelectasis. Unilateral disorders of lung function and hemodynamics manifesting themselves as differences in compliance between right and left lung, elevated dead-space ventilation, elevated intrapulmonary shunt and ventilation/perfusion in homogeneities are accessible to such a direct therapy.

In contrast, East et al. (1982), comparing synchronous with asynchronous SLV in the dog, found no statistically significant differences between the two forms of ventilation.

Clinical Studies

Clinical studies demonstrating the effectiveness of SLV also in the healthy lung are few and far between. Our team has, however, been able to show that ventilation/perfusion changes regularly occuring in ventilated patients in the lateral decubitus position (Kaneko et al. 1966; Rehder et al. 1972; 1973; Trew et al. 1976) can be influenced by SLV in such a manner that the upper lung is perfused more than the lower (Hartung et al. 1982; Weller et al. 1982; Osswald et al. 1983) in contrast to conventional ventilation via an endotracheal tube.

Baehrendtz et al. (1982) were able to confirm this principle in a similarly conducted study with unilateral PEEP ventilation of the dependent lung in lateral decubitus position.

The influence of various respiration parameters on lung mechanics and hemodynamics has been demonstrated by a further study in which unilateral PEEP augmented the pulmonary vascular resistance and led to a reduction in cardiac output rather than to an inverted I/E ratio (Osswald et al. 1983).

Therapeutic Experience

Reports on therapeutic experience with successful application of SLV in both intensive care treatment and anesthesia are available from various authors.

In the case of anesthesiology, the main use of SLV is in intrathoracic operations, where it is in principle a one-lung anesthesia, the contralateral lung not being ventilated. The effects of such SLV with "extreme breathing mode" on cardiorespiratory function have been very carefully investigated by Katz et al. (1982) and Aalto-Setälä et al. (1975) among others. Their results document the fact that oxygen transport is generally adequate but can in individual cases be reduced because of diminished cardiac output, so that careful monitoring is necessary.

Extensive experience of SLV in unilateral lung diseases is available from the sector of intensive care medicine, mainly in the form of case reports of successful therapy with SLV in widely varying clinical situations.

Rafferty et al. (1980) reported on the treatment of bronchopleural fistulas, while Cavanilles et al. (1979) , Gallagher et al. (1980), Glass et al. (1976), and Hillman and Barber (1980) were able to resolve atelectasis in cases remaining resistant to conventional ventilation. Other authors have reported on SLV in pneumonia, pulmonary edema and lung contusions (Carlon et al. 1978a, c; Dueck et al. 1977; Glass et al. 1976; Hartenauer et al. 1981; Hillman and Barber 1980; Miranda et al. 1981; Powner et al. 1977; Rivara et al. 1979). The results obtained revealed marked shunt reductions and rises in PaO_2. In one of the cases of additional preexisting lung disease (fibrosis) there was no improvement in lung function (Hillman and Barber 1980).

Close examination of the case reports fails to yield any grounds for a general statement of an optimum breathing mode such as, for example, best PEEP (Suter et al. 1975) or high PEEP with spontaneous CPAP respiration (Kirley et al. 1975). Neither is there any evidence for an advantage of synchronous over asynchronous SLV. One apparent principle in common is utilization of SLV to supply defined tidal volumes to the most damaged lung with or without PEEP, in order to achieve adequate ventilation and influence on the perfusion. Glass et al. (1976), however, ventilated the healthy side and kept the affected contralateral lung expanded with a continuous flow and PEEP of 20 cm H_2O.

The optimum breathing mode for each individual patient has to be chosen from the large number of possible modes on the basis of the parameter measurements.

Validation and Indications for SLV

The treatment of acute respiratory insufficiency by mechanical ventilation and application of PEEP or maintenance of an inverted I/E ratio can be regarded as an established technique (Cavanilles et al. 1979; Lauer 1973; Pontoppidan et al. 1973; Suter et al. 1975).

Despite the desired effects on gas exchange and compliance, some patients nevertheless exhibit an acute deterioration on application of PEEP under certain conditions, for example [22] unequal distribution of the pathological changes in the lung, (Jardin et al. 1981) such as in unilateral pneumonia, bronchopleural fistulas, unilateral ARDS, or the lung-down-syndrome during and after protracted operations in the lateral decubitus position.

The causes are to be found in lung function and hemodynamics, and include differences in compliance (Glass et al. 1976; Pace et al. 1982; Rivara et al. 1979), between left and right lung, elevated intrapulmonary shunt, and ventilation/perfusion inhomogeneities (Carlon et al. 1978a; Powner et al. 1977; Rivara et al. 1979).

If patients with predominantly unilateral lung conditions are ventilated conventionally with a respirator via an endotracheal tube, the greater proportion of the tidal volume can ventilate the healthy lung while the compliance and function of the affected lung can decrease through further alveolar collapse. In the case of disseminated unilaterial diseases, unchanged alveoli can be overextended, so that perfusion is redistributed into atelectatic areas, with an increase in dead space and shunt volume.

Such pathophysiological features can be better dealt with by separate selective ventilation of each lung (Carlon et al. 1978a; Glass et al. 1976; Hartenauer et al. 1981; Hillman and Barber 1980; Powner et al. 1977; Rivara et al. 1979), and therefore represent one of the most important indications for differential SLV. Separate influencing of perfusion in the two lungs through the ventilation is possible. The validity of this principle has been substantiated by numerous clinical and experimental studies and experiences.

According to the present state of knowledge and experience, the following indications are given for this very laborious ventilation method after the possibilities of conventional forms of ventilation have been exhausted:

1. Unilateral ARDS
2. Treatment of therapy-resistant atelectasis
3. Ventilation during and after lung or intrathoracic surgery
4. Bronchopleural fistulas
5. Prevention of lung-down syndrome

In the appropriate circumstances SLV represents a valuable and effective therapeutic technique.

References

Aalto-Setälä M, Heinonen J, Salorinne Y (1975) Cardiorespiratory function during thoracic anaesthesia: comparison of two-lung ventilation and one-lung ventilation with and without PEEP. Acta Anaesth Scand 19: 287

Baehrendtz S, Hedenstierna G, Santesson J, Bindslev L, Klingstedt C, Dalborn M, Söderberg B, Norlander OP (1982) Perfusion of each lung during differential ventilation with selective PEEP. Anesthesiology 57: A 458

Bender HJ (1981) Implementierung eines rechnergestützten Patientenüberwachungssystems. Inauguraldissertation, Mannheim

Benumhof JL, Rogers SN, Moyce PR, Berryhill RE, Wahrenbrock EA, Saidman LJ (1979) Hypoxic pulmonary vasoconstriction and regional and whole-lung PEEP in the dog. Anesthesiology 51: 503
Björk VO, Carlens E (1950) The prevention of spread during pulmonary resection by use of a double lumen catheter. J. Thorac Surg 20: 151
Carlens E (1949) A new flexible double lumen catheter for bronchospirometry J. Thorac Surg 18: 749
Carlon GC, Ray C, Klein R, Goldiner PL, Miodownik S (1978a) Criteria for selective PEEP and independent synchronized ventilation of each lung. Chest 74: 501
Carlon GC, Kahn R, Baron R, Remaker J (1978b) Pulmonary blood flow distribution during PEEP: a diagnostic test for differential lung ventilation. Crit Care Med 6: 98
Carlon GC, Kahn R, Howlands WS, Baron R, Remaker J (1978c) Acute life-threatening ventilation-perfusion inequality: an indication for independent lung ventilation. Crit Care Med 6: 380
Cavanilles JM, Garrigosa F, Prieto C, Oucins JR (1979) A selective ventilation distribution circuit. Intensive Care Med 5: 95
Dueck R, Wagner PD, West JB (1977) Effects of PEEP on gas exchange in dogs with normal and edematous lungs. Anesthesiology 46: 359
East D, Mebe IV, Westenskow DR, Pace NL (1982) Synchronous versus asynchronous differential lung ventilation following unilateral hydrochloric acid aspiration in the dog. Anesthesiology 57: A 171
Favre JP (1976) Incidents et accident an cours de l'utilisation de la sonde de Carlens. Ann Anesthiol Franc 17: 984
Gallagher TJ, Banner MJ, Smith RA (1980) A simplified method of independent lung ventilation. Crit Care Med 8: 396
Glass DD, Tonnesen AS, Gabel JC, Arens JF (1976) Therapy of unilateral pulmonary insufficiency with a double lumen endobronchial tube. Crit Care Med 4: 323
Hartenauer U, Wendt M, Lawin P, Reinhold P (1981) Treatment of unilateral pulmonary insufficiency with differential lung ventilation via a double lumen endotracheal tube. Crit Care Med 9: 189
Hartung HJ, Bender HJ. Osswald PM, Weller L, Klose R (1982) Alteration of lung parameters by separated lung ventilation. Anaesthesia volume of summaries of 6th European Congress of Anaesthesiology, p 120
Hillman KM, Barber JD (1980) Asynchronous independent lung ventilation. Crit Care Med 8: 390
Jacobaeus JC, Frenckner P, Bjorkman S (1932) Some attempts at determining the volume and function of each lung separately. Acta Med Scand 79: 174
Jardin F, Desfond P, Bazin M et al. (1981) Controlled ventilation with best PEEP and high level PEEP in acute respiratory failure. Intensive Care Med 7: 171
Jenkins AV, Clarke G (1958) Endobronchial anaesthesia with the Carlens catheter. Br J Anaesth 30: 13
Kanarek DS, Shannon DC (1975) Adverse effect of positive PEEP on pulmonary perfusion and aterial oxygenation. Am Rev Respir Dis 112: 457
Kaneko K, Emili M, Dolovich J, Dawson A, Bates VD (1966) Regional distribution of ventilation and perfusion as a function of body position. J Appl Physiol 21: 767
Katz JA, Laverne RG, Fairley B, Thomas AN (1982) Pulmonary oxygen exchange during endobronchial anesthesia. Anaesthesiology 56: 164
Kirby RR, Perry JC, Calderwood HW, Ruiz BC, Lederman DS (1975) Cardiorespiratory effects of high PEEP. Anaesthesiology 43: 533
Kusajima K, Webb WR, Parker FB, Bredenberg CE, Markarian B (1975) Pulmonary responses of unilateral PEEP on experimental fat embolism. Ann Surg 181: 676
Labrousse L, Tenaillon A, Sezille JC, Longchal J, Morin C (1979) Independent lung ventilation: synchronization of two respirators. Abstract. Hopital Bonciant, Paris
Laver MB (1973) Störungen der Lungendurchblutung und des Ventilations-Perfusionsverhältnisses unter spezieller Berücksichtigung von Herzpatienten. In: Wiemers K, Scholler KC (eds) Lungenveränderungen bei Langzeitbeatmung. Thieme, Stuttgart
Mink S, Light RB, Colligan T et al. (1981) The effect of PEEP on pulmonary gas exchange and pulmonary perfusion in canine lobar pneumonia. J Appl Physiol 50: 515
Miranda DR, Stoutenbeck C, Kingma L (1981) Differential lung ventilation with HF PPV. Intensive Care Med 7: 139
Newman RW, Finer GE, Downs JE (1961) Routine use of the Carlens double-lumen endobronchial catheter. J Thorac Cardiovasc Surg 42: 327

Oliveira DM, Sykes MK, Chakrabarti MK, Orchard C, Keslin J (1981) Depression of hypoxic pulmonary vasoconstriction by sodium nitroprusside and nitroglycerine. Br J Anaesth 52: 11
Olsson SG, Fletcher F, Johnson B, wordström L, Prakash O (1980) Clinical studies of gas exchange during ventilatory support – A method using the Siemens-Elema CO_2-analyser. Br J Anaesth 52: 491
Osswald PM, Bender HJ, Hartung HJ, Lutz H, Spier R, Meissner R (1981) Computergestützte Datenpräsentation in der operativen Intensivmedizin. Anästh Intensivmed 22: 145
Osswald PM, Bender HJ, Hartung HJ, Klose R, Olsson SG, Weller L (1983) Die Wirkung von PEEP resp. verlängerter Inspirationszeit auf Lungenmechanik, Gasaustausch und Hämodynamik bei differenter Lungenventilation. Anaesthesist 32: 99
Pace NL, East TO, Mebe IV, Westenskow DR, Lund K (1982) Differential lung ventilation with PEEP following unilateral hydrochloric aspiration in the dog. Anaesthesiology 57: A 460
Pontoppidan H, Geffin B, Lowenstein E (1973) Acute respiratory failure in the adult. Little Brown, Boston
Powner PJ, Eross B, Grenvik A (1977) Differential lung ventilation with PEEP in the treatment of unilateral pneumonia. Crit Care Med 5: 170
Prakash O, Meij S, Zeelenberg C von den Borden B (1982) Computer-based patient monitoring. Crit Care Med 10: 811
Rafferty T, Palma J, Motoyama FK, Schachter N, Ciarcia M (1980) Management of a bronchopleural fistula with differential lung ventilation and PEEP. Respiratory Care 25: 654
Read RC, Riday CD, Eason CN (1977) Prospective study of the Robertshaw endobronchial catheter in thoracic surgery. Ann Thorac Surg 24: 156
Rehder K, Hatch DJ, Sessler AD, Fowler WS (1972) The function of each lung of anesthetized and paralyzed man during mechanical ventilation. Anaesthesiology 37: 16
Rehder K, Wenthe FM, Sessler AD (1973) Function of each lung during mechanical ventilation with ZEEP and with PEEP in man anesthetized with Thiopental-Meperidine. Anaesthesiology 39: 597
Reinhold P, Heller K (1982) "Bronchocath" – ein neuer Doppellumentubus zur seitendifferenten Beatmung. Anästh Intensivther Notfallmed 17: 106
Rivara D, Bourgain JL, Rienf P, Hart A, Lemaire F (1979) Differential ventilation in unilateral lung disease: effects on respiratory mechanics and gas exchange. Intensive Care Med 5: 189
Schaps D, Walterbusch G, Leitz KH, Borst HG (1982) Trachealeinriß durch den Carina Sporn eines White Tubus. Anästh Prax 15: 5
Shapiro S, Watson ChB, Bowe EA, Klein EF (1981) Bronchoscopic placement of the double lumen endotracheal tube for independent lung ventilation. Crit Care Med 9: 189
Suter PM (1983) Non-standard Monitoring während der Beatmung. 4. Internat. Symposium für Anästhesie-, -Reanimations- und Intensivbehandlungsprobleme. Zürs, Austria, 12. – 19. 3. 1983
Suter PM, Fairley H, Isenberg MD (1975) Optimum end expiratory airway pressure in patients with acute pulmonary failure. N Engl J Med 292: 284
Trew F, Warren BR, Potter WA (1976) Differential ventilation of the lungs in man. Crit Care Med 4: 112
Weller L, Bender HJ, Hartung HJ, Osswald PM, Klose R (1982) Veränderungen von Lungenmechanik, Hämodynamik und Gasaustausch bei differenter Lungenventilation während der Narkose. Anaesth Intensivmed Notfallther 17: 332

Automated Anesthetic Record Keeping

N. Ty Smith

The maintenance of an accurate anesthetic record is one of the most important tasks the anesthetist can perform. The development of the anesthesia chart by E.A. Codman and Harvey Cushing represents a major advance in the anesthetic care of the patient. Codman and Cushing, as interns at the Massachusetts General Hospital in 1894–1895, recorded several items on their anesthetic charts, including drugs previously administered on the ward; premedicant drugs; the amount of anesthetic required; and physical signs, such as pupillary size, the rate of pulse and respiration, and the presence of mucous (Beecher 1940). In 1901, Cushing visited Riva-Rocci in Italy to inspect the latter's cuff sphygmomanometer. He recognized its value immediately, and soon introduced it to the wards and operating rooms of his hospital. He was not as successful in the operating room as he might have wished, however. The well known words of the Harvard Medical School Committee set up to examine Cushing's proposal still ring in the ears of those who plan to introduce change in anesthetic records: "The adoption of blood-pressure observations in surgical patients does not at present appear to be necessary as a routine measure." Undaunted, Cushing not only added blood pressure to the anesthetic record, he also published a paper on the subject (Cushing 1903).

The information in anesthetic charts continued to expand over the next two decades, and McKesson's anesthetic record of 1923 (Fig. 1) is difficult to distinguish from a routine anesthetic record of today (Fig. 2). Anesthetic records for patients with significant physiological disturbance or undergoing major operations have changed in form and content over the past decade, however; reflecting the dramatic changes in anesthetic care in these areas occurring during this period. One of the results of these relatively recent changes in anesthetic records is an even greater interhospital variation among anesthetic records than that which existed previously.

The anesthetic record has a wide variety of functions, most of which extend beyond the original intent of Codman and Cushing. An understanding of these functions is important for understanding the design, requirements, and uses of the automated record. The functions are:

1. *A preanesthetic summary.* A large amount of demographic, physical, physiological, pathological, clinical, laboratory and radiological information is summarized on the anesthetic record, usually on the reverse side of the record. Other miscellaneous information, including preanesthetic medication and its impact, patient's preoperative medicines, and direct medicolegal considerations, such as site of surgery and signing of consent form, are also recorded.
2. *A reminder of information to record.* Many anesthetic records are crammed with blank boxes to check and blank spaces to fill out with specific information (Fig. 3). If the anesthetist is reasonably conscientious, this type of record can serve a very useful purpose.

3. *Trends.* If the anesthetic record is filled out during the case as events occur, the anesthetist can detect trends in blood pressure or amounts of drug, for example. From these trends he can make specific diagnoses or decide upon therapeutic maneuvers.
4. *Prediction.* As a corollary of 3, one can predict, with variable accuracy, the intra- and post-anesthetic course of the patient. Unless the trends are clearly presented, however, prediction can be difficult.
5. *An aid in postanesthetic care.* Frequently, decisions made in the recovery room or the intensive care unit are based upon events occurring or agents administered during the anesthetic. For example, in assessing postoperative apnea, it is useful to know whether and how much narcotic and neuromuscular blocking agents were administered.

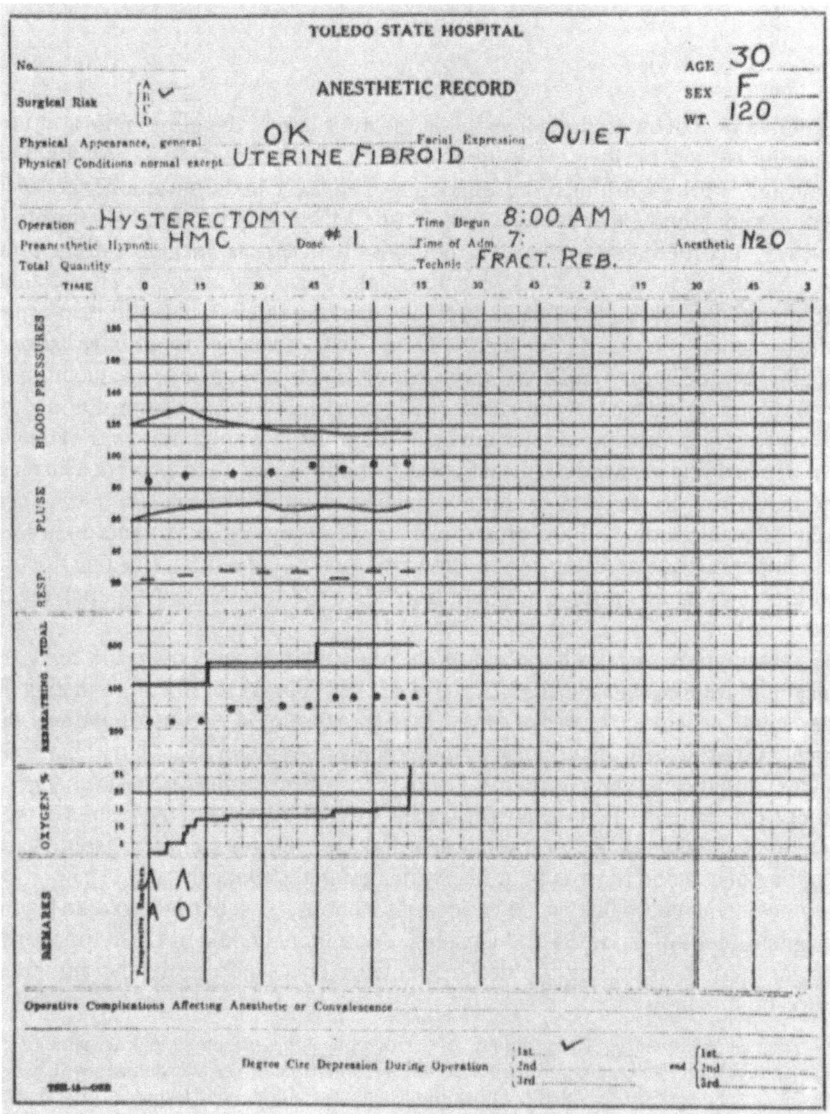

Fig. 1. An anesthetic record from 1923. The record has progressed so that it is very similar to that of today (see Fig. 2)

6. *An aid to the next anesthetist.* If the patient must receive another anesthetic, whether days or years later, the anesthetic record becomes extremely valuable to the subsequent anesthetist. Perhaps of all users of the anesthetic record, the subsequent anesthetist is the most grateful for a complete and accurate record.
7. *Teaching.* The anesthetic record is a useful teaching device, whether during anesthesia, immediately postoperatively, or as a demonstration or a source of information at a case presentation conference.
8. *A database.* The anesthetic record can help implement databases. The potential information available from such databases is vast, including the number or types of cases done during any period, the number of cases done by each anesthetist, the anesthetic agents and techniques used, and the incidence and types of complications.

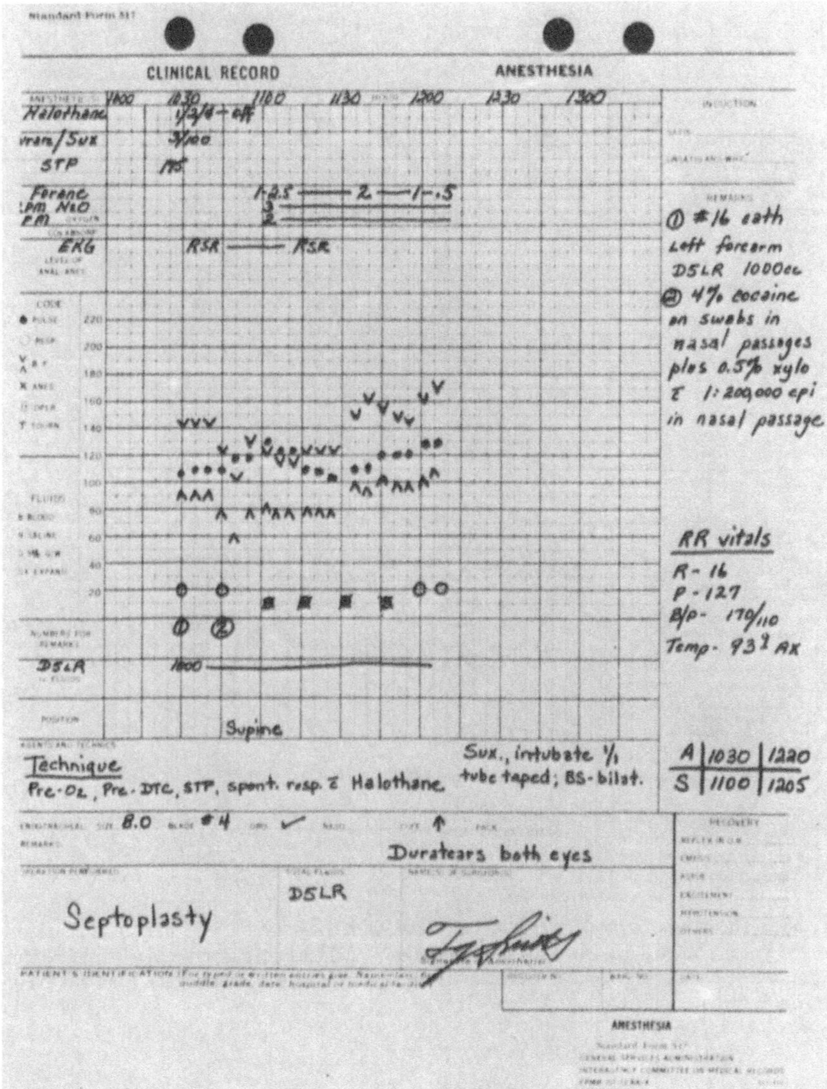

Fig. 2. A record from a routine anesthetic of today (compare Fig. 1)

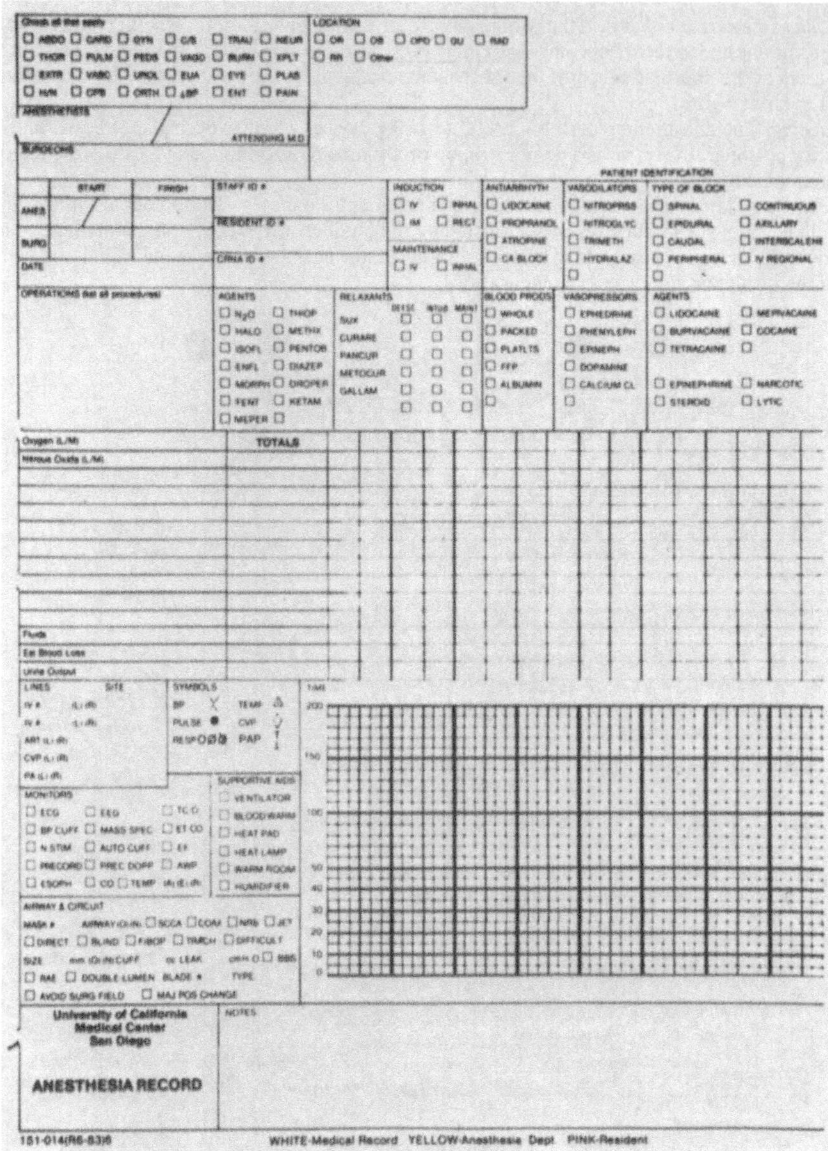

LOCATION

ANESTHETISTS

ATTENDING M.D.

SURGEONS

PATIENT IDENTIFICATION

START

FINISH

ANES

SURG

DATE

STAFF ID #

RESIDENT ID #

CRNA ID #

INDUCTION

MAINTENANCE

ANTIARRHYTH

VASODILATORS

TYPE OF BLOCK

OPERATIONS (list all procedures)

AGENTS

RELAXANTS

BLOOD PRODS

VASOPRESSORS

AGENTS

Oxygen (L/M)

TOTALS

Fluids

Est Blood Loss

Urine Output

LINES

SITE

SYMBOLS

BP

TEMP

PULSE

CVP

PAP

TIME

200

150

100

50

40

30

20

10

0

MONITORS

SUPPORTIVE AIDS

VENTILATOR

HEAT PAD

HEAT LAMP

WARM ROOM

AIRWAY & CIRCUIT

NOTES

University of California

Medical Center

San Diego

ANESTHESIA RECORD

WHITE-Medical Record YELLOW-Anesthesia Dept PINK-Resident

Fig. 3a

Fig. 3a. The front of a modern anesthetic record, with considerable information to check off or fill in. This type of record leaves little to the imagination, but does help guarantee a more nearly complete record. **b** The back of the same anesthetic record as *a*. Again, the record itself is an aid to complete record keeping

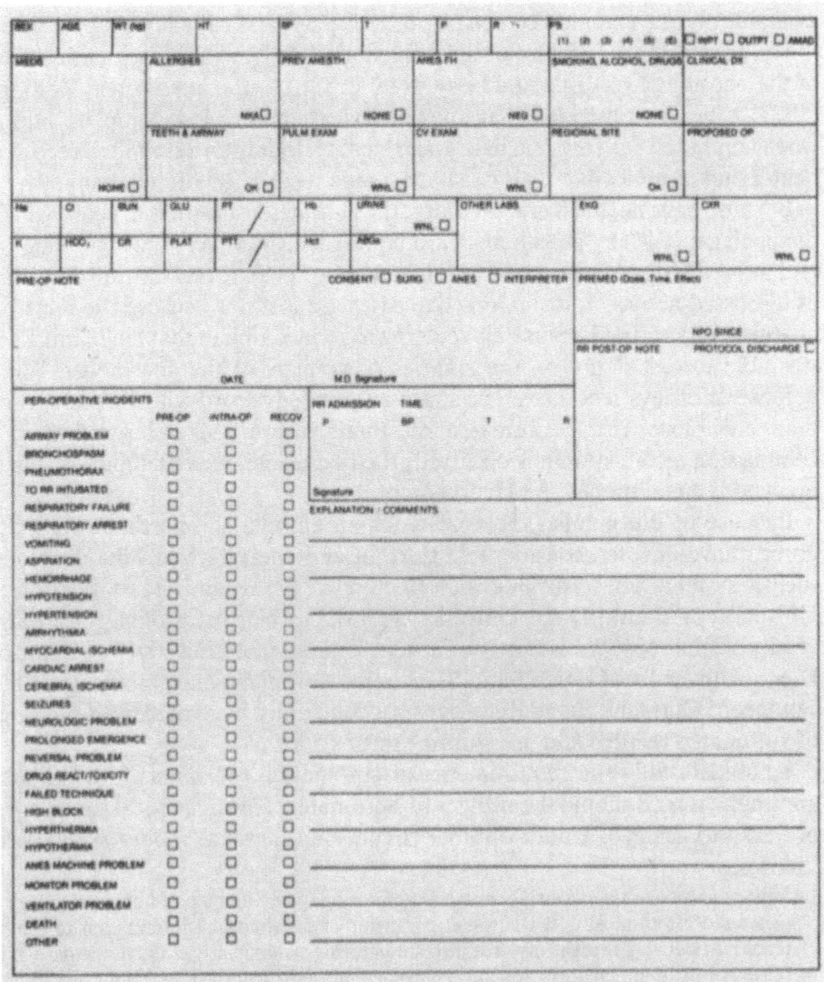

SEX | AGE | WT (kg) | HT | BP | T | P | R | PS (1) (2) (3) (4) (5) (6) | ☐ INPT ☐ OUTPT ☐ AMAD

MEDS — NONE ☐

ALLERGIES — NKA ☐

PREV ANESTH — NONE ☐

ANES FH — NEG ☐

SMOKING, ALCOHOL, DRUGS — NONE ☐

CLINICAL DX

TEETH & AIRWAY — OK ☐

PULM EXAM — WNL ☐

CV EXAM — WNL ☐

REGIONAL SITE — OK ☐

PROPOSED OP

Na | Cl | BUN | GLU | PT / | Hb | URINE WNL ☐ | OTHER LABS | EKG WNL ☐ | CXR WNL ☐

K | HCO₃ | CR | PLAT | PTT / | Hct | ABGs

PRE-OP NOTE — CONSENT ☐ SURG ☐ ANES ☐ INTERPRETER

PREMED (Dose, Time, Effect) — NPO SINCE

DATE — M.D. Signature

RR POST-OP NOTE — PROTOCOL DISCHARGE ☐

RR ADMISSION — TIME — P — BP — T — R — Signature

EXPLANATION / COMMENTS

PERI-OPERATIVE INCIDENTS	PRE-OP	INTRA-OP	RECOV
AIRWAY PROBLEM	☐	☐	☐
BRONCHOSPASM	☐	☐	☐
PNEUMOTHORAX	☐	☐	☐
TO RR INTUBATED	☐	☐	☐
RESPIRATORY FAILURE	☐	☐	☐
RESPIRATORY ARREST	☐	☐	☐
VOMITING	☐	☐	☐
ASPIRATION	☐	☐	☐
HEMORRHAGE	☐	☐	☐
HYPOTENSION	☐	☐	☐
HYPERTENSION	☐	☐	☐
ARRHYTHMIA	☐	☐	☐
MYOCARDIAL ISCHEMIA	☐	☐	☐
CARDIAC ARREST	☐	☐	☐
CEREBRAL ISCHEMIA	☐	☐	☐
SEIZURES	☐	☐	☐
NEUROLOGIC PROBLEM	☐	☐	☐
PROLONGED EMERGENCE	☐	☐	☐
REVERSAL PROBLEM	☐	☐	☐
DRUG REACT/TOXICITY	☐	☐	☐
FAILED TECHNIQUE	☐	☐	☐
HIGH BLOCK	☐	☐	☐
HYPERTHERMIA	☐	☐	☐
HYPOTHERMIA	☐	☐	☐
ANES MACHINE PROBLEM	☐	☐	☐
MONITOR PROBLEM	☐	☐	☐
VENTILATOR PROBLEM	☐	☐	☐
DEATH	☐	☐	☐
OTHER	☐	☐	☐

Fig. 3b

9. *Research.* If properly constructed, the anesthetic database can be a valuable research source. This often requires a record with more detailed requests for information than usual. In addition, the anesthetist must meticulously fill out every detail. Dr. Daniel Moore, in particular, has made very important early contributions to this use of the anesthetic record (Moore 1969; Moore et al. 1968)
10. *Medicolegal.* In the United States, particularly California, the anesthetic record is an important medicolegal document. Lawyers generally agree that defendant anesthetists lose more malpractice cases on the basis of an inadequate or incomplete anesthetic record than from almost all other causes combined.
11. *Financial.* The anesthetic record contains the information necessary for billing the patient, not only for the anesthetic charges but also for many of the hospital charges.

If one takes into consideration these uses for the anesthetic record, it becomes clear why an automated anesthetic record could be very useful. An automated record keeping system provides the benefit of: (a) more accurate data recording (Zollinger et al. 1977) (b) less need for manual charting during crises or other busy periods of anesthetic care; (c) a centralized display on which all data, current and trended, are available on one common screen or other display; and (d) a legible printed record at the end of the case. Because of the obligatory detail and accuracy alone, automation of the anesthetic record could be of great benefit to the anesthetist. Zollinger et al. (1977) have demonstrated that anesthetists' charts are less complete and accurate when compared with the real data generated. Certainly an automated record could be neater and more legible than most anesthetic records generated manually.

Because of its neatness and accurary, the automated anesthetic record will be useful medicolegally. Many anesthetists are concerned, however, that by being objective and more nearly complete, the automated record will reveal any mistakes. Actually, as discussed above, most malpractice cases are lost not because the anesthetist did anything wrong, but because his record was so incomplete that the plantiff's attorney was able to cast doubt on the abilities or veracity of the anesthetist. Thus, many defense attorneys feel that an accurate automated record will win many more cases than it will lose. If the automated anesthetic record does indicate that an error of commission or omission has occurred, the case could be settled out of court, saving everybody time, money, and harassment.

Because of the unmistakable need for an automated anesthetic record, several groups have devoted considerable thought and energy toward the development of such a system. These include investigators at the Miami Heart Institute; Emory University, Atlanta; Duke University, Durham, North Carolina; Ohio State University, Columbus; University of Florida, Gainesville; University of California, San Diego; University of Heidelberg, Mannheim, Germany; and University of Tübingen, Tübingen, Germany. In addition, several companies have perceived the importance of automated records and are working in this area.

To statisfy fully the requirements of automation, all inputs into the automated anesthetic record should themselves be automated. This is an ideal situation, which is not easy to achieve. Under optimal circumstances, these inputs would include the following.

1. *Physiological variables.* During invasive monitoring, when many physiologic variables are being generated electronically, the automatic transfer of physiological information to the anesthetic record is relatively straightforward. If the monitoring is noninvasive, and particularly if it uses the senses of hearing, smell, or touch, it becomes more difficult. An exception is the noninvasive automated blood pressure device, which often has an output of blood pressure and heart rate capable of being transferred to an anesthetic record.
2. *Drugs.* Drugs represent a more difficult situation, and many methods for transferring drug information have been proposed. One of these, described by a group at Duke University is a bar-code method. This does effect electronic transfer. On the other hand, the bar-code system can be difficult to learn, cumbersome to use, and unreliable.
3. *Infusions.* Infusions are somewhat easier to deal with in an automated record system, since there are available infusion devices with an electronic output that supplies the rate of infusion. Obviously, information about the drug, including its concentration, must somehow be entered so that the infusion rate is converted into a drug administration rate, as well as into a cumulative amount.
4. *Anesthesia machines.* Within five yèars microprocessor-controlled anesthesia machines will be available. With these machines, it will be a simple matter to transfer information, such as gas remaining in sources, gas flows, vapor concentration, and disconnects, from the anesthesia machine to the automated record. In the meantime, it will be necessary to transfer this information manually.
5. *Ventilators.* Similarly, ventilators are evolving into microprocessor-controlled devices, which will be able to transfer information, such as rate, I:E ratio, resistance, compliance, pressure or wave form, to the automated record. Once more, until the new ventilators are available, the information must be transferred manually, assuming it is even available to the anesthetist.

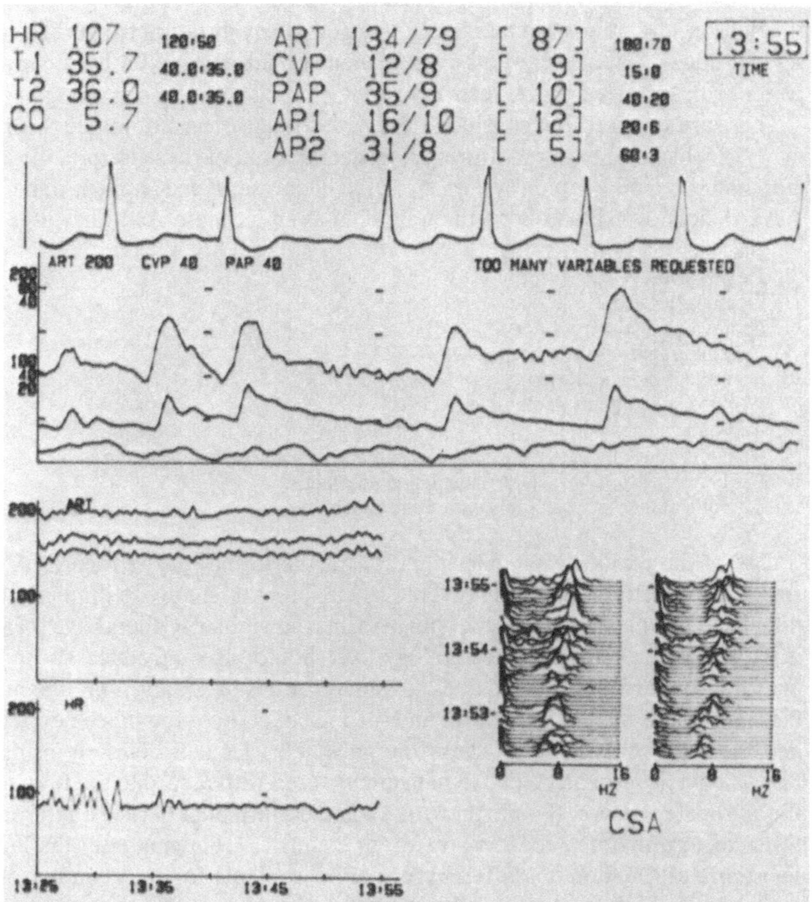

Fig. 4. A (reversed) display form the CICRAM screen. Note the many different types of information which can be displayed on the same screen: (from top to bottom and then left to right) digital of measurements, an on-line, real-time display of some of the continous representation measurements, trend data, and the processed EEG (CSA). The user can magnify any of these sections for greater detail. (Courtesy of Mark Mitchell, M.D.; Dept of Anesthesiology, University of California, San Diego, California.)

6. *Annotations.* There is a considerable amount of miscellaneous material that must be entered into the anesthetic record. This material includes the preanesthetic information described above, as well as a description of anesthetic techniques, such as spinal, the size of the endotracheal tube, the position of the patient, and the onset of anesthesia, surgery, or inflation of a tourniquet. Currently, this information is usually entered manually, either in writing or by keyboard. A local area network connected with a hospital information system could automatically supply much of the preanesthetic information from such diverse places as admissions, the clinical laboratory, the radiology department, and cardiology. Other possible alternatives for entering this information are described below.

There are several design considerations in setting up an automated record system. We shall discuss only a few of these. Given current computer technology, it is possible to use either a screen or hard copy for display to the anesthetist. Although hard copy is more familiar to most anesthetists, currently, the screen is less expensive and more versatile. The screen can display rapidly moving wave forms, as well as trends (Fig. 4).

In addition, the trends can be rapidly changed to any duration from a few minutes to several hours. Theoretically, the anesthetist should not need a hard copy until the patient is transferred to the recovery room.

There are several other considerations in the design of an automated record system, many of which apply to monitoring in general. Some of these criteria for a practical automated record keeping system are self evident; some may appear to be idealistic. Nevertheless, we should keep them in mind as an ultimate goal; they are:

1. Small in size
2. Inexpensive
3. Electrically safe
4. Impervious to electrocautery
5. Easy and rapid set-up
6. Easy and rapid calibration
7. Works on all patients at all times
8. Reproducible results
9. No interference by data collection with surgeon or with surgical procedure
10. Easily read output, with some meaning to anesthetist
11. Output continuous, preferably with trend capabilities

One of the major design considerations is the format of the record. A relatively simple approach, one used by several investigators, is simply to duplicate a conventional manual anesthetic record, both in format and in size. Others have reasoned that if we are introducing new technology, we should also introduce an entirely new anesthetic record, one which takes advantage of this technology. On the other hand, most anesthetists are conservative and the introduction of too much new technology, and too many changes may cause the anesthetist to avoid entirely using the new technology. Several questions remain unanswered with regard to the form and size of the automated record. Should there be a standard format of the anesthetic record for a given region, or for a country, or for all countries, changing only the language as appropriate? Or should a different format be available for each country or even for each hospital? How much information should one attempt to compress into the automatic anesthetic record? Certainly the anesthetist is accustomed to placing a tremendous amount of information on the anesthetic record (Fig. 5), sometimes to the extent that it becomes illegible (Fig. 6). Presumably, the automated record can pack in just as much information, perhaps more, since it is more neatly and clearly printed (Fig. 7). Should the hard copy be larger than the chart size for greater resolution and detail? Then, of course, the consideration becomes how to fit the record into the patient's chart.

If the technology used in an automated anesthesia record keeping system is not very advanced, the automated record may force some sort of standardization upon the anesthetists using it. To put it another way, advanced technology will provide the flexibility to allow the record to adapt to the anesthetist; simple technology will force the anesthetist to adapt to the record. Whether this is good or bad depends on the thought and care with which the format of the automated record has been constructed, and whether one believes that large-area standardization of anesthetic charts is required.

As discussed above, much of the information that is entered into the anesthetic record cannot be automatically entered in the foreseeable future. Currently, this information comprises everything except physiological measurements, and often

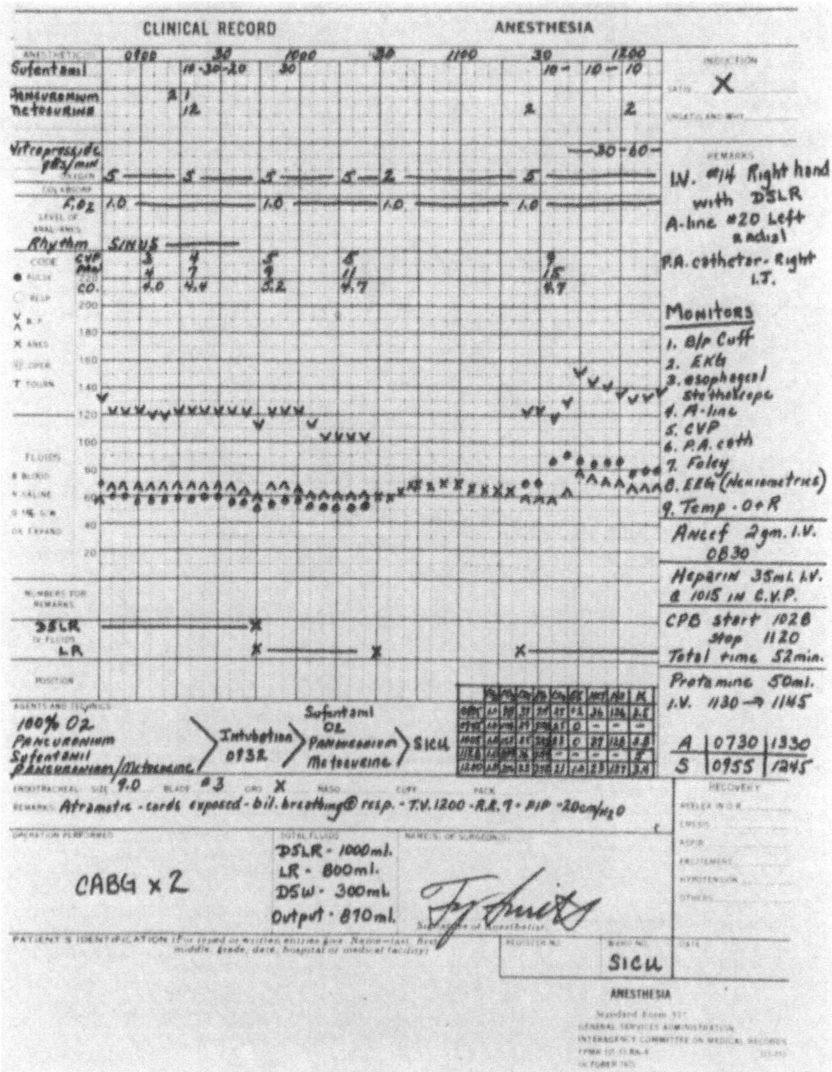

Fig. 5. A manual anesthetic record, packed with information. This record was copied by a non-physician from an original record, and hence is relatively neat and legible

even the latter must be manually entered. The problem for the automated record is to enter the information into the computer that is implementing this automated record. At least four means of information entry have been proposed:

1. The conventional keyboard
2. The special-purpose keyboard with built in function keys for single key-stroke entry for an entire drug name, for example
3. A special pad on which to print manually letters and numbers with the printed characters being entered into the computer
4. Speech recognition by a computer.

We shall briefly examine each of these techniques.

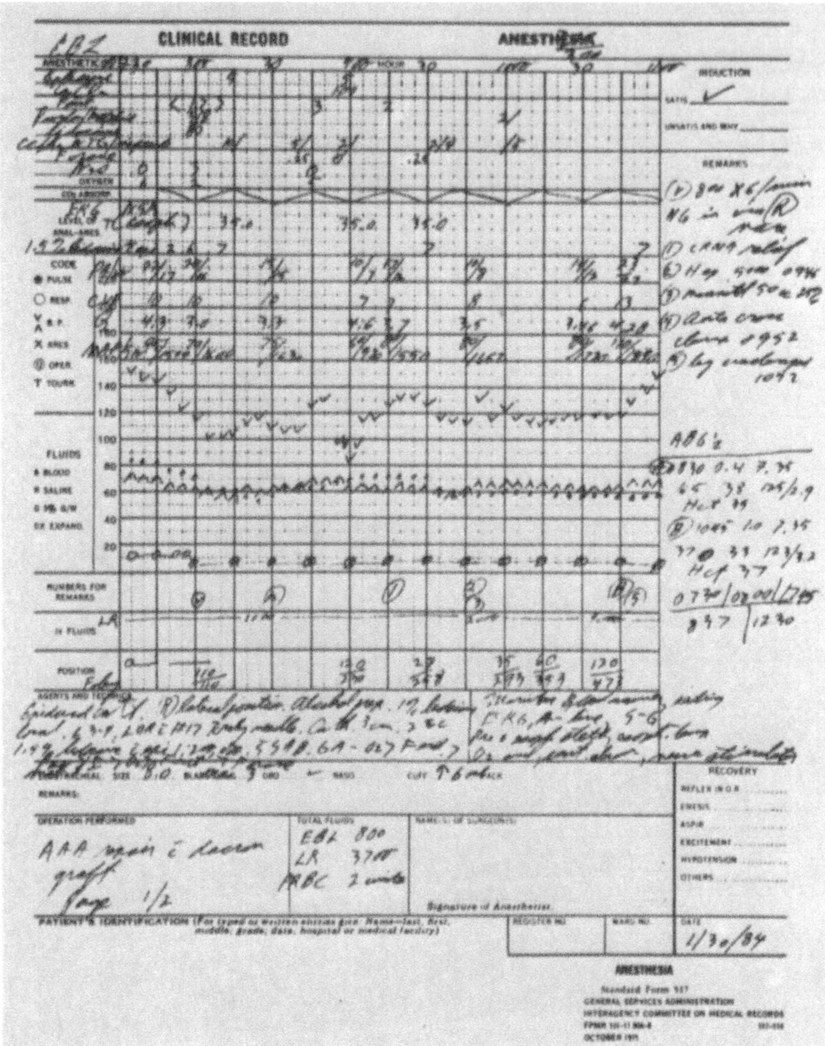

Fig. 6. Compare this crammed anesthetic record with Figs. 5 and 7. The large amount of information is almost counterproductive, in that it leds to illegibility. Note also that the record form does not allow for much of the information needed in the modern complex case, and the anesthetist had to create his own format

The conventional (QWERTY) keyboard would seem to be the most appropriate and useful mode of entry, since an infinite variety of information can be entered with it. Yet there has been a real resistance to its use by clinical anesthetists. The absolute flexibility of the typewriter keyboard is also its disadvantage. Typing is a time-consuming diversion of the clinician's attention from the patient. Certainly its facile use almost requires the use of two hands; most of us can type several times faster with two hands than with one hand. Such distraction of hands or mind can be disruptive,

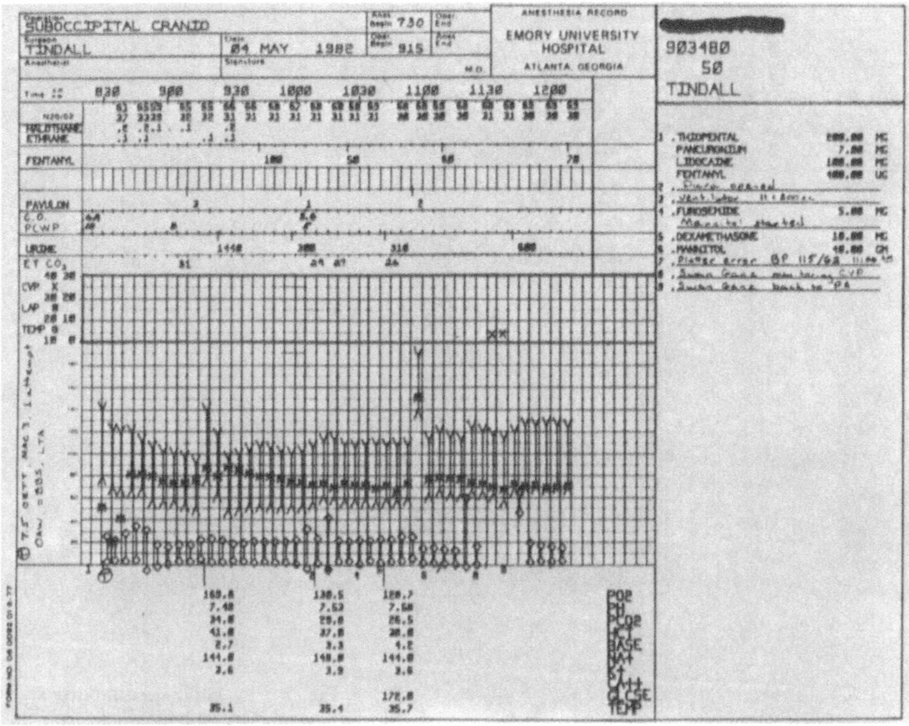

Fig. 7. Examples of outputs from automated recordkeeping systems. A record printed out by a semi-automated system. Note how much more information can be packed into a given area (upper right) than could be in Fig. 5. (Photo courtesy of Wesley Frazier, M.D.; Dept of Anesthesiology, Emory University School of Medicine, Atlanta, Georgia.)

particularly when the patient's condition is unstable, which is, unfortunately, the same time that man-machine communication may be most needed. The use of standard keyboards in experimental computerized monitoring systems in the past has been a major stumbling block to the acceptance of these systems. Nevertheless, the increasing general use and availability of computers, and their keyboards, may bode well for the eventual acceptance of the conventional keyboard. Another encouraging development is that of a new keyboard which permits much more natural and hence rapid typing. Although those accustomed to the QWERTY keyboard may find the new one difficult to adjust to, beginners, or those who have assiduously avoided typing, may find it the stimulus needed to use a full keyboard in everyday, as well as in operating room life. In the other hand, perhaps the typewriter keyboard's use will be reserved for more complicated messages entered at the anesthetist's leisure.

A variation that has been used in several experimental systems with varying degrees of success is the special-purpose keyboard. This keyboard usually has many fewer keys than the standard one, and each key represents an entire entity, such as the name of a drug, or a function (Fig. 8). The concept is to decrease the amount of typing required to send the message to the machine. The special-purpose keyboard would seem to be ideal, since one can enter an entire word or phrase with one key stroke.

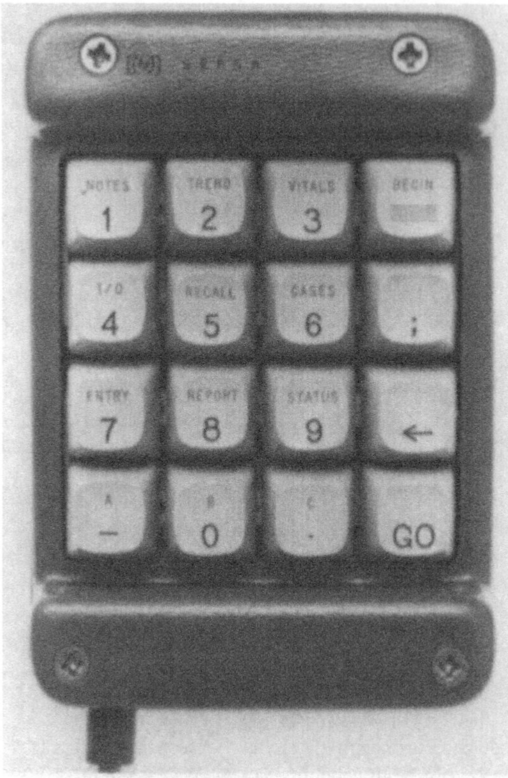

Fig. 8. A simple special-purpose keypad. The cable emerging from the lower left allows remote use of the keypad

However, to incorporate onto one keyboard all the words and phrases necessary or useful to the anesthetist (over 300) is an impossible task. Therefore, one must either severely limit the number of available words, or design for sequental entry. With the latter, one strikes a special key for a class of drugs, for example. Thus one could enter "barbiturates" and obtain a list of barbiturates on the screen. Next, one would enter a number for the appropriate agent, then enter the route and dose. This could require access to and attention to the computer and/or screen, not always a convenient matter. The remote key pad is an elegant solution to this dilemma.

A means to enter directly hand-printed information into the computer would seem to be ideal, since one does not need a complex keyboard, and since one can use a very familiar mode of entry–printing. More importantly, perhaps, one can enter information onto a form very easily, since the entry pad may incorporate a form, and the location of an entry on the pad determines its location on the computer "form" on the screen. However, the system is relatively cumbersome to set up. Furthermore, printing is a laborious task for many, and requires close attention to the special pad and to the screen.

If we agree that one of the main goals of the automated record is to free the hands of the anesthetist to accomplish other tasks, then none of these modes of entry is ultimately statisfactory. Furthermore, the hands of the anesthetist are often occupied during the time that information is being generated at the most rapid rate, for example during induction. We therefore have been evaluating the possibility of using voicerecognition technology to help implement an automated record keeping system. With a voice-recognition system, the anesthetist can enter information, such as a blood pressure value or the insertion of an endotracheal tube while taking the measurement or performing the act, without the necessity of interrupting the routine or act to enter the information. Voice-recognition technology has reached the stage of development that allows us at last to examine the feasibility of its use for the automated record. Unfortunately, any voice-recognition technology which is not prohibitively expensive is very primitive in both concept and design. Most systems must be trained by individual speakers, that is, they are speaker dependent. In addition, they can recognize only a limited number of words, from a list of up to 100 at a time. Thus, many constraints are currently imposed upon the user. The anesthetist must speak one word at a time with a small interval between words. He must speak clearly, in the same type of voice and intonation with which he trained the system. Because of the vocabulary limitations one must set up a special "language for anesthesia record keeping" (LARK), as well as a special syntax. A syntax is a set of formal rules for combining vocabulary words. A vocabulary plus syntax equals a language, which we call EARS (entry into the anesthetic record by speech).

To construct the syntax, we first divided the large word groups into several smaller but still major word groups such as *monitors, drugs, events, and fluids*. This was necessary because of the constraints on the size of the word pool. If the anesthetist says one of these key words, the voice-recognition system will call up another set of words related to this key word. For example, if the word "fluids" is spoken, words such as albumin, normal saline, or liters per minute, will be brought into the recognition memory. After one of these words is spoken, the "number" group of words will be called up. Because of the vocabulary constraints, we can use single digits only; the number hundred ten must be announced as one one zero. Thus, a typical LARK sentence would be "Measurement. Blood-pressure. One one five over seven five."

Most voice-recognition systems advertise at least 99% accuracy, even the less expensive ones. Under fairly ideal circumstances, that is simply repeating words under laboratory conditions outside the operating room, we were able to achieve about 96% accuracy (Sarnat et al. 1981). This may seem adequate, but it must be remembered that the accuracy was estimated for single words. Thus, a sentence containing five words will have an unacceptably high error rate of 20%. Therefore, there must be some way to verify what the computer thought it heard. This is accomplished by having the computer repeat, with a voice synthesizer, the just-entered sentence. To acknowledge that the computer is correct, the anesthetist simply says "yes". If, on the other hand, one or more words is incorrect, a correction must be made. The difficulty of making this correction depends greatly upon the location of the word or words in error.

Thus, the use of speech recognition, although very important for automated record keeping, must wait until technology improves. Four years ago when we began our work on voice recognition, it was estimated by IBM and Bell Laboratories that the next significant step breakthrough in voice-recognition technology would not come for at least ten years. However, technology has been advancing much more rapidly than even these leaders had conceived. Thus this important technology may be soon available, filling a large gap in the final implementation of automated record keeping.

The advantages of displaying information for several body systems together on the same display are many. Primarily, correlations between events (cerebral ischemia) and possible causes (respiratory or circulatory) are more easily made. Although concurrent trending has long been used in physiological and pharmacological laboratories, it has not been available clinically on a widespread basis. A few hospitals, fortunate enough to have strip-chart recorders, have been using these displays for over a decade. Myers et al. (1973) developed a display of arterial pressure, central venous pressure, and compressed special array plotted by an *X-Y* plotter. They called their system VITAC–Vital Indices Transmission and Analysis by Computer. Davis and Klein (personal communication) suggest that the most important systems to chart are central nervous, cardiovascular, respiratory, and neuromuscular. Accordingly, they have plotted variables representing each of these, plus temperature, on a colored display. An attractive feature of their system is that all measurements are noninvasive. Another example of an automatic charting system is the Duke Automated Monitoring Equipment (DAME) system (Burton et al. 1980). The DAME system allows up to 16 types of data to be input simultaneously from a patient. Nonfade displays of current data as well as trends may be produced on a single large monochrome CRT. Information which cannot be transduced is entered via either a bar code reader or a keyboard. The system is equipped with a single sheet of paper containing the most frequently needed bar codes. A booklet contains several hundred additional bar code messages. DAME is actually a computer network consisting of several computers, each performing its own tasks, connected by communications lines and synchronized in the performance of the overall task. Located in each participating operating room is a monitoring cart which contains the various patient monitors and interfaces, a microcomputer, a computer terminal, a large CRT display unit, and the bar code reader. The microcomputer controls the acquisition of all the data in the operating room and maintains the CRT display. Each monitoring cart is connected to a central minicomputer called the data manager, which in turn controls all the carts. The manager provides storage for all patient data during a case and prints the anesthetic record at the end of the case so that the record arrives at the recovery room at about the same time as the patient. The data manager communicates with a larger, faster minicomputer called the host. The host, having a large-capacity remote memory, provides archival storage for the patient data while also serving as the departmental computer resource for research. The network allows communication between the anesthetists in each room with a cart and the central station, so that the need for medical assistance or maintenance may be easily signalled.

Another example of a charting system is the Comprehensive Integrated Clinical/Research Anesthesia Monitor, or CICRAM, developed at the University of California at San Diego (Mitchell et al. 1979). Like the DAME, CICRAM consists of a cart containing all of the appropriate patient interfaces, a computer, and a graphic CRT display. The display used by CICRAM has a very high resolution and can very rapidly update the information on the screen. This allows the system to pack a great deal of data on the screen in a legible fashion. The screen can simultaneously display phasic waveforms, numeric displays of several variables such as blood pressure or heart rate, and trended information, including compressed spectral array displays of the EEG (Fig. 4). The hard copy options include a single-channel strip recorder for phasic waveforms, such as ECG during an arrhytmia, and a plotter with mulicolored pens for producing trend plots and case records. The CICRAM differs from the DAME in that CICRAM is a stand-alone device containing all the intelligence it needs to operate; connection to a network is optional.

In summary, this paper has reviewed the rationale for an implementation of the automated anesthetic record. Extension of computerized trending leads to the concept of automated charting. An automatic charting system creates a fairly complete paper case record which can meet all criteria necessary to be considered the official anesthetic record. These systems are much more than simple trend monitors because much of the information needed on the chart is difficult to acquire automatically. Physiological information is rather easily acquired. However, such information as drug infusion and surgical events are best noted by a human observer and manually communicated to the system. Since there are so many approaches to this common goal, we can only cover some basic principles. It is hoped that the material will serve as a basis for further discussion and investigation.

References

Beecher HK (1940) The first anaesthesia records (Codman, Cushing). Surg Gynecol Obstet 71: 689

Burton LW, Block F, Davis D, et al. (1980) The Duke automatic monitoring system (DAME) and the objective anesthesia record. Scientific Exhibiet, Annual Meeting Am Soc Anesthesiolo, St. Louis, 1980

Cushing HW (1903) On routine determinations of arterial tension in operating room and clinic. Boston Med Surg J 148: 291

Mitchell MM, Meathe EA, Ozaki GT, et al. (1979) Application of computer technology to intra-operative patient monitoring (Abstr). Anestheisiology [suppl] 5: 334

Moore DC (1969) Professional data anesthetic record; an explanation of reasons for development, use and method of coding, 3rd ed. The Mason Clinic, Virginia Mason Hospital, Seattle, Wash.

Moore DC, Bridenbaugh LD, Bagdi PA, Bridenbaugh PO, Stander H, Thomas GB (1968) Tabulation of anesthetic data: an improved system. Anesthesiology 29: 596–599

Myers RR, Stockard JJ, Fleming NI, France CJ, Bickford RG (1973) Remote on-line spectral plotting of electroencephalographic data. Proc SD Biomed Symp 12: 17–23

Sarnat AJ, Quinn ML, Smith NT (1981) A preliminary evaluation of computerized speech recognition for anesthesia (Abstr). Anesthesiology 55: A 128

Zollinger RM, Kreul JF, Schneider AJ (1977) Man-made versus computer-generated anesthesia records. J Surg Res 22: 419–424

Computer Aided Methods to Predict Perioperative Risks

U. Feldmann, P.-M. Osswald, H.-J. Hartung, and H. Lutz

Introduction

Systematic methods for the early detection of risks incurred during illness are necessary in order to prevent these risks by implementing therapy. Many of these methods are based on the evaluation of risk scores; for example, the Apgar-score developed by Virginia Apgar in 1953 is accepted worldwide in assessing the well-being of newborn infants. In anesthesiology, such indices have been in use for a long time. Well known are the ASA-score (1968) based on subjective prognostic criteria and the TISS-score (Keene and Cullan 1983) which orientates itself on objective examination findings.

In 1973, H. Lutz and K. Peter (Lutz and Peter 1973; Peter and Lutz 1973) introduced a preoperative risk checklist containing objective criteria on the preoperative examination findings as well as criteria about the expected operation. The checklist is routinely used in the Department of Anesthesiology and Resuscitation at the Medical School, Mannheim. An attempt is made in this paper to demonstrate the application of computer aided methods in the judgement and validation of existing risk scores, as well as in the evaluation of new scores by using the Mannheim risk score as an example.

Properties of Prognostic Scores

First, some properties of prognostic scores will be graphically displayed and mathematical relationships between prognostic scores and perioperative risks, as well as principles of mathematical decision-making procedures, will be discussed.

Suppose a prognostic score X with integer values $x = 0, 1, 2, 3, \ldots$ is to be validated with respect to a binary risk variable R. The values of the risk variable are $R = r_1$, if a perioperative risk occurs, for example r_1 = "severe complication" and $R = r_0$ in the contradictory case, so that r_0 = "no severe complication." The cohort study is the suitable experimental design to validate a prognostic score in which all operations of a hospital are prospectively recorded within a certain period and the preoperative risk score and the perioperative occurred risk is documented for each patient. As a result, one gets the joint distribution of the relative frequencies

$P(x, r_1)$ of the probands with score $X = x$ and risk $R = r_1$

and the relative frequencies

$P(x, r_0)$ of the probands with score $X = x$ and risk $R = r_0$.

Both distributions are based on the entire sample size of the probands examined. Figure 1 shows these distributions for a hypothetical example. We thereby assume that the base population of all observations was recorded so that the concepts of relative frequency and probability coincide. By summation of the relative frequencies $P(x, r_1)$ over all scores $X = x$, the prevalence $P(r_1)$ of the risk r_1 can be accepted as a measure of risk

$$P(r_1) = \sum_x P(x, r_1)$$

thereby

$$P(r_1) + P(r_0) = 1 \text{ with } P(r_0) = \sum_x P(x, r_0).$$

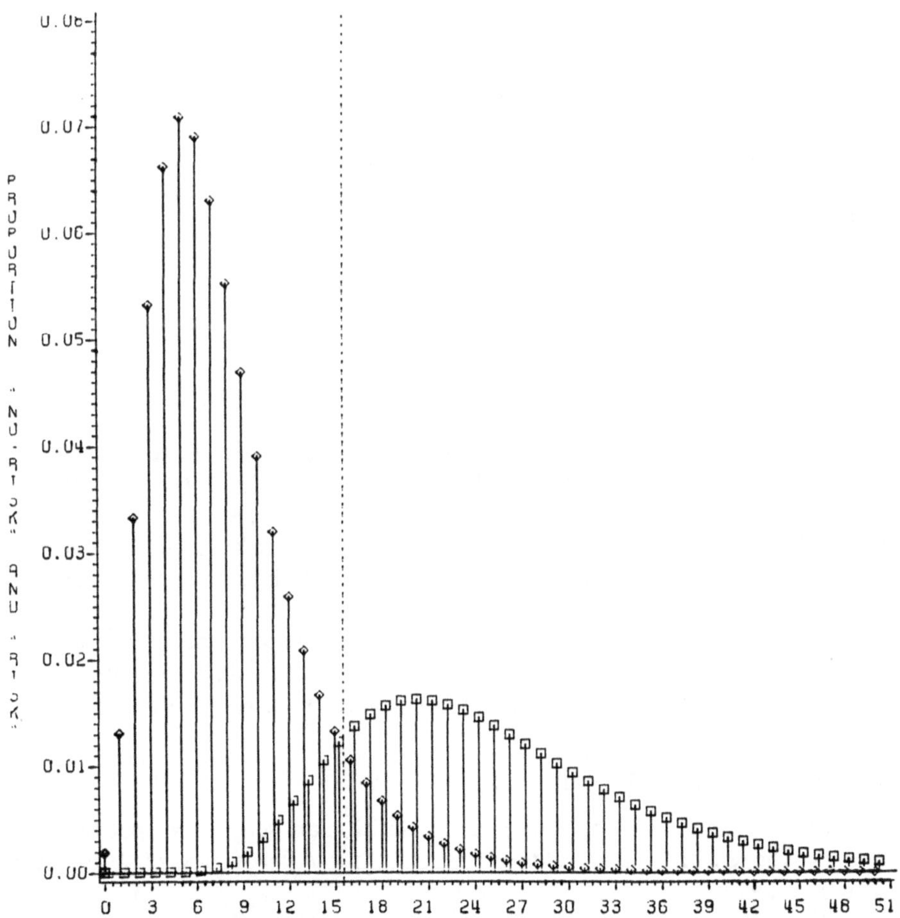

Fig. 1. Example of a joint frequency distribution of a prognostic score X. Proportion of patients ◇ = without, and □ = with, perioperative risk. In all figures proportions are shown, i.e., 0.01 = 1%

For example, the prevalence, often called prior probability, is $P(r_1) = 33\%$ or alternatively $P(r_0) = 77\%$. However, this measure does not take into account the individual score $X = x$ of a patient. In the prediction situation, the individual preoperative findings of the patient are known; however, the future outcome of the operation is unknown and must be estimated.

An adequate quantitative measure for such a prediction is the probabilitiy that risk $R = r_1$ occurs under the condition that the individual risk score value $X = x$ of the patient is known. This is called the posterior probability $P(r_1|x)$. The posterior probability is evaluated as the fraction $P(x, r_1)$ of the risk cases having score value $X = x$ with respect to the total fraction $P(x, r_1) + P(x, r_0)$ of all cases with score value $X = x$.

$$P(r_1|x) = \frac{P(x, r_1)}{P(x, r_1) + P(x, r_0)} \tag{1}$$

Figure 2 shows the posterior probability for $R = r_1$ computed from the data in Fig. 1. The posterior probability for $R = r_0$ to have no risk is then

$$P(r_0|x) = 1 - P(r_1|x). \tag{2}$$

If instead of a cohort study having been carried out for validating a prognostic score, a retrospective case-control study had been conducted, then only the conditional frequency distribubtions $P(x|r_1)$ for the risk group and $P(x|r_0)$ for the no risk group are known and in this case the conditional relative frequencies are related to the special groups

$$\sum_x P(x|r_1) = 1 \quad \text{and} \quad \sum_x P(x|r_0) = 1$$

However, if the prior probabilities are additionally known then:

$$P(x, r_1) = P(r_1) \cdot P(x|r_1) \text{ and } P(x, r_0) = P(r_0) \cdot P(x|r_0)$$

Inserting these expressions in Equ. (1) we get the well known Bayes' formula for evaluating the posterior probability. The posterior probability $P(r_1|x)$ is the most important characteristic measure of a risk score (Fig. 2), since it describes the quantitative relationship between risk score and risk, and makes an individual statement about the probability of a therapeutic success or failure possible. In addition, risk scores should support therapeutic decisionmaking.

At this point it is necessary to assign a certain fixed risk score value $X = x_0$ as a cut-off point and to decide on therapeutic intervention if the individual risk score $X = x$ of the observed patient is greater or equal to the cut-off point x_0. The decision reads:

the risk $R = r_1$ is predicted if $x \geq x_0$.
the risk $R = r_0$ is predicted if $x < x_0$.

As is known, criteria of the goodness of a decision are sensitivity, specificity and accuracy. The sensitivity $S_e(x_0)$ of the decision is the fraction of all correctly predicted risk cases, that is,

$$S_e(x_0) = \sum_{x \geqslant x_0} P(x|r_1)$$

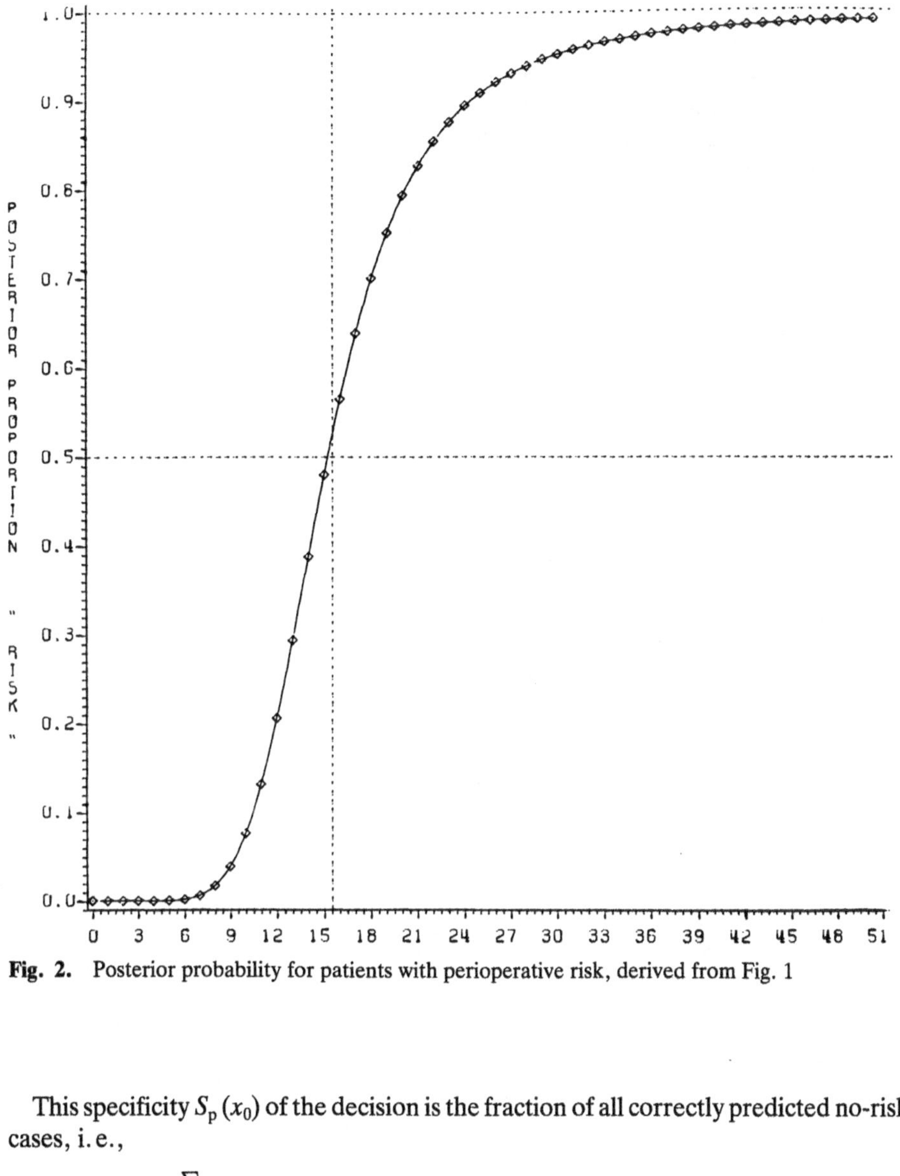

Fig. 2. Posterior probability for patients with perioperative risk, derived from Fig. 1

This specificity $S_p(x_0)$ of the decision is the fraction of all correctly predicted no-risk cases, i.e.,

$$S_p(x_0) = \sum_{x < x_0} P(x \mid r_0)$$

The accuracy $A(x_0)$ of the decision is the fraction of the total of all correctly predicted risk and no risk cases. The accuracy can be computed from sensitivity and specificity as a weighted mean using the prior probabilities as weights, i.e.,

$$A(x_0) = P(r_1) \cdot S_e(x_0) + P(r_0) \cdot S_p(x_0)$$

Figure 3 shows the computed criteria of goodness derived from Fig. 1 for every possible cut-off point $x_0 = 0, 1, 2, 3, \ldots 51$ of the risk scale.

In mathematical decision-making approaches (Wald 1950; Krishnaiah and Kanal 1982) there are essentially two criteria of optimality used for the unambiguous determination of the cut-off point x_0. These decision criteria are:

1. The Minimax rule, to minimize the maximum of the different kinds of error rates. In our case, that means choosing the cut-off point x_0 so that the sensitivity and specificity are equal, with the result (see Fig. 3) $x_0 = 15$.
2. The Bayes rule, to minimize the expected average loss. In our case, this means maximizing the accuracy, thus leading (see Fig. 3) to the result $x_0 = 16$.

Decision rule 2 is strongly related to the posterior probability and is equivalent to the decision to predict a risk $R = r_1$ for the risk score $X = x$ if $P(r_1|x) > 0.5$ (see Fig. 2). The accuracy is the weighted mean of sensitivity and specificity and in case the prior probability $P(r_1)$ is very small then the sensitivity will be underestimated. This

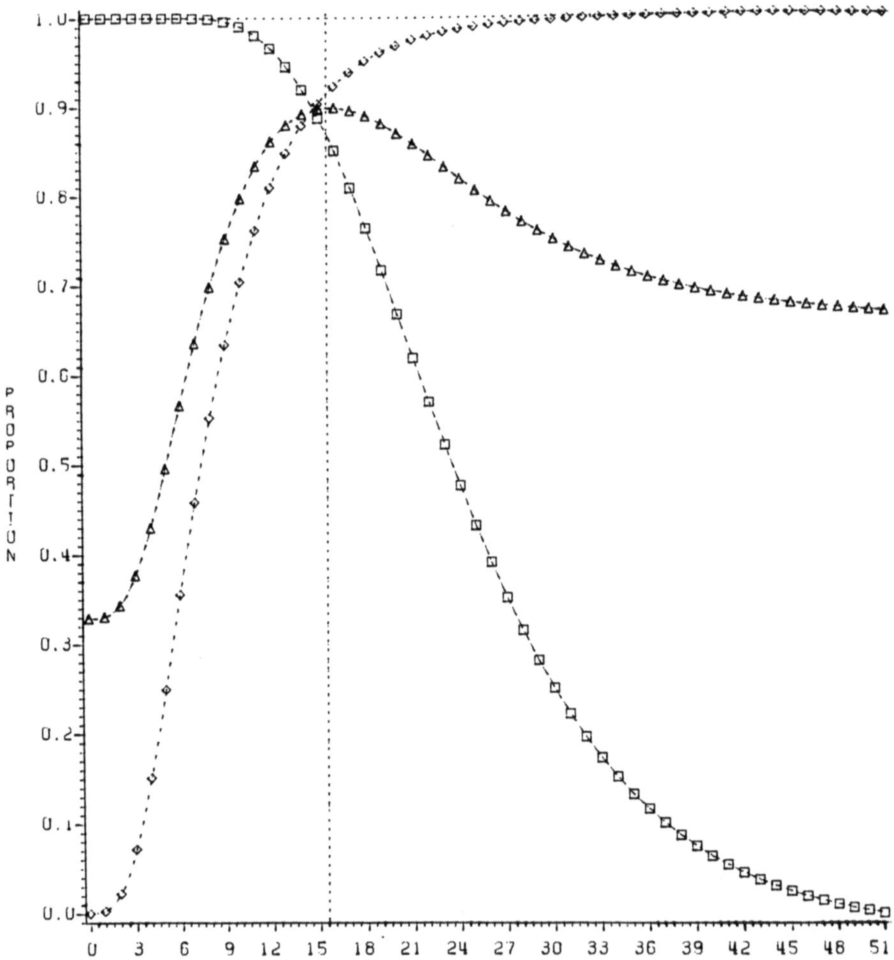

Fig. 3. □ = sensitivity, ◇ = specificity, △ = accuracy, for all possible cut-off points $X=x$, derived from Fig. 1

may occur especially in the prediction of perioperative risks. Therefore, decision rule 2 is often modified in such a way as not to maximize the weighted mean but instead:
3. Maximize the arithmetic mean $\frac{1}{2} S_e(x_0) + \frac{1}{2} S_p(x_0)$ from sensitivity and specificity.

Decision rule 3 is equivalent to deciding to classify a patient with individual risk score $X = x$ into the risk group r_1 if $P(r_1 | x) > P(r_1)$ and this leads to the cut-off point $x_0 = 14$ (see Fig. 2). Thus the knowledge of the posterior probability is obviously sufficient to make optimal decisions in the sense of 2 or 3 as the case may be.

Application to the Mannheim Risk Score

In 1973, H. Lutz and K. Peter (Lutz and Peter 1973; Peter and Lutz 1973) developed a preoperative checklist (Table 1) that is routinely used in the Medical School at Mannheim to quantify the preoperative examination findings for every surgical patient with a special risk score. The checklist has practical consequences with respect to the planning and preparation of the anesthesia. For example, the selection of the anesthetist and his assistants, the selection of the operating theater, the monitoring, and the postoperative planning in the recovery room.

In order to validate this checklist, a cohort study was carried out and in a period of six weeks each operation in four operating theaters was prospetively recorded. The preoperative status of the patient and the complications arising intraoperatively, in the recovery room, and during the stay in hospital, were documented. A total of $n =$ 700 operations were analysed.

Severe complications occurred in the case of $n_1 = 178$ patients, where severe complication is defined as a remaining organ damage (122 cases) or fatal outcome (56 cases). Figure 4 shows the frequency distributions for severe and not severe complications according to the Mannheim risk score. Furthermore, in Fig. 4 the endpoints $x_0 = 2, 5, 10, 20$ of the five risk groups I to V (see Table 1) defined by the Mannheim risk score are stated.

The usefulness of the Mannheim risk score as an instrument to predict severe complications is shown in Fig. 5. The posterior frequencies of the severe complications increase with growing risk score, but a high score values Fig. 5 does not show a very uniform behaviour. The question of which of the five risk groups predicts a severe complication becomes clear by computing sensitivity, specificity and accuracy (Fig. 6). The cut-off point $x_0 = 11$ shows a sensitivity of 81%, a specificity of 78% and an accuracy of 79%. Thus the risk groups IV and V of the Mannheim risk index are shown to be excellent indicators in the prognosis of serious complications. From the total number of 700 patients, 140 cases with severe complications were correctly predicted by the risk groups IV and V and 414 cases without severe complications were correctly assigned to the groups I to III. The cut-off point maximizing the total number of correctly predicted severe and non-severe complications is $x_0 = 13$ (see Fig. 6). Here sensitivity decreases to 69% while specificity is 88% and accuracy is 82%.

Table 1. Preoperative risk check-list developed by H. Lutz, K. Peter for use at the Medical School, Mannheim

0	1	2	4	8	16	Score
Routine elective operation	More urgent planned operation	Urgent non planned operation	Immediate intervention			
Superficial surgery	Extremities	Opening of abdominal carity	Opening of thorax or skull	Opening of two carities	Polytrauma/ shock	
Age 1–39 years	0–1 years 40–69 years	70–79 years	> 80 years			
Anticipated operating time < 60 min	< 120 min	< 180 min	> 180 min			
Weight normal ± 10%	– 10%–15%	+ 10%–30% – 15%–25%	> + 30%			
Blood pressure normal < 160/95 mmHg	Treated hypertension (controlled)	Untreated or short-term treated hypertension	Treated hypertension (uncontrolled)			
Cardiac performance normal	Recompensated cardiac insufficiency	Angina pectoris			Decompensated cardiac insufficiency	
ECG normal	Moderate changes	Pacemaker ECG	Sinus arrhythmia >5 ventr. extrasyst./min			
No myocardial infarction	> 2 years	> 1 year	> 6 months	> 3 months	< 3 months	
Breathing normal	Obstruction (treated)	Obstruction (untreated)	Broncho-pulmonary infections pneumonia	Restriction	Obvious insufficiency; cyanosis	
Liver function (lab. tests) normal	Slight changes	Severe changes				
Kidney function (lab. tests) normal	Slight changes	Severe changes				
Acid-base and electrolyte levels normal	Slight changes	Severe changes				
HB >12,5 g%	10–12,5 g%	< 10 g %				
Burns index (% body area × age)	⩽ 20	⩽ 40	⩽ 60	⩽ 80	> 80	
					Total score	

Risk group	I	II	III	IV	V
Score	0–2	3–5	6–10	11–20	> 20

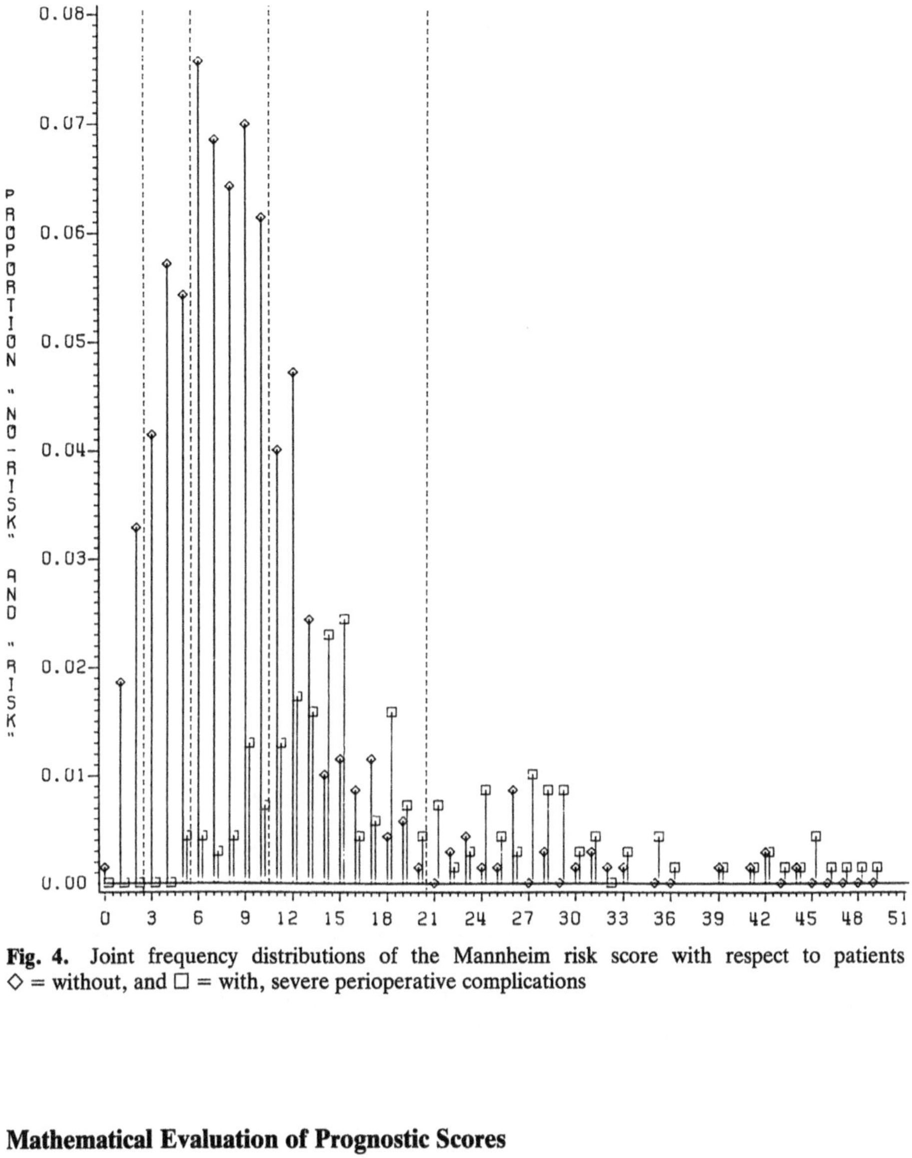

Fig. 4. Joint frequency distributions of the Mannheim risk score with respect to patients ◇ = without, and □ = with, severe perioperative complications

Mathematical Evaluation of Prognostic Scores

In medicine, the use of mathematical methods, especially methods of discriminant analysis for deriving prognostic scores is increasing (Afifi et al. 1971; Crandon et al. 1980a, b; Goldman et al. 1977; Titterington et al. 1981; Wassner and Timm 1976). Possibly, the best analyzed study is the head injury study by Titterington et al., which investigates the feasibility of prediction and the degree of recovery that individual patients would attain. Here several techniques of discriminant analysis are compared using criteria of prognostic success and reliability. The state of the art for the application of mathematical decision procedures in medicine is collected in the proceedings edited by De Dombal and Gremy (1976).

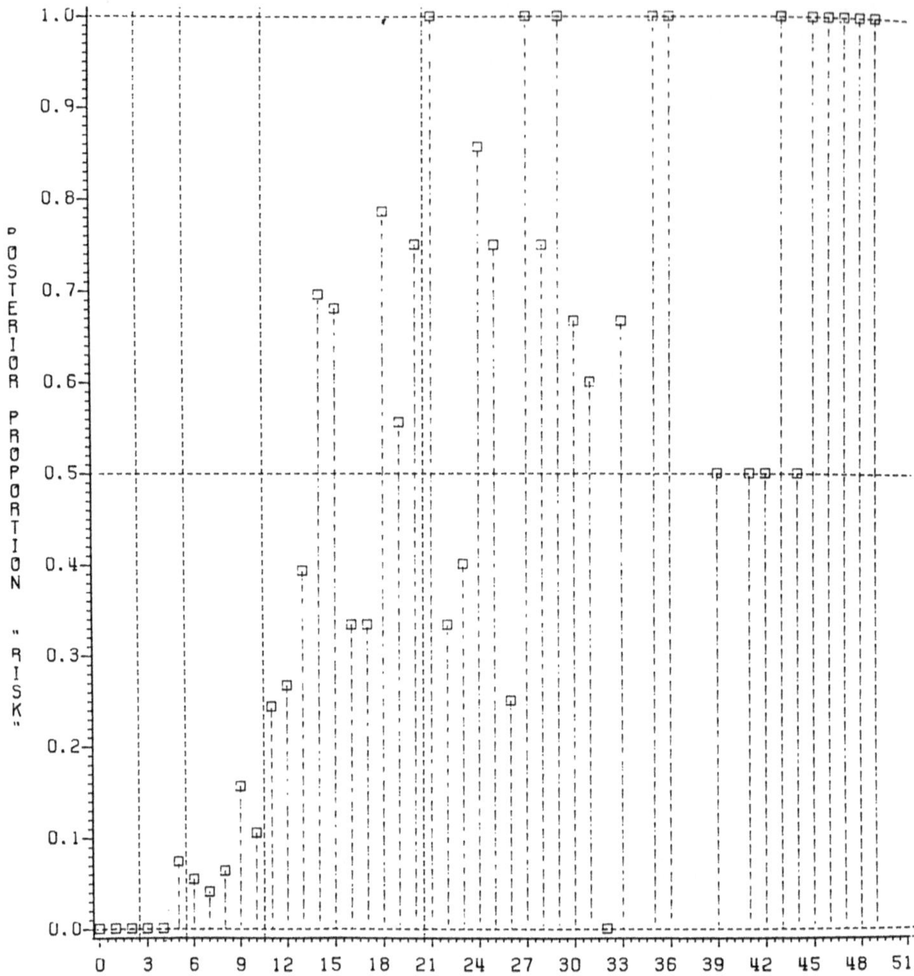

Fig. 5. Posterior frequency distributions of the Mannheim risk score with respect to patients with severe perioperative complications, derived from Fig. 4

The main purpose of this paper is to evaluate a linear risk score to predict perioperative complications. Many techniques of discriminant analysis lead to non-linear and even non-parametric discriminant scores which can only be solved with the aid of computers. Linear discriminant scores result from the well known linear discriminant analysis (Lachenbruch and Goldstein 1979) as well as from the more recently developed logistic discriminant analysis (Anderson 1982) and probit discriminant analysis (Wassner and Timm 1976). We use logistic discrimination (see also the work of Crandon et al. 1980a, b) as an example of a mathematical approach to predict perioperative risk with linear risk scores. While in the case of logistic discrimination a

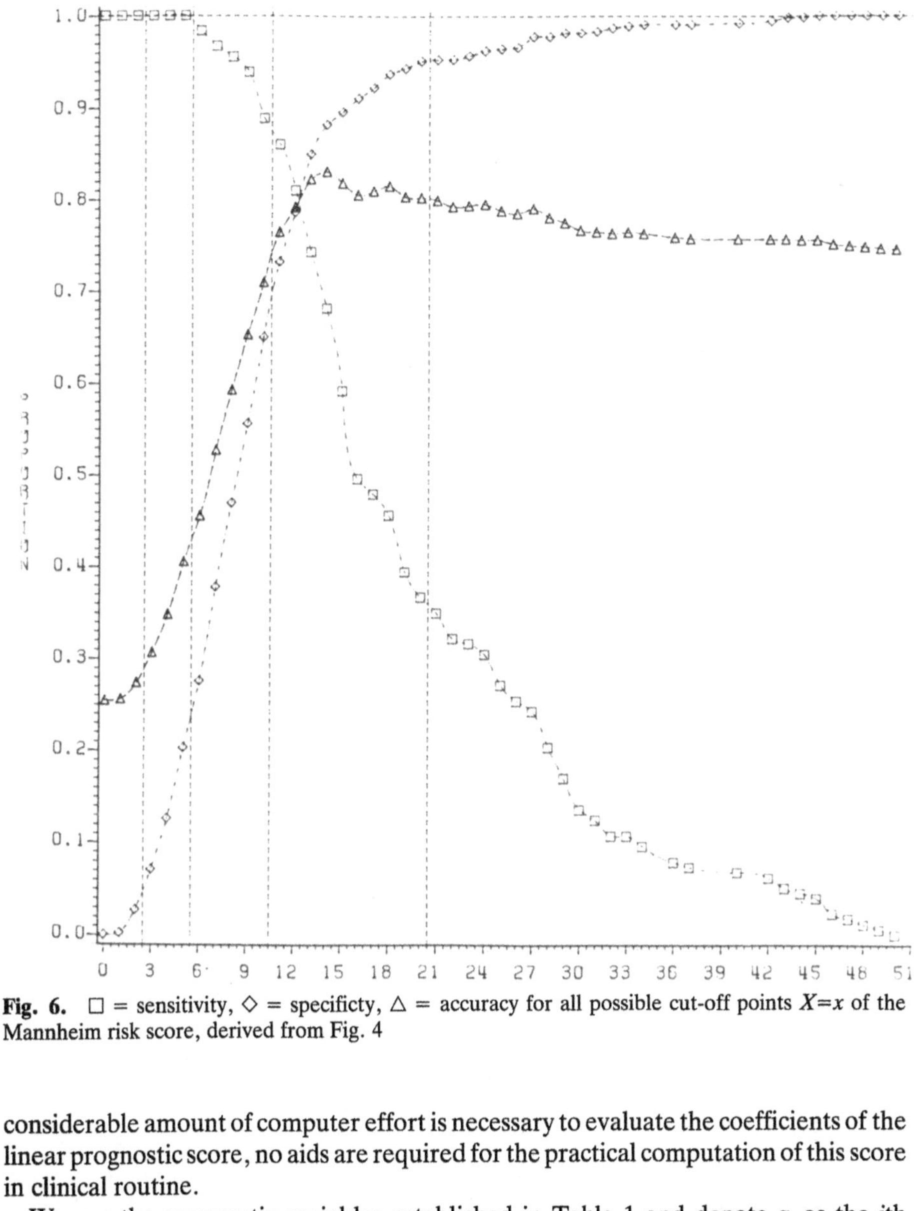

Fig. 6. □ = sensitivity, ◇ = specificty, △ = accuracy for all possible cut-off points $X=x$ of the Mannheim risk score, derived from Fig. 4

considerable amount of computer effort is necessary to evaluate the coefficients of the linear prognostic score, no aids are required for the practical computation of this score in clinical routine.

We use the prognostic variables established in Table 1 and denote z_i as the ith variable. Using the dataset mentioned in the previous section, logistic discriminant analysis evaluates a coefficient of regression b_i for every prognostic variable z_i by the maximum likelihood method (according to Anderson, cited in Krishnaiah and Kanal 1982) and leads (see Table 3) to the logistic score

$$x = \sum_i b_i z_i$$

and to the intercept x_0.

Figure 7 shows the joint frequency distribution for risk and no risk cases computed by the logistic risk score. The linear logistic discrimination assumes the log-likelihood ratio to be a linear function of the risk score:

$$\ln \left(\frac{P(x, r_1)}{P(x, r_0)}\right) = c\,(x_0 - x)$$

Thereby

$$x = \sum_i b_i z_i$$

is the logistic risk score, x_0 is the intercept and c is a scale factor chosen ($c = 2.17$) to give the logistic risk score the same range as the Mannheim risk score. From the

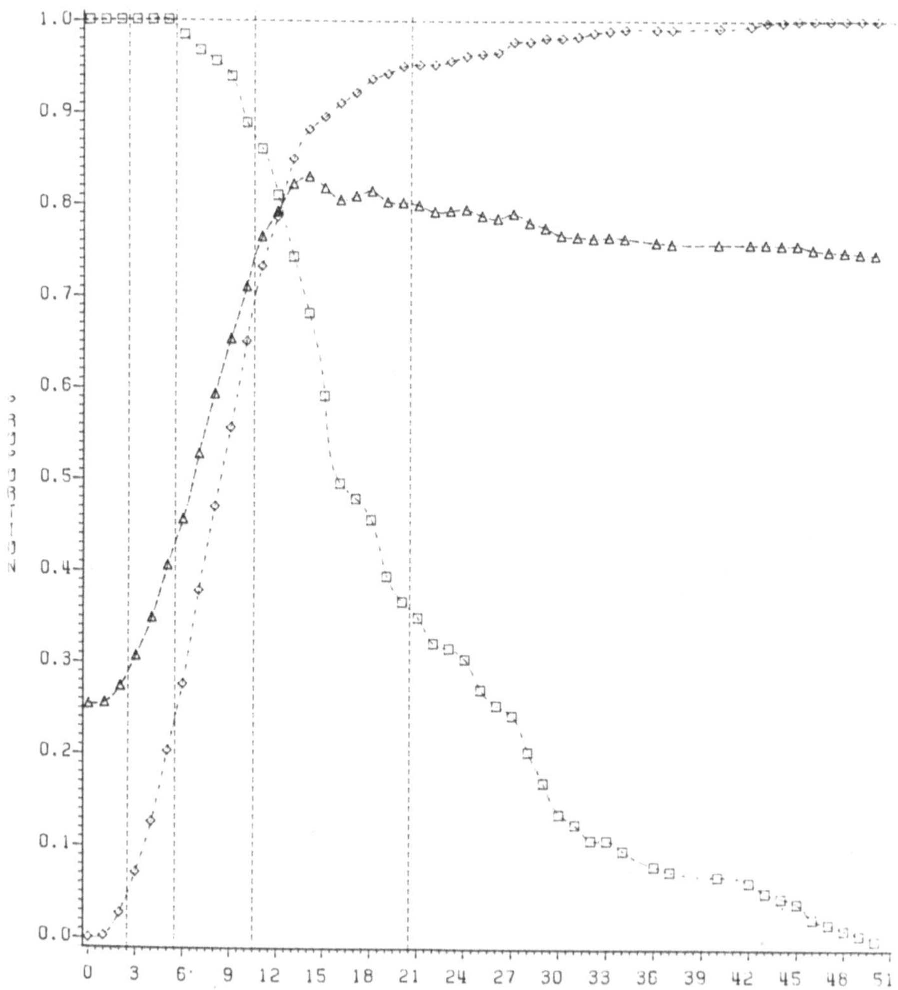

Fig. 7. Joint frequency distribution of the logistic risk score with respect to patients □ = without, and △ = with, severe perioperative complications

definition of posterior probability, given in the second section, the probability of risk $R = r_1$ follows as:

$$P(r_1|x) = \frac{\exp[c \cdot (x_0 - x)]}{1 + \exp[c \cdot (x_0 - x)]} \tag{3}$$

In Fig. 8 the estimated posterior probability (Eq. [3]) and the corresponding observed posterior frequency are displayed.

The estimated posterior probability of risk is a mathematical function called a logistic function, which permits the estimate of the expected probability of risk (Fig. 8) for any arbitrary score value $X = x$. The logistic function shows an excellent adaptation to the observed frequency distribution. $P(r_1|x_0) = 0.5$ is valid for the computed intercept $x_0 = 21$. This intercept optimizes the expected accurary according

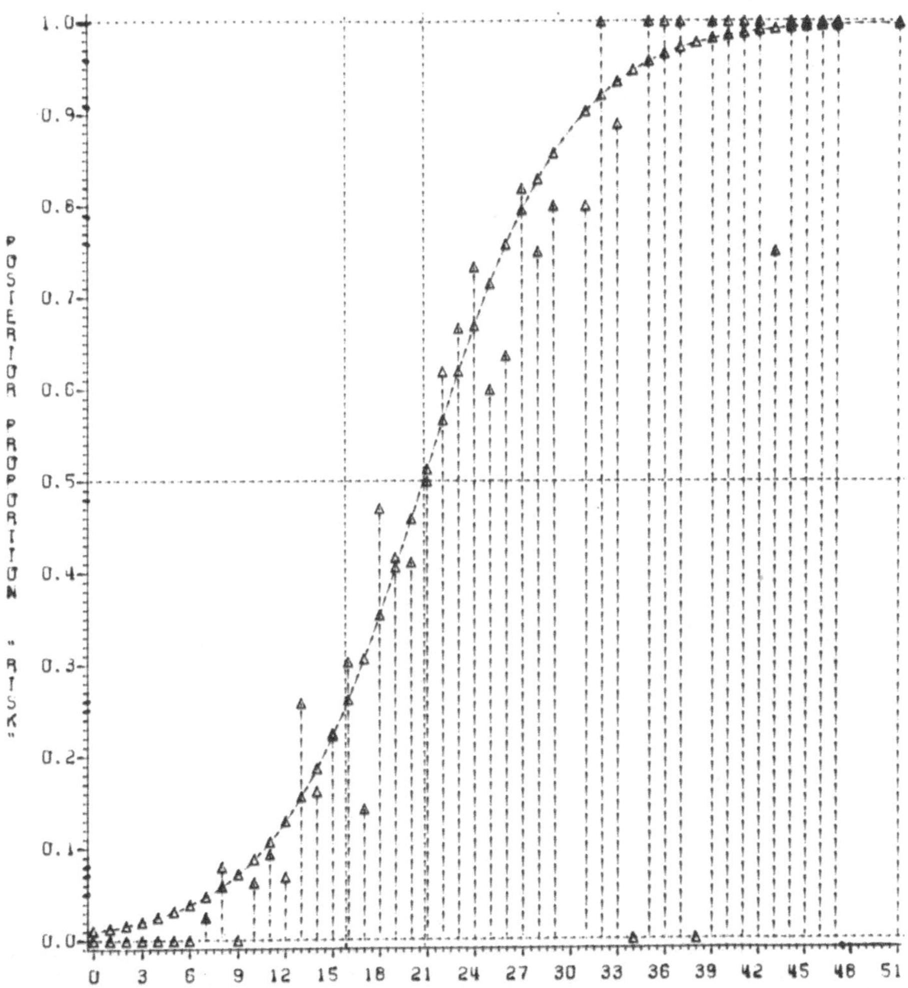

Fig. 8. Posterior frequency distribution (dashed) and expected posterior (splined) probability of the Logistic risk score with respect to patients with severe perioperative complications

to the criterion of optimization 2 in the second section. However, since prior probability of severe complications only amounts to $P(r_1) = 25.4\%$, we use the argument given in that section and chose the criterion of optimality (3) in making the decision. This leads (see Fig. 8) to the cut-off point $x_0 = 15$ and maximizes the arithmetic mean from expected sensitivity and specificity.

In Fig. 9 the observed sensitivity, specificity and accuracy are shown. The cut-off point $x_0 = 15$, which is not estimated from observed frequencies but from expected posterior probability Eq. (3) leads (Fig. 9) to the observed sensitivity of 81%, the observed specificity of 77% and the observed accuracy of 76%. This result hardly differs from that obtained from the Mannheim risk score (see previous section) and as far as a decision criterion for severe complications is concerned the Mannheim risk score could even be preferred. However, the advantage in using methods of

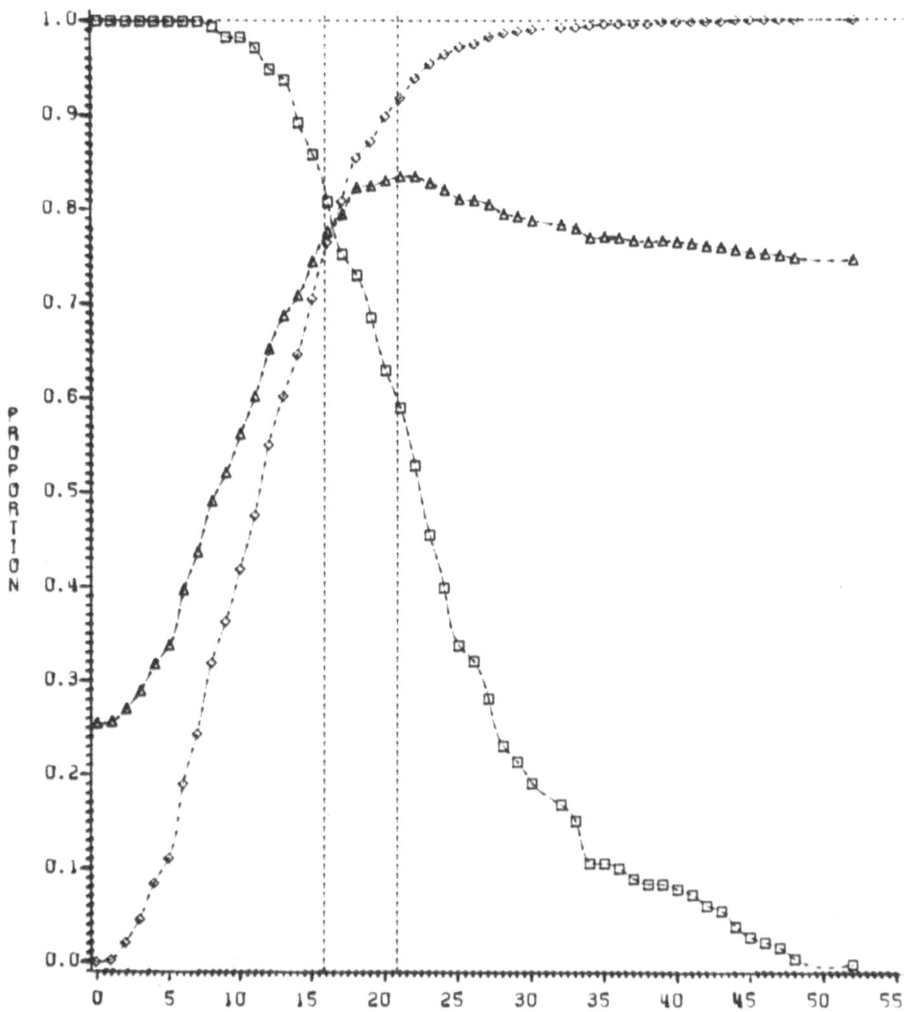

Fig. 9. □ = sensitivity, ◇ = specificity, △ = accuracy, for all possible cut-off points $X{=}x$ of the logistic risk score

mathematical discrimination is that Eq. (3) unambiguously establishes a functional mathematical relationship between prognostic score and estimated posterior probability of risk and so allows for individual prognosis.

A further advantage of mathematical procedures, which we will discuss in the penultimate section, is that the prognostic relevance of the prognostic variables can be determined.

Prediction with Ordered Risk Categories

In the case of almost all risk scores which are used in medicine (see also Table 1), ordered risk categories, mainly the categories I to V are subsequently formed. This may be a reference to the Apgar score (Agpar 1953) or the ASA score (1968) which have five categories to assess the severity of a future risk. In risk scores, these categories are not constructed to predict the manner of risk but to allocate the degree of severity of risk by one of the five ordered risk categories. Attempts are often made to determine such categories even in the case where only a binary risk variable is measured for validation. This leads to defining severity of risk by the posterior probability.

However, in order to asses the risk categories to the degrees of severity of risk, it is necessary to define a clinical criterion for this kind of severity and to validate this in a cohort study. The following clinical complication rating was designed:

I.	No complication	($n = 115$)
II.	No organ damage	($n = 221$)
III.	Questionary organ damage	($n = 186$)
IV.	Remaining organ damage	($n = 122$)
V.	Fatal outcome	($n = 56$)

This postoperative clinical categorizing of the risk occurred results from necessary consideration of the preoperative findings for the patient, for instance, age carries the possibility of various types of morbidity. Since preoperative and perioperative examination findings are necessary to carry out the staging of complication groups the problem of reliability of allocation arises, which, however, should not be discussed here.

For perspicuous presentation of data we use three ordered complication categories in this paper:

r_0 = mild complications	(complication I/II)	($n_1 = 336$)
r_1 = moderate complications	(complication III)	($n_2 = 186$)
r_2 = severe complications	(complication IV/V)	($n_3 = 178$)

The joint frequency distributions $P(x, r_0)$ and $P(x, r_1)$ and $P(x, r_2)$ of the Mannheim risk score are shown in Fig. 10 for the three defined risk groups of the risk variable R. The corresponding posterior distributions

$$P(r_k \mid x) = P(x, r_k) \;/\; (P(x, r_0) + P(x, r_1) + P(x, r_2))$$

with

$$k = 0, 1, 2$$

are presented in Fig. 11.

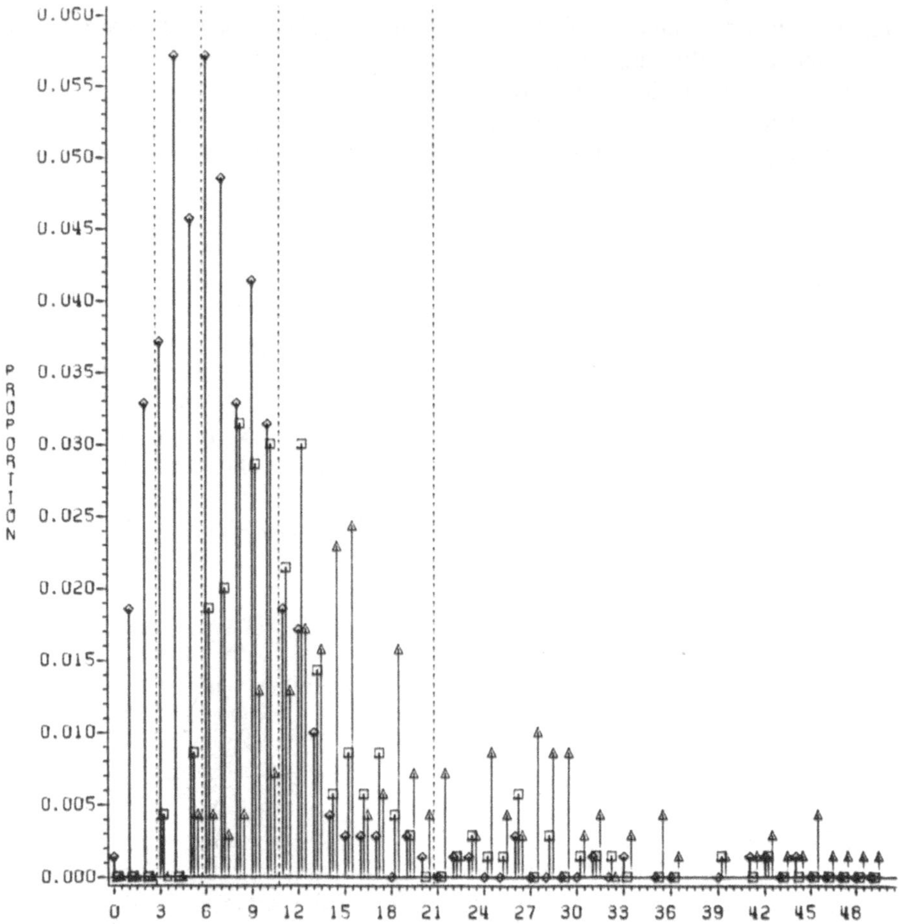

Fig. 10. Joint frequency distribution of the Mannheim risk score with respect to patients with ◇ = mild, □ = moderate, and △ = severe, perioperative complications

To establish an unambiguous relationship between preoperative risk score and postoperative observed complication, the risk score has to be divided into groups corresponding to the measureable complication categorization. For our purposes, we must define two cut-off points x_0 and x_1 with $x_0 < x_1$ which result in three intervals for a decision:

the risk $R = r_0$ is predicted if	$x < x_0$
the risk $R = r_1$ is predicted if	$x \leq x < x_1$
the risk $R = r_2$ is predicted if	$x \geqslant x_1$

The presentation of criteria of goodness for this decision, namely the proportions of the respective correctly predicted risks r_0, r_1 and r_2 is possible in the form of a classification matrix (Table 2), not, however, in the form of a two-dimensional plot.

In order to validate the Mannheim risk score with respect to the defined ordered complication groups, we use the risk groups in Table 1 and divide them into three

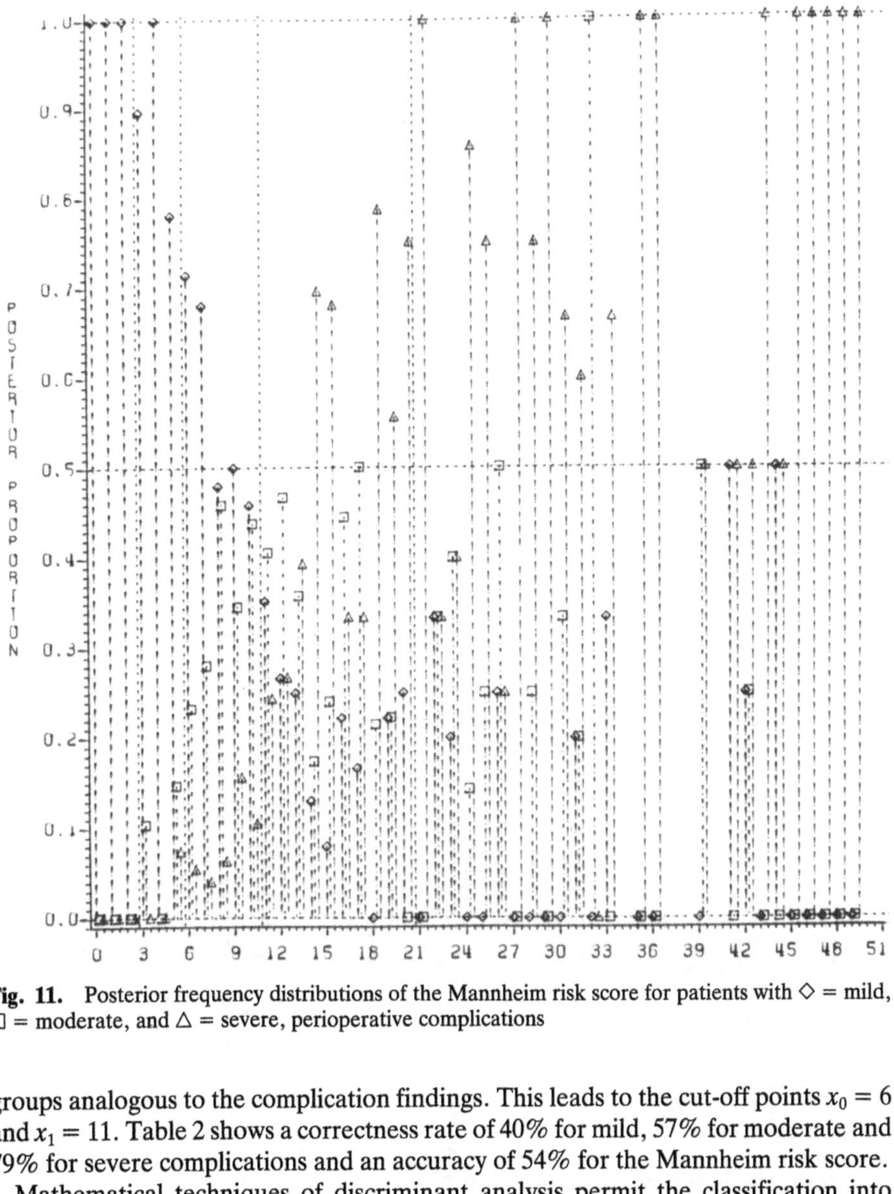

Fig. 11. Posterior frequency distributions of the Mannheim risk score for patients with ◇ = mild, □ = moderate, and △ = severe, perioperative complications

groups analogous to the complication findings. This leads to the cut-off points $x_0 = 6$ and $x_1 = 11$. Table 2 shows a correctness rate of 40% for mild, 57% for moderate and 79% for severe complications and an accuracy of 54% for the Mannheim risk score.

Mathematical techniques of discriminant analysis permit the classification into more than two categories. However, these are usually nominally scaled categories which predict the kind of risk and which require several discriminant scores for such a prediction. Only very few discriminant procedures (Anderson and Philips 1981; Feldman et al. 1984) exist to classify ordinal scaled categories like the severity of complications. In this case, the evaluation of only one risk score is necessary. We use the method of ordinal logistic discrimination described in Feldman et al. (1984). With the aid of the maximum likelihood method the coefficients of regression b_i and the intercepts x_0 and x_1 are evaluated from the dataset described in the third section and shown in Table 3. This leads to the logistic risk score $x = \sum b_i z_i$.

Table 2. Classification matrices of the prediction with ordered risk categories

Mannheim risk score	Complications			
	Mild	Moderate	Severe	Total
$0 \leq x \leq 5$	*135*	9	3	147
$6 \leq x \leq 10$	163	*107*	35	305
$11 \leq x$	38	70	*140*	248
Total	336	186	178	700
Correct	40%	57%	79%	54%

Logistic risk score	Complications			
	Mild	Moderate	Severe	Total
$0 \leq x \leq 9$	*202*	24	3	229
$10 \leq x \leq 17$	98	*89*	38	195
$18 \leq x$	36	73	*137*	246
Total	336	186	178	700
Correct	61%	48%	77%	61%

Table 3. Coefficients of regression b_i, their asymptotic standard deviations s_{b_i}, levels of significance P and their ranks k for the binary and ordinal scaled logistic discrimination

Prognostic variable	Logistic discriminant analysis							
	Dichotomous				Ordinal			
i Z_i	b_i	s_{b_i}	P%	k	b_i	s_{b_i}	P%	k
Expected surgery condition								
1 Urgency of surgery	1.33	0.57	2.01	9	0.98	0.48	4.21	10
2 Localisation of surgery	0.95	0.19	0.01	1	0.95	0.16	0.01	3
3 Age	1.77	0.54	0.10	6	1.68	0.42	0.01	6
4 Surgery time	1.64	0.41	0.01	4	1.83	0.33	0.01	2
5 Body weight	1.12	0.43	0.88	8	0.83	0.32	0.87	9
Cardio-circulatory conditions								
6 Blood pressure range	1.58	0.39	0.01	3	1.90	0.32	0.01	1
7 Cardial efficiency	2.90	0.78	0.02	5	3.01	0.63	0.01	5
8 ECG	1.44	0.71	4.23	10	1.86	0.59	0.05	8
9 Myocardial infarction	0.08	0.29	–	13	0.12	0.16	–	14
10 Condition of respiration	0.62	0.19	0.12	7	0.55	0.15	0.02	7
Blood chemistry								
11 Liver status	0.52	0.83	–	11	0.42	0.59	–	13
12 Kidney status	0.25	1.00	–	14	1.28	0.89	–	11
13 Acid-base status	0.54	1.14	–	12	0.93	0.91	–	12
14 Hemoglobin	3.63	0.87	0.01	2	3.55	0.69	0.01	4
15 Burn-index	–	–	–	–	–	–	–	–
Intercept x_0	21.4	1.75			11.9	1.21		
Intercept x_1	–	–			18.8	1.67		
Scale factor c	2.17				1.65			

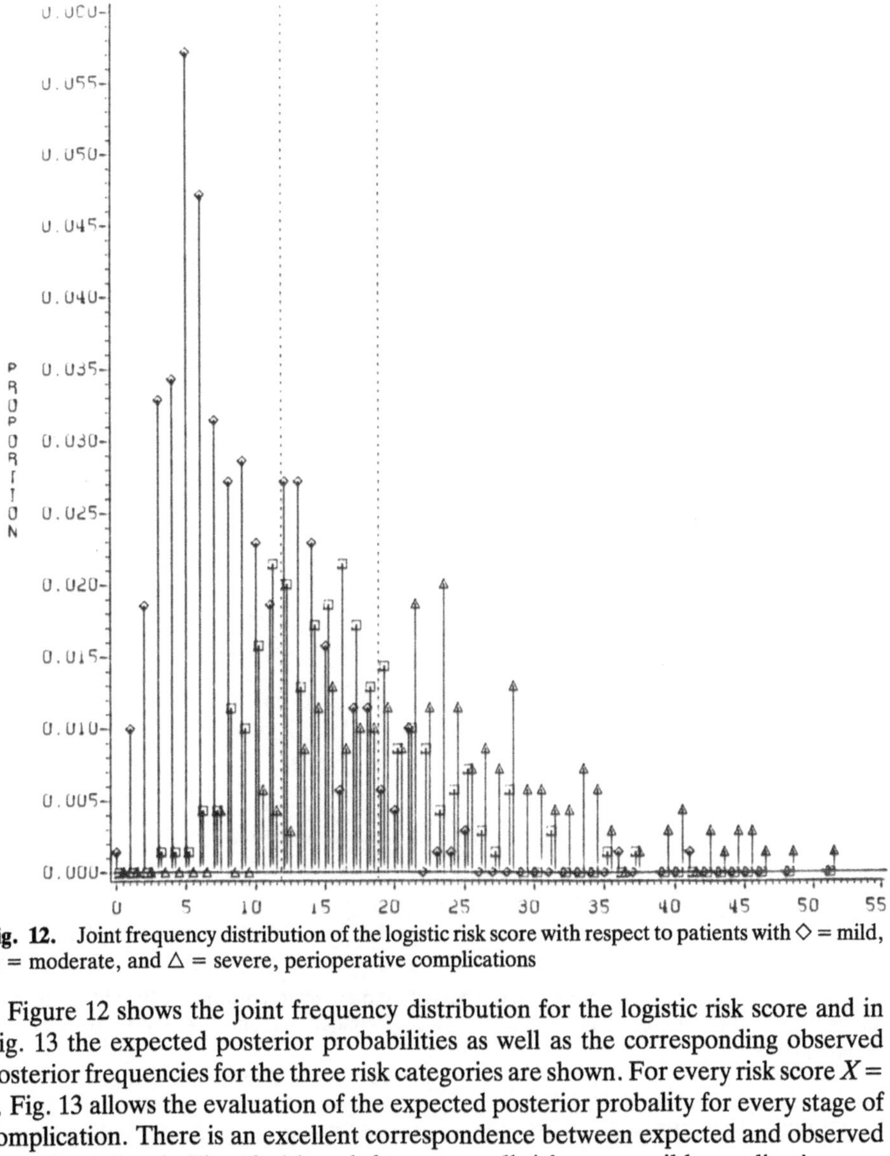

Fig. 12. Joint frequency distribution of the logistic risk score with respect to patients with ◇ = mild, □ = moderate, and △ = severe, perioperative complications

Figure 12 shows the joint frequency distribution for the logistic risk score and in Fig. 13 the expected posterior probabilities as well as the corresponding observed posterior frequencies for the three risk categories are shown. For every risk score $X = x$, Fig. 13 allows the evaluation of the expected posterior probality for every stage of complication. There is an excellent correspondence between expected and observed posterior values in Fig. 13 although for very small risk scores mild complications are slightly underestimated while moderate ones are overestimated.

Even though a two-dimensional graphic presentation of the criteria of goodness of decision is impossible in the event of more than two complication categories, optimal decisions can still be made using the expected posterior probabilitis shown in Fig. 13.

Depending on the desired criterion of optimality (see second section), the cut-off points x_0 and x_1 can be chosen from Fig. 13. If accuracy is to be maximized the cut-off points are ascertainable from the expected posterior probabilities

$$P(r_0 | x_0) = P(r_1 | x_0)$$

and

$$P(r_1 | x_1) = P(r_2 | x_1)$$

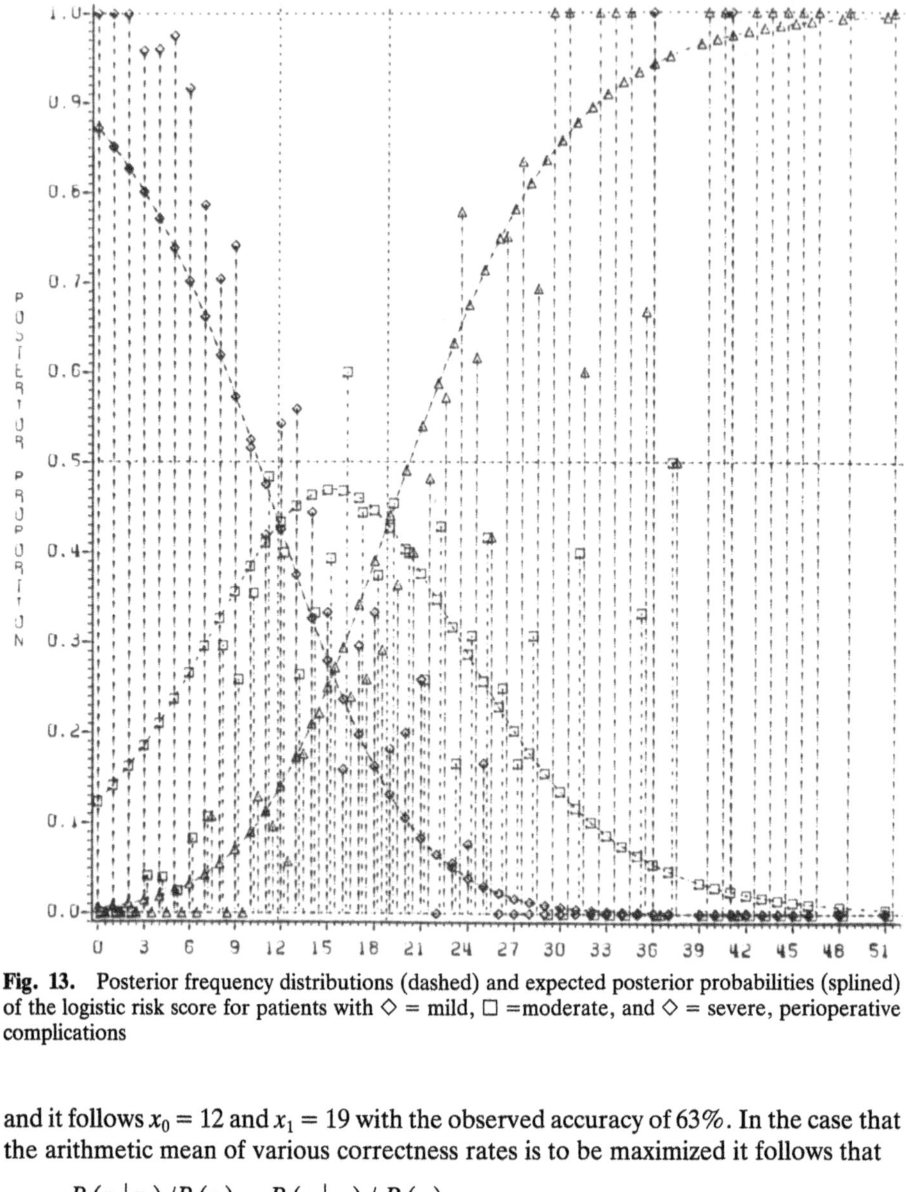

Fig. 13. Posterior frequency distributions (dashed) and expected posterior probabilities (splined) of the logistic risk score for patients with ◇ = mild, □ =moderate, and ◇ = severe, perioperative complications

and it follows $x_0 = 12$ and $x_1 = 19$ with the observed accuracy of 63%. In the case that the arithmetic mean of various correctness rates is to be maximized it follows that

$$P(r_0|x_0)/P(r_0) = P(r_1|x_0)/P(r_1)$$

and

$$P(r_1|x_1)/P(r_1) = P(r_2|x_1)/P(r_2)$$

This leads (see Fig. 13) to the cut-off points $x_0 = 10$ and $x_1 = 18$. The corresponding classification matrix is shown in Table 2. One gets an observed correctness rate of 61% for mild, 48% for moderate, 77% severe complications and an accuracy of 61%.

In ordinal classification, the logistic risk score shows a better performance than the Mannheim risk score, especially in the separation of mild and moderate complications.

Selection of Relevant Prognostic Variables

An advantage in applying mathematical procedures to the field of prognostics and diagnostics consists in the presentation of strategies for selecting the relevant prognostic variables. Such methods allow the relevant variables to be chosen from a set of possible prognostic variables without loss of information for the prognostic statement. This reduction of dimensionality of the variable space reduces the diagnostic effort and allows optimal decisions to be made with a minimal use of resources. The application of such selection procedures is intended to make the underlying prognostic process more objective and therefore possibility lead to a better understanding of this process. With regard to Habbema and Gelpke (1981), in order to perform a selection of variables at least four choices must be made: the strategy of selection; the criterion of optimality for selecting variables; the rule for terminating selection; and the statistical assumption about the probality distributions of underlying data. We want to apply such stragegies of selection using the preoperative Mannheim checklist.

Table 3 shows the coefficients of regression b_i as well as their asymptotic standard deviations s_{b_i} according to the logistic risk score with binary and ordered complication rating. Since the estimation was carried out with aid of the maximum likelihood method, the coefficients of regression can be regarded as asymptotically normally distributed. Therefore, using simple Student's t-tests, the hypothesis can be proven whether the true coefficients of regression differ from zero. The tests of all coefficients of regression with ranks 1 to 10 lead to significant results, using a significance level of $\alpha = 5\%$ (see table 3). However, taking into account the problem of multiple comparison, we must apply the sequential Bonferroni-Holm procedure Holm 1979. If we fix the overall significance level $\alpha = 5\%$, this then leads to the result that only the variables with ranks 1 to 9 make a contribution to the prognosis.

The described procedure for selection of relevant prognostic variables can be applied only to the logistic discriminant analysis since only here the standard deviations (and correlations) of the regression parameters can be evaluated. The usual procedure of variable selection (Habbema and Gelpke 1981; Krishnaiah and Kanal 1982) is the stepwise selection approach which is performed either forwards or backwards. If we use the maximum likelihood function as a criterion of optimality, all stepwise selection procedures conclude that variables with the ranks 10 to 14 (see Table 3) do not show a significant ($\alpha = 5\%$) increase of the likelihood function. Therefore, they make no contribution to the improvement of the goodness of adaptation of the expected posterior probability to the observed data. Without significant loss of information, it suffices to use only the variables with the ranks 1 to 9 for purposes of preoperative prognostics of perioperative risks. The most important prognostic variables (see Table 3) are blood pressure range, expected surgery time, localisation of surgery, hemoglobin, cardiac efficiency, condition of respiration, and age. No contribution to the goodness of prediction is made by the kidney status, the liver status, the acid-base status and myocardial infarction time.

The last finding is noteworthy. It was found that of the 700 observed patients only a very few cases occurred having had a myocardial infarction within the last two years ($n = 8$), the last year ($n= 2$), the last six months ($n = 4$) or the last three months ($n = 5$) before the operation. Since the collected data came from four general surgery theaters, it is possible that cardiac infarction patients, as well as burn patients ($n = 5$), are not adequately represented in the present dataset.

Here the general problem of the probability of risk scores between several hospitals arises. Since every hospital, due to its specific diagnostic and therapeutic program shows a specific patient structure, it is necessary to adapt the risk score individually to these features and validate it for each hospital. Therefore, a computer aided evaluation and validation of prognostic risk scores is only significant if a respesentative recording of all operations in a hospital is carried out within the framework of a cohort study.

To avoid parameter estimation bias when using techniques of discrimination, one part of the dataset should be regarded as a training sample for selection of variables and evaluation of posterior probability and the part other of the dataset should be treated as a test sample to validate the evaluated risk score.

Conclusion

Since hardly any methodical literature exists on the principles of evaluation and validation of perioperative risk scores this paper attempts to show some mathematical basis of computer aided prognosis and to illustrate them using the preoperative risk checklist at Mannheim as an example.

The posterior probability of the risk is identified as the most important criterion for individual prognostic assertions as well as for objective therapeutic decision-making support. It seems to be necessary, in the evaluation and validation of perioperative risk scores to show the observed posterior frequency distribution along with the observed joint distribution of the score values in order to be able to judge whether a risk score has good prognostic properties.

The application of techniques of discriminant analysis in the evaluation of prognostic scores was shown to be successful in prediction performance as well as in decision performance whereby, a simple functional relationship between risk score and expected risk is established.

The advantage in using computer aided methods in a prognistic framework is especially seen in the prediction of ordinal scaled risks a well as in the selection of relevant prognostic variables.

References

Afifi AA, Sacks ST, Liv VY, Weil MH, Schubin H (1971) Accumulative prognostic index for patients with barbiturate, glutethimide und meprobamete intoxication. N Engl J Med 285 27: 1497–1502

Anderson JA, Philips PR (1981) Regression, discrimination and measurement models for ordered categorical variables. Appl Stat 33: 22–31

Apgar V (1953) A proposal for a new method of evaluation of the newborn infant. Curr Res Anaesth Analg 32: 260–267

ASA (1968) New classification of physical status. Anesthesiology 24: 11

Crandon AJ, Peel KR, Anderson JA, Thompson V, McNicol GP (1980a) Postoperative deep vein thrombosis: identifying high-risk patients. Br Med J 2: 343–344

Crandon AJ, Peel KR, Anderson JA, Thompson V, McNicol GP (1980) Prophylaxis of postoperative deep vein thrombosis: selective use of low-lose heparin in high-risk patients. Br Med J 2: 345–347
DeDombal FT, Gremy F (eds) (1976) Decision making and medical care. North Holland, Amsterdam
Feldmann U, Osswald MP, Johann A (1984) Einsatz der logistischen Diskriminanzanalyse zur Prognostik postoperativer Komplikationen mit ordinaler Risiko-Skalierung. In: Wagner G (ed) Der Beitrag der Informationsverarbeitung zum Fortschritt der Medizin. Springer, Berlin, Heidelberg, New York (Med. Informatik und Statistik, vol 50) 267–280
Goldmann L, Caldera L, Nussbaum SR et al. (1977) Multifactorial Index of cardiac risk in noncardiac surgical procedures. N Engl J Med 297 16: 845–849
Habbema JDF, Gelpke GJ (1981) A computer program for selection of variables in diagnostic and prognostic problems. Comput Programs Biomed 13: 251–170
Holm S (1979) A simple sequentially rejective multiple test procedure. Scand J Statist 6: 65–70
Keene AR, Cullan DJ (1983) Therapeutic intervention scoring system, Update 1983. Crit Care Med 11: 1–3
Krishnaiah PR, Kanal LN (eds) (1982) Handbook of statistics, vol 2. Classification, pattern recognition and reduction of dimensionality. North Holland, Amsterdam
Lachenbruch PA, Goldstein M (1979) Discriminant analysis. Biometrics 35: 69–85
Lutz H, Peter K (1973) Das Risiko der Anästhesie unter operativen Bedingungen. Langenbecks Arch Chir 334: 671–679
Peter K, Lutz H (1973) Präoperative Befunderhebung. Langenbecks Arch Chir 334: 681–687
Titterington DM, Murray GD, Murray LS, Spiegelhalter DJ, Skeene AM, Habbema JDF, Gelpke GJ (1981) Comparison of discrimination techniques applied to a complex data set of head injured patients (with discussion). J Stat Soc Series A 144: 145–175
Wald A (1950) Statistical decision functions. Wiley, New York
Wassner UJ, Timm J (1976) Zur präoperativen Ermittlung der Wahrscheinlichkeit einer pulmokardialen Insuffizienz nach Lungenresektion. Chirurg 47: 602–605

New Tasks for Medical Informatics?

C. O. KÖHLER

Theses

1. The *interdependence* of all fields of sciences is growing stronger and stronger.
2. Further progress in medicine can no longer be envisaged without *interdisciplinary work* (medicine, biology, chemistry, physics, biochemistry, informatics, mathematics).
3. The main problem of further progress is the *recognition of structures,* i.e., of biological structures as well as of transitionary structures of our knowledge.
4. The *detailed knowledge* of biological-medical facts and functions is growing larger and larger. Combining this knowledge and forming a new, overriding knowledge will be an essential task for the future (Köhler 1982).

Introduction

To be a researcher with comprehensive knowledge, as we knew them in the past, is no longer feasible today. Due to the immense growth of detailed knowledge (thesis 4), no researcher, however eminent, can do without the help of specialists from his own or from other fields of science. Research work is developing into team work to an ever increasing extent. This is not only a statement but also a request, for valuable research work would be wasted if every scientist had to acquire detailed knowledge from the necessary marginal fields.

By way of example I want to cite the development of the computer tomograph. Without the detailed knowledge of physicians, physicists, engineers, information scientists and mathematicians, working together in a team, such a device could not have been developed and constructed. Further progress in medicine can only be attained by interdisciplinary work in such a team. This statement can be illustrated by a further example, the data processing of biosignals (as required in intensive care, for instance).

What has been said for CT and biosignal data processing applies to practically any field of medicine, be it virology, urology or cardiology, to name but a few, and from which examples of very interesting interdisciplinary work are known to me. Prosthetics and endoprosthetics, for instance, are a promising field for the future. Here I want to cite as a relatively simple example the development of prostheses for joints. Next to orthopedists and ceramics experts, engineers, information scientists and other medical specialists have worked on the development of such relatively simple prostheses as, for example, the hip joint. The problem of developing an artificial knee joint – another seemingly simple example – forms a transition to thesis No. 3: the recognition of structures.

Structures and Their Recognition

Let me, to begin with, say a few general words on the subject of "structure". What does "structure" mean or, better, what actually is a "structure"? "Texture", "construction," "internal classification," "order," all these are explanations from the dictionary but none of them, in my opinion, in itself sufficiently describes the actual meaning of the word "structure." By "structure" I myself also understand the "purposeful order," the "purposeful texture," but, of course, one can engage into long deliberations and discussions about the concept "purposeful." Purposeful, for whom or for what? Who presents the criteria for "purposeful?" Is it possible that the semantic contents of "purposeful" may change in the course of time? It would be presumptuous of me to even begin to try and answer these questions in the short time of my lecture. In order to create a basis for further deliberation, let me define the concept "purposeful" "as not accidental, and obeying and overriding purpose".

Structure – especially in the biological and medical field – is thus a non-accidental texture obeying an overriding purpose totally and in all its parts. However, it must be doubted whether with the complete recognition of all biological and medical structures "the experience of life as such and thus also its mental significance" can be explained. This somewhat modified sentence by Schipperges (1983a) may be drastically clarified by a citation from Lichtenberg (1970): "The most perfect ape cannot draw an ape; this can only be achieved by man, but only man considers this to be an advantage."

Structure must also be seen in the course of time. Structure can, so-to-speak, be considered as being four-dimensional. In biology all processes are controlled by one and one only quite definite three-dimensional structure. Thus, new or already existing three-dimensional structures are created again and again. These structural transitions and structural linkages are energy dependent. It will, of course, have to be taken into consideration that energy in all its manifestations, in particular for instance in the form of binding energy in molecules, of which little is known so far, is considered as belonging to the four dimensions.

In biological systems, too – not to mention physical and chemical systems (Prigogini 1979) – it is frequently the case that under certain parameter constellations, structures are formed as pulsating processes. In medicine many such rhythms are known (Gai 1981). "Life is rhythm," this sentence by Heraklit can be applied to biochemical processes (e.g., circadian rhythms), to physiological processes (e.g., heart beat) as well as to being born, dying and possibly reincarnation.

Medicine and biology as sciences are as yet far from being able to recognize all the structures at work in them. Neither is it possible to name the percentage of structures already known since not even the total quantity of all structures can be summed up. The ascent of Mount Everest might be used as an analogy to the solution of this task, when one may find oneself at the first 10 cm or the first 10 m without even knowing whether one is ascending the right mountain.

Taking into account this somewhat provocatice, pessimistic attitude, it can be understood how demanding my request actually is, even if we are optimistic enough to believe that we have already reached a hight of 4000 m. Perhaps we share the fate of the Chinese who believed themselves to be quite close to the peak several thousand years ago. Seen from the present western point of view, it was but a side peak.

Scientific progress has always caused us to change our opinion as it had been taught us. Le me give you an example from my own specialty: Charles Babbage, (1864) who was first to invent a computer, in his memoirs *Passages from the Life of a Philosopher* wrote in the middle of the last century, contrary to the general opinion of this contemporaries, that he was not afraid to lose his reputation to those who came 50 years after him. He judged the development too optimistically. It took almost 100 years before we were able to put his epoch-making ideas into practice.

The starting point of general deliberations about "structures" was the development of an artificial knee joint. You all know that we are as yet far from being able to produce a satisfactory substitute. Why not? Our technology has reached such a state of excellence. Obviously because we have not yet fully recognized the procedural and static structures of the knee joint and their functions. Almost all the structures of the build-up of the knee and the process of its functions are on a macroscopic level, but how is the situation on the microscopic level and even on finer structures? I already mentioned the example of the recognition and explanation of the binding energy in molecules. Even if we already had at our disposal assumptions or sufficient approaches in the form of algorithms or mathematical models for the solution of this set of problems, none of today's computers would be in a position to calculate these even approximately. Specialists have worked out that, with today's algorithms and computers, many centuries would be required for the solution of such problems (Hossfeld 1983).

In thesis 3 I also used the word "transitionary structures of our knowledge." What do I want to imply by this? Research cannot surrender, if faced by seemingly unsoluble tasks. It never did. Otherwise we would still find ourselves in the stone age. Therefore, we are forced to pretend with our present state of the art that the known structures are "true" and consider them as standards for our further work. I call these structures "transitional structures." The problems of "standards" and of "standardization" are to be briefly touched upon.

Standardization

While in the first part "structure" was discussed as an object concept, this paragraph uses the corresponding term "standard" in its dynamic, i.e., to be executed, form "standardization." This linguistic dissonance is intended. Structure is something that exists, "structurization" is not given to man. We can only describe already existing structures if we have recognized them previously. However, we are able, with more or less difficulty, to set up standards and to exercise standardization. We even have to do so.

What does "standard" mean? "Standard" is "average pattern," "normal measure." What is "normal" in medicine? This is a question which has occupied generations of physicians at many meetings, but they have not come much closer to answering this question after so many years. "Standardization" is "unification according to patterns." According to which "patterns?" According to the pattern of a structure, and then – see above.

Standardization would, therefore, no longer be necessary if all structures were known. Standardization is but an aid for the time when we are still forced to work with patterns set up by ourselves and more or less in keeping with reality (transitional structures of our knowledge). If the pattern is no longer correct, standardization will have to begin all over again. The problem is that there is surely an infinite number of patterns with differing grades of recognition in the scientific world. Here, too, "general opinion" plays a decisive part. Of course, we will land in chaos if we do not attempt to create any order at all. Hermann Hesse (1972) says in this connection: "Chaos will have to be recognized, will have to be lived before it can be turned into a new order." The time to do so should have come by now. If we agree on one (or few) standard(s) in order to create the "new order", this does not by any means imply that these must be the "true ones." The word "agree" contains the dynamite already broached in the discussion on structure. One can only reach "agreement" on matters, facts, patterns or structures which have a high degree of probability of being "correct" (Popper 1979). The degree of probability cannot be measured: it is but an assumption by those who want to or should reach an agreement. Would it be measurable, we would know all we are seeking. And then an agreement would no longer be necessary but only "understanding." Accordingly, standardization is merely *one* aid for the recognition of structure. The future will show how effective this aid was or is.

Future Tasks

With regard to theses 1 and 3, I briefly broached the fundamental problems to be solved interdisciplinarily. As far as thesis 4 is concerned, the understanding of the problem is only now slowly being awakened. A complete combination of the ever growing detailed knowledge to attain an overriding knowledge of structure is hardly feasible with today's methods of science and research. Even for the preparatory work for the development of new methods of research the above mentioned scientists are called upon. Economists, sociologists and psychologists should join in this. These probably quite newly conceived methods or tools, of which the contours can partly be recognized but partly have not even been thought of, can also be developed only by interdisciplinary cooperation. Tools already in use but definitely not yet perfect, which, for instance, have also been developed by economists, are methods of "system or problem analyses" respectively of different kinds. Since (rightly so) some of these approaches also consider human behaviour, the way of human thinking (which cannot yet be explained), the forms of cooperation and the strategies in the exchange of knowledge, ideas (as prestages of knowledge) and again strategies themselves, sociologists and psychologists also play a part.

A further approach to new tools are the "expert systems." Naturally, expert systems can only be built up by experts from several specialities of special science (who set up the "rules") and by informaticians (who develop the algorithms for processing these rules). And there are, of course, the information scientists who build the required computers.

Let me, on the basis of what is known so far (or at least known by the direction of development), speculate a little as to what might result in the future. This is certainly utopia at the present time, but electricity, aeroplane, computer and nerve-controlled prosthesis (to mention only a few) were also utopia at one time ore other. I can imagine that, for instance, there will in future be systems which will develop the "rules" – premised in the exact systems – independently. Such systems will be able to draw the necessary knowledge from facts (published in whatever way). The great problem will be to decide which facts are to be used. The valuation of facts in the medical-biological field has so far been governed by "general opinion." I have remarked on this before. One will have to endeavour to objectify general opinion, again with the aid of systems. Such interlocking and interconnected systems would be able to combine the latest detailed knowledge into structure of overriding knowledge continuously.

A further possibility could be to show to researchers, on the basis of the above mentioned systems, new problems resulting for one thing from the present state of the art, but which also (due to this knowledge) may be successfully solved. Moreover, such a system might also suggest ways to a solution. The decision as to which way the solution should be chosen is up to the researcher, but here, too, he could employ the above mentioned systems. This is then a strongly recursive process as already is used in informatics today.

There are surely many more approaches which are not yet entirely feasible today. We can only arrive at new lines of thought and thus at new methods and thus at new knowledge if we continue to use our imagination (or do so again?). In my opinion, in today's research, be it at the university, in big science institutions, in large industrial undertakings, the forms of organization and thus research itself have become far too encrusted and burdened by problems of quantity (e.g. the number of students at the universities, but also by the mere number of occuring problems).

It will probably be necessary for us to arrive at new configurations in the forms of organization of research. Trends can be seen in the USA as well as in Europe. A. Toffler (1981) showed the way, which we will probably go in the future sociologically and thus also in research. In my opinion, we will need far more people like Toffler and Illich who will show us the roads we can tread with greater effectiveness, with greater efficiency but also with greater humanity. The new forms of organization and rule required are again based not last on a further knowledge of the structures in natural sciences and sociology. Let me conclude my lecture with a quotation from Lichtenberg (1970) again:

"Before God there are only rules (structures), actually only one rule (structure) and no exceptions. Because we do not know the uppermost rule (structure), we create general rules (structures) which are not rules (structures); it might even be possible that what we call rules (structures) can be exceptions for finite beings."

References

Babbage C (1864) Passages from the life of a philosopher. Longman and Green, London

Gai S (1981) Rhythmen in Biologie und Medizin. Diplom-Arbeit, Fachbereich Medizinische Informatik, Univ. Heidelberg / FH Heilbronn

Hesse H (1972) Schriften zur Literatur, vol 2 Suhrkamp, Frankfurt
Hossfeld (1983) Die Zukunft der Datenverarbeitung. Vortrag anläßlich der Inbetriebnahme des Vektorrechners der Universität Karlsruhe im Rechenzentrum der Universität Karlsruhe
Köhler CO (1982) Ziele, Aufgaben, Realisation eines Krankenhaus-Informationssystems. Springer, Berlin Heidelberg New York
Lichtenberg GC (1970) Ausgewählte Werke. (ed by Johann E) Gutenberg, Frankfurt
Popper KR (1979) Die beiden Grundprobleme der Erkenntnistheorie. Mohr, Tübingen
Prigogine I (1979) Vom Sein zum Werden. Piper, Munich
Schipperges H (1983a) Information, Intelligenz, Intuition. Zum semantischen Bezugsfeld der Datensprache. In: Köhler CO, Böhm K, Thome R (eds) Aktuelle Methoden der Information in der Medizin, vol 2, Informationsverarbeitung im Gesundheitswesen. ecomed, Landsberg, pp. 49–58
Schipperges H (1983b) Epidemiologisches und Epistemologisches. In: Köhler CO, (ed) Gustav Wagner -65. pp 29–34, DKFZ, Heidelberg
Toffler A (1981) The third wave. Bantam Books, New York
Wolff HP (1983) Wenn der Tod als Betriebsunfall verdrängt wird. Frankfurter Allgemeine Zeitung 3 September 1983

Artificial Intelligence: the Expert Systems Approach to Medical Consultation

E. H. Shortliffe and L. M. Fagan

Introduction

For over two decades, the field of artificial intelligence (AI) has focused on developing symbolic models of human inference. Recently these computing techniques and themes have come together to form what is now known as "expert systems research" (Buchanan 1982; Duda and Shortliffe 1983). This brief report reviews AI and expert systems to acquaint the reader with the field and to suggest advantages that these techniques may offer to computer systems for advanced medical monitoring.

Knowledge Engineering

Artificial intelligence is the subfield of computer science devoted to developing programs with an ability to reason symbolically (rather than by combining numbers statistically or by using other numerical manipulations). Related assumptions are that such programs should ultimately be able to acquire new knowledge and to apply it appropriately. They should also be able to manipulate and communicate ideas.

The AI subfield of particular relevance to the study of medical decision making is the construction of expert advice systems that provide consultations using knowledge acquired from experts in a domain. Computers have long been used to store data, but isolated data points do not become knowledge until they have been analyzed and summarized. Factual knowledge that may be derived from data is only one kind of knowledge required for expert problem solving, however. Also required is judgmental knowledge – the kind that experts recognize is based on their own experience but which may be difficult to verify without complex and time-consuming studies. In addition, expert decision makers use common sense knowledge that is symbolic in nature and reflects simple shared world experience. Also pertinent is strategic or heuristic knowledge – the kind of knowledge that often distinguishes an expert from a well trained novice. Examples include an anesthesiologist's favorite method for selecting an optimal anesthetic agent for a compromised patient or a cardiologist's favorite technique for choosing the diagnostic tests by which to assess a patient with a new complaint of chest pain. Expert judgment, combined with a "strategic plan", can accordingly be used to adapt a program to idiosyncratic situations. The challenge is to build expert advice systems that contain and utilize all the types of knowledge outlined here.

An expert system, then, is a computer program that contains and can apply specialized knowledge. It uses this knowledge to make suggestions to users who may not have the full range of expertise available to the system. An expert system functions as an interface between the intended user of the system and the domain expert (or experts) who collaborated in its construction. Building such programs is known as "knowledge engineering" (Feigenbaum 1977; Michie 1973) and typically requires close collaboration between human experts in a field and computer scientists familiar with expert systems research.

Issues in Knowledge Engineering

Knowledge Representation

We have mentioned at least four kinds of knowledge that an expert system requires to provide specialized consultation. An active area of AI research is the development of new techniques to encode and manipulate such symbolic knowledge. Common methods for knowledge representation include production rules, frames, semantic networks, and combinations of these (Winston 1977). Most knowledge can be encoded in whatever formalism a designer wishes. However, the last decade's research has taught us that, whatever representation technique is used, it should ideally do the following:

- Provide explanations that convey a line of reasoning that a user can understand and critique.
- Separate domain knowledge from the program itself so that knowledge can be revised without making changes to the computer program.
- Assure transparency and a level of performance such that an expert can easily identify and correct faults in the knowledge.
- Adopt an inferential method such that the system reliably reaches excellent decisions by using its knowledge appropriately.

Many medical expert systems have taken advantage of the expressive power of a representation technique known as production rules (Davis and King 1976). A production rule is a conditional statement that indicates the circumstances under which a particular conclusion may be drawn. One system known as MYCIN (Davis et al. 1977; Shortliffe 1976), used about 500 such rules dealing with the diagnosis and treatment of bacteremia and meningitis to give advice about antimicrobial therapy. The rules were encoded in a stylized language that the computer could interpret. In addition, routines were written to translate the rules into English so that they could be used to explain system decisions to the users.

As is true in other complex domains, human actions and beliefs in medicine interact with common sense and with precise knowledge in ways that defy simple delineation. The challenge at this stage in the development of expert systems is, therefore, to constrain the task realistically so that the program is tenable but still allows useful decisions for solving real problems. For example, we have found that production rules need substantial modification to deal with decisions in settings like medical monitoring where parameters change rapidly and analyses of temporal trends are crucial (Fagan 1980).

Knowledge Acquisition

As researchers gain experience in constructing consultation systems, identifying and encoding expert knowledge has been perceived as one of the most complex and arduous tasks encountered. Experts often have difficulty distilling their knowledge, and, because there are other major problems in identifying and encoding knowledge, the most appropriate domains for expert systems research at this time may therefore be fields in which the knowledge is already highly structured and well specified.

Models of Reasoning

Once knowledge has been captured from experts, books, or other sources, and once it has been encoded, the program must have an effective method to search through the knowledge base for relevant facts and to tie them together in ways that simulate human reasoning. Two issues result: control of the reasoning process and management of uncertainty.

Control of the Reasoning Process

Reasoning methods in artificial intelligence systems fall into several categories (Nilsson 1980; Shortliffe 1984). *Goal-directed reasoning* is the term for the control process used in many rule-based systems, including MYCIN (Buchanan and Shortliffe 1984). The approach is called "goal-directed" because predefined goals provide the initial focus, and rules are involved or questions asked in an effort to achieve a specific goal. The conditional statements in the rules initially invoked define a new set of subgoals, and additional rules may then be invoked in an effort to achieve these subgoals. The process is applied recursively, and entire reasoning networks can accordingly be generated from a single initial goal.

When reasoning is based on observations rather than goals, problem solving proceeds forward – from data to conclusions – in what is known as *data-driven reasoning*. Many expert systems use this alternative approach, and there are psychological data to suggest that "forward reasoning" more closely approximates the way human beings solve complex problems. As data become available to the reasoning system, the observations evoke certain inference rules which, if they succeed, allow new conclusions to be reached. The resulting conclusions may themselves evoke additional rules, and so on. No specific goal guides the reasoning process; the data that are entered "drive" the rules and, at completion, the system can make available whatever conclusions have been reached. This form of reasoning is particularly relevant for medical monitoring applications in which physiological data are routinely acquired from sensors and can be used to drive the inference process.

Another reasoning strategy more closely parallels the form of problem solving demonstrated by human decision makers when they are observed in psychological experiments. This approach, known as *hypothesis-directed reasoning,* begins with data-directed inference based on initial case descriptors. This initial data set "evokes" a set of hypotheses that are then used to guide data collection. The well-known INTERNIST program for medical diagnosis uses a reasoning strategy of this type (Miller et al. 1982).

Management of Uncertainty

When individual inference steps are not certain, a level of complexity is added to the interpretation of conclusions reached by an intelligent program. Not only are conventions needed to assign weights to the rules, but also, when two or more pieces of evidence support the same conclusion, some mechanism is needed to determine the net strength of the hypothesis. Expert system researchers have found that formal probability theory is less than satisfactory for these purposes, although some have attempted to adapt it to symbolic reasoning systems (Duda et al. 1978). In rulebased systems the need to combine pieces of evidence regarding a single hypothesis, but derived from a number of different rules, may require a numeric system to capture and represent an expert's measure of belief regarding the inference stated in the rules. Conditional probabilities were not adequate for this purpose in MYCIN, for example. That program accordingly used a specialized scoring scheme of numerical weights called certainty factors to encode the strengths of the conclusions in rules (Shortliffe and Buchanan 1975).

Generation of Good Advice

The ultimate test of the validity of the model of reasoning used in an expert system is its ability to reach accurate conclusions and thereby to give valuable advice. Some researchers do not believe it will be possible for computer-based consultants to function at the level of human experts until we better understand and model the inferences used by intelligent problem solvers. Others argue that the details of a reasoning model are not important as long as the system reaches good decisions and can explain its reasoning in understandable terms. However, psychological studies of human problem solving, e.g., Elstein's work in the field of medicine (Elstein et al. 1978) are being studied increasingly by knowledge engineers as they attempt to develop systems that are more robust.

Explanation of Decisions

As we have stressed, a crucial aspect of the interaction between an expert and his client is the ability of the non-expert to request explanations regarding the recommendation received. Our group recently surveyed several hundred physicians and found that they cited explanation as a principal requirement for a clinically acceptable computer-based consultation (Teach and Shortliffe 1980). In fact, most physicians felt that explanation is more important than absolute accuracy, presumably because they believed the latter is unrealistic. If a program can explain the basis for its conclusions, users can examine the reasoning carefully and decide for themselves whether to follow that advice. We believe this is important for an expert system in medicine; consultation programs are *tools* for use by individuals who are highly trained and unwilling to turn over their decisions to a computer program, regardless of how well it has been validated.

Validation

As expert systems have begun to mature, techniques have become necessary to demonstrate that they can perform as an expert in the field. One lesson of early evaluation experiments has been that the design of such experiments is itself an area of research interest; a number of specific points are pertinent.

First, any evaluation is difficult because there is so much difference of opinion in medicine, *even among experts*. Hence, it is unclear how to select a standard by which to measure the system's performance. Actual clinical outcome cannot be used because each patient is treated in only one way and because a poor outcome in a gravely ill patient cannot necessarily be ascribed to poor selection of therapy.

Second, evaluations of systems like MYCIN have suggested that it is important to control for any bias that evaluators may harbor against computer-based decision aids. One approach is to design studies in which evaluators are unaware which recommendations were offered by an advice system and which came from expert physicians (Yu et al. 1979). This approach eliminates the bias and provides a more useful estimate of how the computer's performance compares with that of the domain experts.

Eventually, other questions must be answered regarding medical expert systems. Each question requires its own evaluation. Is the system used? If so, do the users follow the system's advice? If so, does the user benefit from the encounter with the system? Will the system be costeffective? What are the legal implications in the use of, or failure to use, such systems? The answers to these questions are years away for most consultation systems but ultimately are just as important as whether the methodology leads to accurate and reliable advice.

Generalization

We mentioned earlier the importance of separating the knowledge in an expert system from the program that processes that knowledge and generates the advice. One reason for this separation is the ease with which information can be added or corrected. Many expert systems include "editors" that allow a knowledge engineer to modify the knowledge base without having to change the program in any way.

There is a second advantage. One can imagine the development of interchangeable knowledge bases, each driven by the same program. Each knowledge base would have to be structured in accordance with the conventions required by the program, but once this were accomplished, a single program could generate advice in a number of different domains. This area of active research is known as "generalization" or the development of "system building tools" (Nii and Aiello 1979; van Melle 1980). The key idea is to develop a general purpose program that can be used by knowledge engineers to build an expert system in a new domain. Such programs must define conventions for the representation of knowledge and for the inferential models. The builders of systems must in turn comply with these conventions.

Relevance of Expert Systems for Medical Monitoring Applications

Patient monitoring applications have only recently begun to look to artifical intelligence techniques for useful methodologies. An early example was the Ventilator Manager (VM) program (Fagan 1980; Fagan et al. 1980) which monitored physiological parameters from post-surgical patients and provided advice on how best to wean them from ventilatory support. The VM work suggests that symbolic processing approaches are highly relevant for applications in critical care monitoring settings. A major challenge, however, is to develop improved methods for managing temporal inference and for recognizing trends, simultaneous events, or patterns that occur repetitively or sequentially.

Setting a Context for Data Interpretation

The Ventilator Manager program was designed to provide a context in which numeric data from monitoring devices could be interpreted flexibly. For example, a model of "ventilatory mode" was developed and used to guide the system's interpretation of parameters such as heart rate, end-tidal CO_2, and tidal volume. Assessing context is problematic, however, when one has to assume that only a small amount of descriptive non-numeric information about a patient will be available (as is generally the case in a monitoring environment where personnel are not likely to keep the system constantly informed about those patient data that are unavailable directly from the monitoring devices). The context, therefore, must be inferred from some of the numerical information which is, in turn, used to interpret the remaining data. For example, certain sudden changes in airway parameters can generally be interpreted as the context "suctioning the patient" and the interpretation of cardiac and hemodynamic parameters are then interpreted in light of this new clinical situation. This high level model of the patients' current state can be used to help in the analysis of trends in measurements. e. g., to provide a basis for predicting difficulties, to allow for selective tracking of "problems" as opposed to measurements, and to provide a more clinical orientation for subsequent collection of data.

Simulating the Flexibility of Expert Reasoning

Symbolic processing can merge mathematical analysis with judgment or "intelligence" similar to that of an expert. For example, the VM program often throws out data because a sensor is operating outside its limits of reliability or is improperly connected. When the trend concerning a suspect time period is examined, the unreliable data are ignored, much as they would be by an experienced clinician observing the same trend information. Similarly, recognition that the clinical situation drastically changed in the immediate past can be used to tag as dubious any conclusions made by an averaging function applied to current data. VM determines the utility of "recent" measurements based on how quickly the clinical situation is changing.

Facilitating Statements Of Expectations

The ultimate goal of a computer-based monitoring system is to predict problems before they happen rather than to "alarm" as difficulties arise. As noted above, providing a context is the first step towards reaching that goal. A system like VM can be provided with a mechanism for adjusting the acceptable limits for one or more variables based on recent events interpreted by the program. Other AI programs also address this problem, e.g., programs for military signal analysis and speech understanding can set up "future expectations" and then perform an analysis that is triggered when future expectations are not realized.

Providing an Ability to Select Relevant Data for Analysis

AI allows for a selective evaluation of measured data. Many approaches to the interpretation of data have concentrated on selecting the "most important variable" or on creating a "figure of merit index" that tries to summarize difficulties into one specific number. Symbolic reasoning approaches can allow the expert physician to specify a wide variety of relations between variables, or between variables and other available information. As always, using knowledge about the current clinical context can be used to guide the evaluation of rules and, thereby, to draw attention to specific relations only when they are important. A single index can be replaced with specific subtopics, e.g., "hemodynamic status", and with their relations to therapeutic goals, e.g.,"the hemodynamics have not been stable long enough to suggest removing ventilatory support." A central goal is to turn a large amount of data into useful diagnostic conclusions supported by logically referenced specific numerical data.

Summary

A decade's experience with medical expert systems research has led to an understanding of additional requirements for symbolic processing approaches to medical decision making. These include extending the knowledge base beyond the facts necessary for expert performance, providing a superstructure for organizing large numbers of inferential rules, and extending the inferential aids to include assistance throughout the patient's clinical course. For medical decision aids in critical care environments or other dynamic situations, programs cannot depend on interactions with the clinical users. Furthermore, they must handle data that are changing over time and may be episodically absent or spurious. Such systems must also be able to track the patient's status during the course of disease or in response to therapy. Although major research issues remain, recent experiments have suggested that knowledge engineering techniques can be adapted to dynamic clinical settings such as monitoring patients in the intensive care unit.

Acknowledgment. This paper is an abridged and updated version of a longer article that appeared under the title "Expert systems research: modelling the medical decision making progress" in *An Integrated Approach to Monitoring* (J. S. Gravenstein, R. S. Newbower, A. K. Ream, and N. T. Smith, eds.), pp. 183–200, (Woburn, M. A.: Butterworth's), 1983.

References

Buchanan BG (1982) Research on expert systems, In: Machine intelligence, Hayes J, Michie D, Pao YJ (eds) Howard, Chichester, Ellock EW, Michie D (eds)
Buchanan BG, Shortliffe EH (1984) Rule based expert systems: The MYCIN experiments of the Stanford heuristic programming project. Addison-Wesley, Reading MA
Davis R, King J (1976) An overview of production systems. In: Machine representation of knowledge. Wiley and Sons, New York
Davis R, Buchanan BG, Shortliffe EH (1977) Production rules as a representation for a knowledge-based consultation program. Artif Intell 8: 15–45
Duda RO, Shortliffe EH (1983) Expert systems research. Science 220: 261–268
Duda RO, Gaschnig J, Hart PE et al. (1978) Development of the PROSPECTOR consultation system for mineral exploration. Final report SRI Projects 5821 and 6415. SRI International
Elstein AS, Shulman LS, Sprafka SA (1978) Medical problem solving: an analysis of clinical reasoning. Harvard University Press, Cambridge, Mass
Fagan, LM (1980) Representing time-dependent relations in a clinical setting. PH. D. Thesis, Heuristic Programming Project, Stanford University
Fagan LM, Shortliffe EH, Buchanan BG (1980) Computer-based medical decision making: from MYCIN to VM. Automedica 3: 97–106
Feigenbaum EA (1977) The art of artificial intelligence: themes and case studies in knowledge engineering. Proceedings of the 5th International Joint Conference on Artificial Intelligence, Cambridge, Massachusetts, 1977, pp 1014–1029
Michie D (1973) Knowledge engineering. Cybernetics 2: 197–200
Miller RA, Pople HE, Myers JD (1982) INTERNIST-1: An experimental computer-based diagnostic consultant for general internal medicine. N Engl J Med 307: 468–476
Nii HP, Aiello N (1979) AGE (Attempt to Generalize): A knowledge-based program for building knowledge-based programs. Proceedings of the 6th International Joint Conference on Artificial Intelligence, Tokyo, August 1979, pp 645–655
Nilsson NJ (1980) Principles of artificial intelligence. Tioga Menlo Park
Shortliffe EH (1984) Reasoning methods in medical consultation systems: artificial intelligence approaches. Comput Prog Biomed 18
Shortliffe EH (1976) Computer-based medical consultations: MYCIN. Elsevier/North Holland, New York
Shortliffe EH, Buchanan BG (1975) A model of inexact reasoning in medicine. Math Biosci 23: 351–379
Teach RL, Shortliffe EH (1980) An analysis of physician attitudes regarding computer-based consultation systems. Comput Biomed Res 14: 542–558
van Melle W (1980) A domain-independent system that aids in constructing knowledge-based consultation programs. Ph. D. Thesis, Stanford University (Technical Memo HPP-80-11, Heuristic Programming Project)
Winston PH (1977) Artificial intelligence. Addison-Wesley Reading
Yu VL, Fagan LM, Wraith SM et al. (1979) Antimicrobial selection by a computer: a blinded evaluation by infectious disease experts. JAMA 242: 1279–1282

Expert Consultation Systems in Medicine

P. L. Miller

Introduction

An expert medical consultation system is a computer program designed using artificial intelligence (AI) techniques, usually with the goal of assisting a physician with decisions involving patient care.

Research on expert systems (Duda and Shortliffe 1983; Hayes-Roth et al. 1983) is a subfield of artificial intelligence (Winston 1977), a discipline which has been growing and evolving over the past twenty five years. Work on AI has received substantial coverage in the popular press, and has also recently been attracting a great deal of industrial interest for commercial applications.

Over the years, AI techniques have been applied to a wide range of problems, including playing sophisticated games such as chess, "understanding" spoken and written language, robotics, and visual recognition of objects in a scene. Basic research areas in AI also include (a) how best to represent complex real-world knowledge in a machine, (b) how to incorporate "common sense" into computer systems, (c) learning, and (d) the modeling of cognitive processes.

It is difficult to define AI precisely. Usually it is described as the science of developing computer systems which behave or respond in a manner that appears to exhibit intelligence. Implicit in this definition, however, is the understanding that programs which perform purely *numerical* computation, such as scientific computations, do not constitute AI. The type of problems which AI adresses usually involve symbolic (non-numeric) computation.

Expert system research has evolved as subfield of AI over the past fifteen years. An expert system is a computer system designed to operate in a complex, real-world domain. Example domains are geologic analysis (Campbell et al. 1982), computer system design (McDermott 1982), and medicine.

To construct an expert system, a human expert in the field typically interacts with computer specialists over a period of time. During this interaction, he works to make his knowledge ("expertise") explicit to that it can be incorporated into the computer. The ultimate goal is to develop a system which can make expert level judgements and recommendations.

It is interesting that much of the initial research on expert systems was performed in medical domains. In fact, in the mid-1970s the majority of expert systems were medical. In recent years, however, the technology developed building these systems has spread rapidly to many other areas. As a result, medical systems now represent only a modest fraction of expert systems currently being implemented.

Expert Systems in Medicine

Over the past decade a number of expert-systems have been developed in different areas of medicine. (Shortliffe et al. 1979; Kulikowski 1980; Szolovits 1982; Clancey and Shortliffe 1983) These include systems which deal with both diagnosis and medical management. Most of these projects are currently still in the research and development stages. This section gives an overview of a number of wellknown medical expert systems.

Dendral

DENDRAL (Buchanan and Feigenbaum 1978; Lindsay et al. 1980) is a non-clinical expert system which served as a precursor to certain later lines of expert system research. Dendral was developed at Stanford to analyze mass spectrographic and nuclear magnetic resonance data to help in identifying chemical compounds. Since it is able to hypothesize all plausible interpretations of the data, DENDRAL finds structures in a systematic, comprehensive way which humans cannot easily equal.

The MYCIN Systems

Certain of the approaches developed in the DENDRAL project were further refined in MYCIN (Shortliffe 1976; Buchanan and Shortliffe 1983), a consultation system developed in the domain of infectious disease. MYCIN explored the use of "production rules" as a medium for knowledge representation, as discussed more fully in a later section entitled "Flexibility of Knowledge Representation". The domain-independent core of MYCIN was then packaged into EMYCIN ("empty" MYCIN) a system for building expert systems (van Melle 1979). One system built using EMYCIN was PUFF (Aikins et al. 1983), currently in use for interpreting pulmonary function tests.

Two additional projects used the MYCIN infectious disease knowledge base to investigate fundamental aspects of expert system design. The GUIDON/NEOMYCIN project (Clancey and Letsinger 1981; London and Clancey 1982) developed an "expert teaching system" which used MYCIN's knowledge base to explore epistemological issues of sophisticated computer-aided teaching. TEIRESIAS (Davis and Lenat 1982) used MYCIN's rule-based knowledge as a domain to explore issues of knowledge acquisition. This research involved giving a system "meta-knowledge" about its own knowledge, so it could actively help a domain expert update its knowledge base. "Knowledge acquisition" is discussed later.

CASNET and EXPERT

Another center of expert system development is at Rutgers. This work started with CASNET (Kulikowski and Weiss 1971), a system which performed diagnosis in ophtalmology. Next EXPERT (Weiss et al. 1978; Weiss and Kulikowski 1979) was developed, a rule-based system designed to facilitate the development of expert systems in different domains. By incorporating appropriate rules, EXPERT has been applied in diverse areas including endocrinology, and in two systems developed collaboratively at the University of Missouri, AI/COAG (Kingsland et al. 1982) whose domain is coagulation/hematology, and AI/RHEUM (Lindberg et al. 1980; Kingsland and Lindberg 1983) which deals with rheumatology.

A recent interesting extension of EXPERT is a "compiler" which allows the system's rules to be translated onto a microchip. (Weiss et al. 1981) Using this process, SPE, a modest-sized rule-based system which interprets serum protein electrophoresis data, has been incorporated into the hardware of a commercial laboratory instrument.

INTERNIST/CADUCEUS

By far the most ambitious project is the INTERNIST/CADUCEUS system (R. Miller et al. 1982) under development at the University of Pittsburg, which attempts to embrace the whole of internal medicine. Experimental evaluation of the first developmental prototype (INTERNIST-1) using clinicopathological cases from the *New England Journal of Medicine* demonstrated impressive performance. The evaluation, however, also demonstrated the need to incorporate deeper types of knowledge (anatomy, physiology, etc.) into the diagnostic reasoning process. The project is now at work exploring these issues (Pople 1982).

PIP and the Digitalis Advisor

Another varied set of systems has been developed at MIT in conjunction with Tufts Medical School, and other nearby medical centers. PIP (Pauker et al. 1976) explored diagnostic issues in the domain of renal disease. The Digitalis Advisor (Gorry et al. 1978) focused on medical management in the domain of digitalis therapy. ABEL (Patil et al. 1981) has explored acid base and electrolyte disorders, attempting to develop appropriate deep models of underlying processes to guide the system's analysis.

Several Management Systems

Most of the work outlined above has focused primarily on medical diagnosis. Several systems, however, have dealt with medical management, an area which may prove to be particularly fertile for computer assistance. In addition to the Digitalis Advisor mentioned above, two systems which have focused on management are VM (Fagan et al. 1979) which deals with the ventilatory management of a patient receiving respiratory support, and ONCOCIN (Shortliffe et al. 1981) which helps implement oncology protocols. Both of these systems extend the rule-based approach developed in diagnostic systems into medical management.

Also included are two critiquing systems: ATTENDING (Miller 1983a, b) which critiques anesthetic management, and HT-ATTENDING (Miller and Black 1984) which critiques the pharmacologic management of essential hypertension. These two systems are described further in the section on "Critiquing."

Expert Systems: Desired Capabilities

This section discusses the question of how expert systems differ from other computer programs which deal with medical problems. A wide range of computer systems are under development to assist the physician in many areas of medicine. Some of these are based on probabilistic techniques. Most are written using conventional programming techniques, i. e., the step-by-step programming of computer instructions based on flowchart logic.

Expert systems differ from these other, non-AI, systems in a number of ways. The easiest way to characterize the differences is to discuss three design goals which are central to expert system research: (1) flexibility of knowledge representation, (2) explanation capabilities, and (3) knowledge acquisition capabilities.

Flexibility of Knowledge Representation

Perhaps the most important design goal is that an expert system have a very flexible, manipulable knowledge representation. Many expert systems achieve this flexibility by storing their knowledge in the form of "production rules". Such systems are therefore called "rule-based." The wide use of such rules may create the impression that an expert system *must* be based on rules. This is certainly not the case, but nevertheless, many expert systems do indeed use production rules to store their knowledge of their domain.

The following example rule, taken from the MYCIN system (Shortliffe 1976, p. 71) serves to illustrate the flexibility that rules allow. The rule is stored internally as follows:

Premise: (and (Same CNTXT GRAM GRAMPOS)
(Same CNTXT MORPH COCCUS)
(Same CNTXT CONFORM CLUMPS))
Action: (Conclude CNTXT ident STAPHYLOCOCCUS TALLY.7)

An English translation of the rule is shown below:

If: 1. The stain of the organism is GRAMPOS, and
2. the morphology of the organism is COCCUS, and
3. the growth conformation of the organism is CLUMPS
Then: There is suggestive evidence (.7) that the identity of the organism is STAPHYLOCOCCUS.

As can be seen, the rule consists of two parts: a premise and an action. Such a rule can be used to make *inferences*. For instance, if the three conditions in the premise are found to hold, the inference implied by the action can be made. Other rules may include the inference made by this rule as part of their premise. In this way, a chain of inferences can be built up by successive rules, until the system's final conclusions are reached.

A rule-based system contains many such rules. Each rule can be thought of as a "chunk" of knowledge. There are several advantages to structuring knowledge in this form.

Ease of Understanding. As can be seen in the example, the English translation of the rule is relatively easy to infer from the rule's internal form. As a result, a medical collaborator could hope to inspect the system's knowledge himself and help debug it, even if he knew little about computer programming. Were the knowledge "procedurally embedded" in a conventional programming language, it would be much less accessible.

Accessibility of the System Itself. With its knowledge stored in this standardized flexible form, not only is it more accessible to the designers, it is also possible for the system to inspect and manipulate the knowledge itself. In this way, as discussed below, not only can the rules be used to make inferences, they may also greatly facilitate explanation and knowledge acquisition. Thus, flexibility of knowledge representation is central to expert system design.

Explanation

The second desired capability is that an expert system should be able to explain its internal logical processes to the user (Swartout 1981; Scott et al. 1983). In particular, it should be able to explain: (a) why it is pursuing a certain line of questioning, and (b) why it has made a certain recommendation.

In fact, a recent study (Teach and Shortliffe 1981) investigated physician attitudes toward medical consultation systems. The conclusions of this study were interesting in that the physicians queried did not insist that the computer always be right. They apparently felt that this was too much to ask of any expert, human or otherwise. They did feel, however, that it was critical that the computer be able to explain its recommendations so that the physician could evaluate the advice he was given.

There are a number of possible ways to approach the design of such an explanation capability. In a rule-based system, the rules can be used directly for this purpose.

1. In a rule-based system, the rules are frequently used to direct the questioning of the user. As a result, were the physician to query why a certain question was asked, the system could reply with the English translation of the rule involved. ("I am asking this question because if [premise of the rule], then [action of the rule].")
2. Similarly, if the physician queried one of the system's inferences, the system could justify it by quoting the English translation of the rule which yielded that inference. Indeed, if necessary, the physician could start with the system's final conclusions and ask successively "why... why... why..." and in this way trace back through the entire chain of inferences which had been made.

As can be seen, this form of explanation allows a physician to ask *why* the system has made a particular conclusion or recommended a particular approach. It does not, however, lend itself as well to letting him ask *why not* take a different approach. Questions as to "why not" may be very important to the physician. The section on "Critiquing" discusses a different approach to computer advice, a *critiquing* approach, which may prove helpful in this regard.

Knowledge Acquisition

The third desired capability is that an expert system be able to assist in the modification of its own knowledge (Davis and Lenat 1982). In the long run, this may prove to be a critical capability. Real-world expertise has a number of very interesting characteristics which make such "knowledge acquisition" important.

Completeness may only be approached asymptotically. No human expert or group of experts can ever know everything about their domain of expertise. As a result, no expert system can be expected to know everything either, especially since there are practical limits on the extraction of knowledge from a human expert. At some point, the law of diminishing returns sets in. As a result, one may periodically come upon additional knowledge which must be added to the system. Completeness of an expert system's knowledge base can probably only be approached asymptotically.

Medical knowledge evolves. This practical barrier to making an expert system's knowledge complete is heightened by the fact that medical knowledge is *not static*. New drugs, tests, and procedures frequently become available. New studies are performed evaluating the relative efficacy of different approaches to a problem. An expert system must therefore be updated as the field itself evolves.

As a result of this evolution of real-world expertise, an expert system differs greatly from a more conventional program. The expert system's knowledge must constantly evolve to reflect the evolution of human knowledge. This requirement, in turn, places demands on the system's design.

Whenever a programmer leaves any programming project, the software he has created is immediately placed in jeopardy. Other programmers may find it difficult to understand it well enough to modify it. The ultimate solution to this problem is to have the computer help update itself. Work on such knowledge acquisition aids is currently still largely developmental. It is clear, however, that a flexible knowledge representation, such as production rules, can greatly facilitate the process.

Critiquing

The previous section described three general capabilities which researchers are working to incorporate into expert systems. This section focusses on one particular capability being developed in several recent medical systems: a critiquing capability. The critiquing approach to computer advice may prove particularly well suited to the clinical environment.

Most expert systems have tried to simulate a expert's decision making process. They gather information and attempt to come to similarly expert conclusions. From a clinical standpoint, such a system has the effect of trying to tell the physician what to do.

In contrast, a critiquing system assumes that the physician has already evaluated his patient, and has already formulated certain thoughts about management. Rather than duplicate this process, the system critiques it, thereby tailoring its advice around the physician's proposed plan.

There are several potential advantages to critiquing as a modality for computer advice. (a) It casts the computer in the role of the physician's ally, rather than a competitor. It may therefore prove more acceptable. (b) There is a great deal of subjectivity in medical decisions. Seldom is one approach "right" and all others "wrong." As a result, it makes sense to let the physician lead the way, and have the computer play a secondary role. (c) It makes both medical and medicolegal sense to leave the major responsibility and decision-making with the physician. The computer can help the physician evaluate and optimize *his* plan.

Two systems which implement the critiquing approach are discussed below, along with excerpts from critiques which they produce.

ATTENDING: Anesthesiology

ATTENDING (Miller 1983a, b), designed to critique anesthetic management, was the first system to implement the critiquing approach. In the excerpt below, a patient has four medical problems: chronic renal failure, a prior stroke, a penetrating eye wound, and a full stomach. A physician has suggested an anesthetic management which includes intubation by rapid-sequence technique, using the muscle relaxant succinylcholine.

> Intubation of this patient is certainly necessary because of a full stomach. Rapid sequence intubation is a reasonable approach. The choice of succinylcholine, however, could have two possible risks. First, there is the risk that this could cause eye morbidity from increased intraocular pressure. Second, if the stroke is recent and involves hemiparesis, there is the risk of life-threatening hyperkalemia. An alternative would be high dose pancuronium. Here, however, in a patient with chronic renal failure, there is the risk of prolonged postoperative paralysis due to compromised renal excretion. Thus there is no ideal way to perform rapid sequence intubation. An alternative approach, perhaps, to rapid sequence intubation would be intubation after mask induction with cricoid pressure.

Each underlying medical problem implies risks for a patient's anesthetic management. Certain anesthetic techniques may increase a particular risk, other techniques may decrease it. In complicated patients with several problems, there are frequently risk trade-offs where techniques good for one problem are bad for another, and vice versa. In planning such a patient's management, a physician must weigh the various risks against one another. As illustrated above, ATTENDING is designed to help in this process, discussing the relative merits of the physician's plan as compared with alternatives which might be reasonable or preferred. The physician is then free to do as he chooses. ATTENDING is currently being used for teaching anesthesia residents using hypothetical cases.

HT-ATTENDING: Essential Hypertension

HT-ATTENDING (Miller and Black 1984) is being developed to critique the pharmacologic management of essential hypertension. In the following excerpt, a hypertensive patient with gout is being started on antihypertensive treatment. A physician has proposed using hydrochlorothiazide 50 mg bid, a not uncommon initial regimen.

> In the United States, diuretics are recommended by most authorities as initial or step one therapy. Since the initiation of diuretic therapy may precipitate a gouty attack, you may wish to start prophylactic treatment when beginning a diuretic in a patient with gout.
>
> A thiazide diuretic or similar acting agent is the drug of choice for most patients. Hydrochlorothiazide is a commonly used thiazide diuretic. Chlorthalidone or metolazone are alternative

agents worth considering since they are long-acting and can be given once a day. We usually start treatment with a lower dose than the dose you propose. We now recommend treatment with hydrochlorothiazide 25 mg qd or bid. Recent work by Materson (1) has shown that low doses of diuretics may be as effective as higher doses yet cause less hypokalemia.

There is a bewildering, changing array of drugs available for treating hypertension. It is difficult for the physician to keep abreast of all the various alternatives, each with its own set of indications, contraindications, and relative merits in different patients. HT-ATTENDING is designed to give a physician feedback as to how his approach to a particular patient fits in with current thinking in the field and the current spectrum of agents available for treatment.

Summary

The field of expert system research is a dynamic area of Artificial Intelligence. A number of very different expert systems are currently under development in different areas of medicine. These differ from more conventionally programmed systems in a number of ways. Of particular significance are the sophisticated capabilities which researchers would like to incorporate: flexibility of knowledge representation, explanation, and knowledge acquisition. Critiquing is another interesting capability which may prove particularly well suited to the clinical environment. Although most expert systems in medicine are still developmental, their promise for the future is clear.

References

Aikins JS, Kunz JC, Shortliffe EH, Fallat RJ (1983) PUFF: An experimental system for interpretation of pulmonary function data. Comput Biomed Res 16: 199–208

Buchanan BG, Feigenbaum EA (1978) DENDRAL and Meta-DENDRAL: Their applications dimension. Artif Intell 11: 5–24

Buchanan BG, Shortliffe EH (1983) Rule-based expert systems: The MYCIN experiments of the Heuristic programming project. Addison-Wesley, Reading

Campbell AN, Hollister VF, Duda RO, Hart PE (1982) Recognition of a hidden mineral deposit by an artificial intelligence program. Science 217: 927–929

Clancey WJ, Letsinger R (1981) NEOMYCIN: Reconfiguring a rule-based expert system for application to teaching. Proceedings of the Seventh International Joint Conference on Artificial Intelligence, Vancouver, pp 829–836

Clancey WJ, Shortliffe EH (1983) Readings in medical artificial intelligence: the first decade. Addison-Wesley, Reading

Davis R, Lenat DB (1982) Knowledge-based systems in artificial intelligence. McGraw Hill, New York

Duda RO, Shortliffe EH (1983) Expert systems research. Science 220: 261–268

Fagan LM, Kunz JC, Feigenbaum EA, Osborn JJ (1979) Representation of dynamic clinical knowledge: measurement interpretation in the intensive care unit. In: Proceedings of the Sixth International Joint Conference on Artificial Intelligence, Tokyo, pp 260–262

Gorry GA, Silverman H, Pauker SG (1978) Capturing clinical expertise: a computer program that considers clinical responses to digitalis. Am J Med 64: 452–460

Hayes-Roth F, Waterman DA, Lenat DB (1983) Building expert systems. Addison-Wesley, Reading

Kingsland LC, Lindberg DAB (1983) Research methods in AI model building: The history of a project. In: Proceedings of AAMSI Congress-83, San Francisco, pp 76–80

Kingsland LC, Gaston LW, Vanker AD, Lindberg DAB (1982) A knowledge-based consultant system for problems in human hemostasis. In: Proceedings of the American Medical Informatics Association Congress 82, San Francisco, pp 325–329
Kulikowski CA (1980) Artificial intelligence methods and systems for medical consultation. IEEE Trans PAMIPAMI-2: 464–476
Kulikowski CA, Weiss S (1971) Computer-based models for glaucoma. CBM-TM-MS1, Dept. of Computer Science, Rutgers University
Lindberg DAB, Sharp GC, Kingsland LC, Weiss SM, Hayes SP, Ueno H, Hazelwood SE (1980) Computer based rheumatology consultant. Proc MEDINFO 080: 1311–1315
Lindsay RK, Buchanan BG, Feigenbaum EA, Lederberg J (1980) Applications of artificial intelligence for organic chemistry: The DENDRAL project. McGraw-Hill, New York
London R, Clancey WJ (1982) Plan recognition strategies in student modelling: prediction and description. In: Proceedings of the American Association for Artificial Intelligence, Pittsburgh, pp 335–338
McDermott J (1982) R1: A rule-based configurer of computer systems. Artif Intell 19: 39–88
Miller PL (1983a) Critiquing anesthetic management: the "ATTENDING" computer system. Anesthesiology 53: 362–369
Miller PL (1983b) ATTENDING: critiquing a physician's management plan. IEEE Trans PAMI PAMI-5: 449–461
Miller PL, Black HR (1984) Medical plan-analysis by computer: critiquing the pharmacologic management of essential hypertension. Comput Biomed Res (in press).
Miller RA, Pople HE, Meyers JD (1982) Internist-I, an experimental computer-based diagnostic consultant for general internal medicine. N Eng J Med 307 (8): 468–476
Patil RS, Szolovits P, Schwartz WB (1981) Causal understanding of patient illness in medical diagnosis. In: Proceedings of the Seventh International Joint Conference on Artificial Intelligence, Vancouver, pp 893–899
Pauker SG, Gorry GA, Kassirer JP, Schwartz WB (1976) Towards the simulation of clinical cognition: taking a present illness by computer. Am J Med 60: 981–996
Pople HE (1982) Heuristic methods for imposing structure on ill-structured problems: The structuring of medical diagnostics in artificial intelligence in medicine. In: Szolovits P (ed) Artificial Intelligence in Medicine. Westview, Boulder
Scott AC, Clancey WJ, Davis R, Shortliffe EH (1983) Explanation capabilities of production-based consultation systems. In: Clancey WJ, Shortliffe EH (eds) Readings in medical artificial intelligence: the first decade. Addison-Wesley, Reading
Shortliffe EH (1976) Computer-based medical consultations: MYCIN. American Elsevier, New York
Shortliffe EH, Buchanan BG, Feigenbaum EA (1979) Knowledge engineering for medical decision making. A review of computer-based clinical decision aids. Proc IEEE 67: 1207–1224
Shortliffe EH, Scott AC, Bischoff MB, Campbell AB, Van Melle W, Jacobs CD (1981) An expert system for oncology protocol management. In: Proceedings of the Seventh International Joint Conference on Artificial Intelligence, Vancouver, pp 876–881
Swartout WR (1981) Explaining and justifying expert consultation programs. In: Proceedings of the Seventh International Joint Conference on Artificial Intelligence, Vancouver, pp 815–822
Szolovits P (ed) (1982) Artificial intelligence in medicine. Westview, Boulder
Teach RL, Shortliffe EH (1981) An analysis of physician attitudes regarding computer-based clinical consultation systems. Comput Biomed Res 14: 542–558
van Melle W (1979) A domain-independent production-rule system for consultation programs. In: Proceedings of the Sixth International Joint Conference on Artificial Intelligence, Tokyo, pp 923–925
Weiss S, Kulikowski C (1979) EXPERT: A system for developing consultation models. In: Proceedings of the Sixth International Joint Conference on Artificial Intelligence, Tokyo, pp 942–950
Weiss S, Kulikowski C, Amarel S, Safir A (1978) A model-based method for computer-aided medical decision-making. Artif Intell 11: 145–172
Weiss S, Kulikowski C, Galen R (1981) Developing microprocessor based expert models for instrument interpretation. In: Proceedings of the Seventh International Joint Conference on Artificial Intelligence, Vancouver, pp 853–855
Winston PH (1977) Artificial intelligence. Addison-Wesley, Reading

The Importance of Using a Computer to Provide Pediatric Anesthesia and Emergency Drug Information and Treatment Regimens in the Clinical Setting

D. J. Essin, D. L. Warner, M. Jagodowicz, and S. N. Steen

The delivery of accurate drug dosages is the responsibility of every individual who is involved in the administration of drugs and of the facility where the care is delivered. Most commonly dosages are computed mentally or with scratch-pad arithmetic. Occasionally a facility will require that the dose of an especially hazardous drug (e. g., digoxin) be checked by a second individual prior to administration. Several recent studies (Koren et al. 1983; Jagodowicz et al. 1984) have demonstrated that errors occur in approximimately 5%–15% of dosage calculations done both in a neonatal intensive care unit and in preparation for surgery. The risk to children is proportionately greater because virtually every drug dose administered to a child requires a calculation; there are very few dosages which can be standardized as can be done for adults.

The operating room and the intensive care unit are two areas within the hospital where emergencies occur frequently. In the midst of an emergency, the time available to compute drug doses is severely reduced, increasing the potential risk. A computer program has been developed to assist the anesthetists and intensivists in the management of the pediatric patient.

Materials and Methods

The computer program has two components, one of which produces an anesthesia reference sheet and the other an intensive care unit reference sheet. It is entitled PAEDIATRICS (Pediatric Anesthesia and Emergency Drug Information and Treatment Regimens in the Clinical Setting). The program was written in BASIC + 2 and runs on a PDP 11/34-A minicomputer (Digital Equipment Corp., Maynard, Mass.). A teleprinter has been installed in a location convenient to the operating theater and the pediatric intensive care unit and is continuously available to the medical staff of the Pediatric Pavilion of the Los Angeles County/University of Southern California Medical Center.

In operating, the program requires only that the user choose which sheet is desired and then enter the patient's identifying information, age, and weight. All calculations and decision points are based on this information. The dosages per unit weight are those favored by the medical staff. The emergency drug doses are based on the recommendations of the American Heart Association.

```
PATIENT: SAMPLE PATIENT                                DATE:  24-Jun-84
 1  month of age                                       WEIGHT:    4.3KG (    9lb)

                    THE FOLLOWING VALUES SERVE AS GUIDELINES. THEY
                  SHOULD NOT TAKE PRECEDENCE OVER CLINICAL JUDGEMENT.

Estimated endotracheal tube size use 3.5 mm I.D.
Ventilator TIDAL VOLUME (10 ml/kg) =  43 ml
AIR/O2 GAS MIXTURE (L/MIN) = % O2:
3.5  air/ 0.5  O2 = 30% O2                             3  air/ 1  O2 = 40% O2
2.5  air/ 1.5  O2 = 50% O2                             2  air/ 2  O2 = 60% O2

estimated BLOOD VOLUME (80 ml/kg) =  344 ml
estimated 10% of BLOOD LOSS (8 ml/kg) =  34 ml
IV - Maint.(2 L/sq m)=   18 ml/hr; Operative (4-10 ml/kg/hr)=   17-   43 ml/hr

                        -----INDUCTION DRUG DOSAGES-----

THIOPENTAL (4mg/kg)       =  17.2 mg I.V.         (soln. 25mg/ml) =  0.7 ml
ATROPINE (0.01mg/kg)      =   0.04 mg I.V.       (soln. 0.4mg/ml) =   0.11 ml
SUCCINYLCHOLINE (1mg/kg) =   4.3 mg I.V.        (soln. 20mg/ml) =   0.22 ml
                (2mg/kg) =   8.6 mg *I.M.*      (soln. 20mg/ml) =   0.43 ml

                        -----ADDITIONAL DRUG DOSAGES-----

PANCURONIUM (0.04-0.1mg/kg)=  0.17-  0.4 mg I.V.(soln. 1mg/ml)=  0.17-  0.4 ml
CURARE (0.2-0.4mg/kg)=  0.9 -  1.7 mg I.V.       (soln. 3mg/ml)=  0.3-  0.6 ml
PROSTIGMINE (0.04mg/kg) =  0.17 mg I.V.           (soln. 1mg/ml) =  0.17 ml
METHOHEXITAL (1.5mg/kg) =  6.5 mg I.V.           (soln. 10mg/ml) =  0.6 ml
             (5.0mg/kg) = 21.5 mg *I.M.*         (soln. 50mg/ml) =  0.4 ml
KETAMINE (1mg/kg) =   4 mg I.V.                  (soln. 10mg/ml) =  0.4 ml
         (5mg/kg) =  22 mg *I.M.*                (soln. 50mg/ml) =  0.4 ml
MAX. LOCAL LIDOCAINE (5mg/kg)=  22 mg              4.3 ml of 0.5%
                                                   8.6 ml of 0.25%
MAX. LOCAL BUPIVACAINE (2mg/kg) =   9 mg           1.7 ml of 0.5%
                                                   3.4 ml of 0.25%
MAX. LOCAL EPINEPHRINE (3ug/kg) =  13ug            1.3 ml of 1:100,000
                                                   2.6 ml of 1:200,000
                                                   5.2 ml of 1:400,000

                   -----EMERGENCY DRUGS (I.V. DOSAGE)-----

COUNTERSHOCK for V FIB (2joules/kg)=   9 joules. IF INEFFECTIVE DOUBLE DOSE
DANTROLENE for MH (2-10mg/kg)=   9 -  43 mg      (soln. 20mg/60ml sterile H2O)
EPINEPHRINE (0.1ml/kg)=  0.4 ml                  (soln. 1:10,000) =  0.43 ml
ATROPINE (0.01mg/kg)=  0.04 mg  - - - - - -      (soln. 0.4mg/ml) =  0.11 ml
                                                 (soln. 0.1mg/ml) =  0.4 ml
CALCIUM CHLORIDE 10% (5mg/kg)=  22 mg  - - -     (soln. 100 mg/ml)=  0.2 ml
SODIUM BICARBONATE (1mEq/kg)=  4.3mEq            (8.4% soln.=1mEq/ml)=  4.3 ml
                                                 (7.5% soln.=.9mEq/ml)= 4.8 ml
LIDOCAINE 1% BOLUS(1mg/kg) =   4 mg  - - - -     (soln. 10mg/ml)=  0.4 ml
LIDOCAINE(20-50ug/kg/min)=  86 - 215ug/min       (1gm in 500ml D5W=2mg/ml)
BRETYLIUM (5-10mg/kg)=  22 -  43 mg              (soln.50mg/ml)= 0.4 -  0.9 ml
PROCAINAMIDE (1mg/kg) =  4.3 mg                  (soln. 100mg/ml)=  0.04 ml
DOPAMINE (2-20ug/kg/min)=  8.6- 86.0ug/min       (50mg in 500ml D5W=100ug/ml)
ISOPROTERENOL (0.1ug/kg/min)=  0.4ug/min         (1mg in 500ml D5W=2ug/ml)
VERAPAMIL (0.1mg/kg)=   0.4 mg over 1 min.       (soln. 2.5mg/ml)=  0.17 ml
NITROPRUSSIDE (.5-10ug/kg/min) =  2.2- 43.0ug/min(50mg in 500ml D5W=100ug/ml)
DEXTROSE 25% (2ml/kg) =   9 ml              (dilute D50/W 1:1 with sterile H2O)
NALOXONE (0.01mg/kg) =  0.04 mg                  (soln. 0.4mg/ml)=  0.11 ml
FUROSEMIDE (1mg/kg) =  4.3 mg                    (soln. 10mg/ml)=  0.4 ml
MANNITOL 20% (0.25-0.5g/kg) =  1.1-  2.2g        ( 0.2g/ml)=  5.4- 10.8 ml
PROPRANOLOL(0.005-0.01mg/kg)=  0.02-  0.04 mg  (soln. 1mg/ml)=  0.02-  0.04 ml
HYDROCORTISONE (4-75mg/kg) =  17- 323 mg       (soln. 50mg/ml)=  0.3-   6.4 ml
```

Fig. 1. Anesthesia reference sheet

SAMPLE PATIENT — PF #: 000-00-00 — DATE: 24-Jun-84
1 month~~s~~ of age — WEIGHT: 4.3 kg (9 lb)

THE FOLLOWING VALUES SERVE AS GUIDELINES. THEY
SHOULD NOT TAKE PRECEDENCE OVER CLINICAL JUDGEMENT.

Estimated endotracheal tube size use 3.5 mm I.D.
COUNTERSHOCK VENT. FIB.(2joules/kg)= 9 joules. IF INEFFECTIVE DOUBLE DOSE

estimated BLOOD VOLUME (80 ml/kg) = 344 ml
estimated 10% of BLOOD LOSS (8 ml/kg) = 34 ml

*** EMERGENCY DRUGS ***

DRUG	INITIAL DOSE	CALCULATED DOSE	FREQUENCY
EPINEPHRINE (1:10,000)	0.1ml/kg	0.43 ml	q 5 min.
NaHCO3 (7.5%)	1ml/kg	4.3 ml	q 10 min.
CALCIUM CHLORIDE (10%)	10 mg/kg	0.4 ml	q 10 min.
ATROPINE (0.1mg/ml)	0.01 mg/kg	0.43 ml	q 5 min.
(0.4mg/ml)	0.01 mg/kg	0.11 ml	q 5 min.
LIDOCAINE (1%)	1.0 mg/kg	0.43 ml	q 3 min.
(2%)	1.0 mg/kg	0.22 ml	q 3 min.
VERAPAMIL (2.5mg/ml)	0.12-0.25 mg/kg	0.22- 0.43 ml	q 30 min.
PROPRANOLOL (1mg/ml)	0.01 mg/kg	0.04 ml	PRN X 3
DEXTROSE (50% soln.)	0.25 gm/kg	2.15 ml	PRN
NARCAN (0.4mg/ml)	0.01 mg/kg	0.11 ml	PRN
(0.02mg/ml)	0.01 mg/kg	2.15 ml	PRN
FUROSEMIDE (10mg/ml)	1.0 mg/kg	0.43 ml	PRN
MANNITOL 20%	0.25-0.5 gm/kg	5.4- 10.8 ml	PRN
VALIUM (5mg/ml)	0.1-0.3 mg/kg	0.09- 0.26 ml	q 2-5min.

****

DOPAMINE (200mg/250ml)			NITROPRUSSIDE (50mg/250ml)			ISUPREL (2mg/100ml)		
UG/KG/MIN	ML/KG/HR	ML/HR	UG/KG/MIN	ML/KG/HR	ML/HR	UG/KG/MIN	ML/KG/HR	ML/HR
1	0.075	0.32	1	0.3	1.3	0.1	0.3	1.3
2	0.150	0.65	2	0.6	2.6	0.2	0.6	2.6
3	0.225	0.97	3	0.9	3.9	0.3	0.9	3.9
4	0.300	1.29	4	1.2	5.2	0.4	1.2	5.2
5	0.375	1.61	5	1.5	6.5	0.5	1.5	6.5
6	0.450	1.94	6	1.8	7.7	0.6	1.8	7.7
7	0.525	2.26	7	2.1	9.0	0.7	2.1	9.0
8	0.600	2.58	8	2.4	10.3	0.8	2.4	10.3
9	0.675	2.90	9	2.7	11.6	0.9	2.7	11.6
10	0.750	3.23	10	3.0	12.9	1.0	3.0	12.9

Based on Protocols from the American Heart Association and LAC-USC Pediatric ICU

Fig. 2. Intensive care unit reference sheet

Results

Examples of a completed reference sheet of each type have been prepared and appear in Fig. 1 and 2.

Discussion

This computer program is designed to support the decision – making activities of specialists in anesthesia and intensive care. It does not make suggestions regarding which drug to administer nor does it critique the choice of the physician. Its sole purpose is to reduce morbidity and mortality by allowing the correct dosage of a drug to be immedidately available. The concept of using a computer to perform calculations of this type is not unique to us. A number of practicing anesthetists and intensivists have written programs for their own use which run on a variety of programmable calculators and personal computers. These individuals have recognized that morbidity reduction extends beyond arriving at correct dosages into the realm of stress reduction and elimination of distraction when managing a complex and emergent situation.

The unfortunate aspect of many of these programs is that they represent the efforts of one person to solve an individual problem. Considering the potential for errors if the hand calculation method is employed, a computerized verification of anesthetic and emergency dosages should be performed for every pediatric patient. To accomplish this goal, a verification system of this type must be provided and supported by each facility caring for children.

In addition to the potential impact of this program on patient care, some consideration should be given to the consequences of providing a continuously available computer tool to physicians. It is not uncommon to encounter resistance from physicians to technological innovations. The increased complexity of medicine can lead to anxiety and indecision in the face of an emergency. The result may be a focusing of hostility on the new apparatus, engendered by the difficulty of dealing with a more complex environment.

The program presented here and its attendant hardware are technically simple. They represent the "trailing edge" of the new technology. In addition the product of the program is information which can reduce stress during an emergency. We believe that frequent exposure to simple, useful computer applications is necessary to pave the way for general acceptance of applications currently considered to be on the "leading edge".

Summary

In order to improve the treatment of children in critical care settings, a computer program has been developed to assist in the preparation of correct drug and anesthetic doses during surgery and while managing emergencies in the intensive care unit. The availability of this information, in addition to reducing the likelihood of dosage errors, removes an important source of distraction of the physician in attendance.

Acknowledgments. Supported in part by the Anesthesia Development Fund of the Department of Anesthesiology, University of Southern California/Los Angeles County Hospital and the Los Angeles County Lung Association.

References

Koren G, Barzilay Z, Modan M (1983) Errors in computing drug doses. Can Med Assoc J 129: 721–723

Jagodowicz M, Warner DL, Essin DJ, Steen SN (1984) A pediatric anesthesia and emergency drug computer program. 22nd Annual Western Anesthesia Resident's Conference, 27–29 April 1984, University and California, Irvine Medical Center, Orange, California 92668, USA.

Computer Systems in Artificial Ventilations (New Techniques)

W. Koller, A. Aloy, N. Mutz, and G. Pauser

Computer monitoring, surveillance, and therapy of artificially ventilated patients requires a quantity and quality of machine-configuration (e.g., on-line real-time data processing and multidirectional data traffic) which are not available today. Earlier hopes for the machine-controlled respiratory-controlled respiratory-therapeutic loop – although software, hardware and peripheral monitoring devices are developing rapidly – must remain a dream. In 1975, Baum et al. presented a concept that also could not be realized. One of the unfulfilled needs for this concept was exact on-line monitoring of arterial oxygenation and CO_2 elimination. Furthermore, end-expiratory CO_2 levels are not applicable as primary parameters for respirator settings because of secondary influences from pulmonary perfusion and metabolic state. A computer that initiated the respiratory regimen on the respirator would therefore lack basic data and would remain widely disorientated (Fig. 1). Application of ventilatory support has two major goals:

1. to achieve adequate gas exchange for O_2 and CO_2; and
2. to hold lung-mechanics parameters within a suitable range.

Influenced by these two parameters other systems of the organism must be continuously monitored and sometimes an adequate therapeutic regimen must be decided and applied. The age of growing computer technology in critical care medicine has led to a more and more sophisticated application of the systems, even during respiratory therapy.

In our intensive care unit (ICU) two different computer systems are avialable for monitoring and treatment during artificial ventilation [2, 3]. Our bedside monitoring, controlled by a PDP 11 computer, allows a very comprehensive surveillance over off-line data, adjusted to respiratory treatment needs as well as accompanying therapy. Table 1 provides a summary of respirator settings and gas checks plus calculated parameters. Considering the elaborate format for data on flowcharts, this mode of presentation became an important part of clinical routine, it saves time and offers excellent possibilities for surveillance. Influenced by our specific respirator settings (inspiratory reserve volume, IRV) hemodynamics have to be observed very closely. For this purpose the system can be used on-line and therefore produces continuously observable data, which can be correlated with the above mentioned respiratory data.

Hemodynamic data, for example, can be produced for different time intervals and for any combination of the available parameters; Figs. 2 and 3 demonstrate this. This way of looking at a large amount of data is extremely helpful for making therapeutic

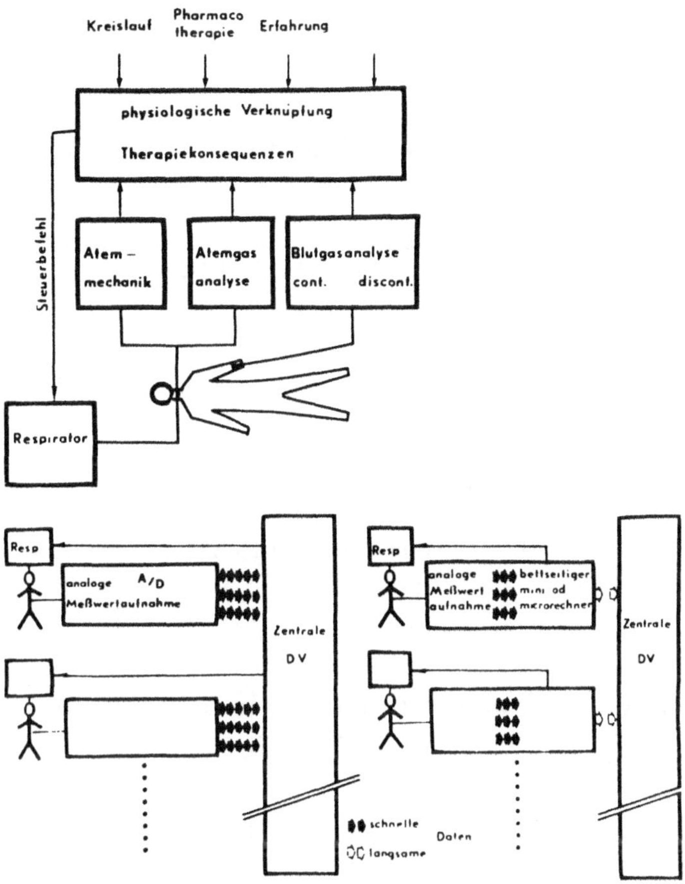

Fig. 1. Computer controlled respiratory concept (Baum et al. 1975)

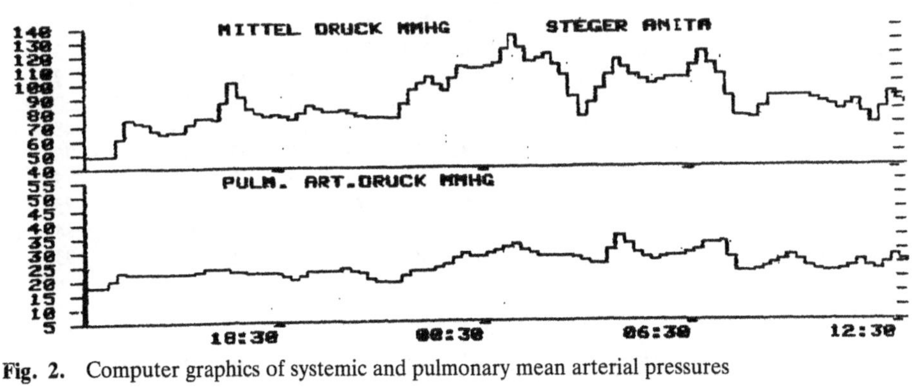

Fig. 2. Computer graphics of systemic and pulmonary mean arterial pressures

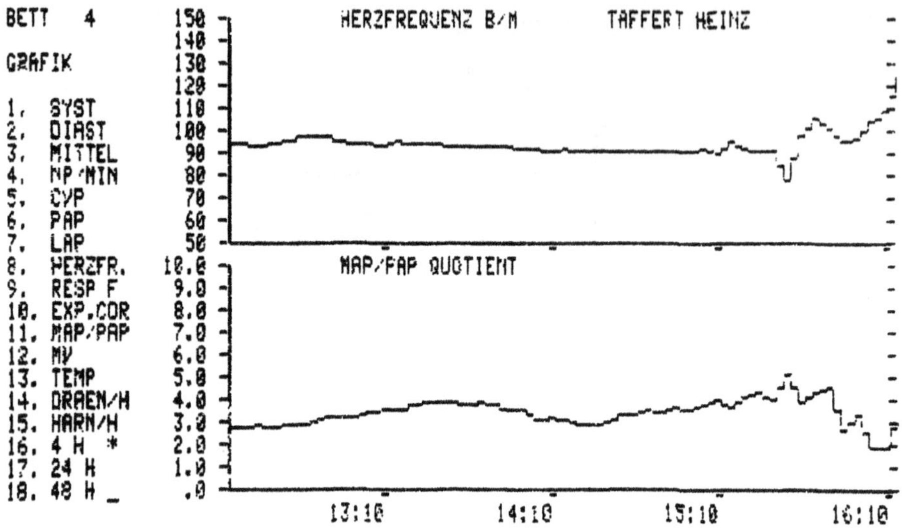

Fig. 3. Computer graphics of heart rate and MAP/PAP-quotient

Table 1. Computer prints of respiratory settings and blood gas analysis

Respirator	UV1		UV1	UV1	UV1	UV1	UV1			UV1		
Status	CMV		CMV	CMV	CMV	CMV	CMV			CMV		
P-max	58	58	50	62	34	52	50			48		
P-end insp.	52	52	46	58	34	48	42					
Peep	10		10	10	11	10	10			10	8	
Tidal vol.	900		900	900	500	900	900			800	800	
Minuten vol.	10.5		10.5	10.5	12.0	10.5	11.0			11.0	11.0	
Resp. freq.	12		12	12	22	12	12			14	14	
I : E (num)	21		21	21	21	21	21			31	31	
FIO_2	.80		.80	.75	.75	.75	.75	.75	1.00	.75	.75	1.00
Art.-Ven.-Cap.	Art.	Art.	Art.	Art.	Art.	Art.	Art.	Art.	Art.	Art.	Art.	Art.
Bar. Druck	758	758	758	758	758	758	758	758	760	760	754	754
Pat. Temp.	37.0	37.0	37.0	37.0	37.0	37.0	37.0	37.0	37.0	37.0	37.0	37.0
Hemoglobin	10	10	10	10	10	11	11	11	11	11	9	9
PH TK.	7.35	7.29	7.30	7.36	7.33	7.33	7.22	7.37	7.36	7.40	7.30	7.30
PCO_2 TK.	52	55	56	51	54	54	63	47	48	46	48	45
PO_2 TK.	72	77	73	63	52	63	53	63	72	70	76	75
BE	2.1	–.4	.8	2.4	1.5	1.4	–3.5	1.9	.9	3.1	–2.5	–3.8
FIO_2	.80	.80	.80	.75	.75	.75	.75	.75	.75	.75	.75	.75
HCO_3	27.8	26.2	27.3	27.9	27.6	27.6	24.9	26.9	26.2	27.6	23.4	21.9
Sättigung	93	93	93	90	83	90	78	91	93	93	93	93
O_2-Content	13.1	13.1	13.1	12.6	11.6	13.9	12.0	14.1	14.4	11.8	11.8	11.8
O_2-Utili.												
A-ABO_2	455	447	450	428	436	425	426	433	424	428	416	420
Quotient	.86	.85	.86	.87	.89	.87	.88	.87	.85	.85	.84	.84

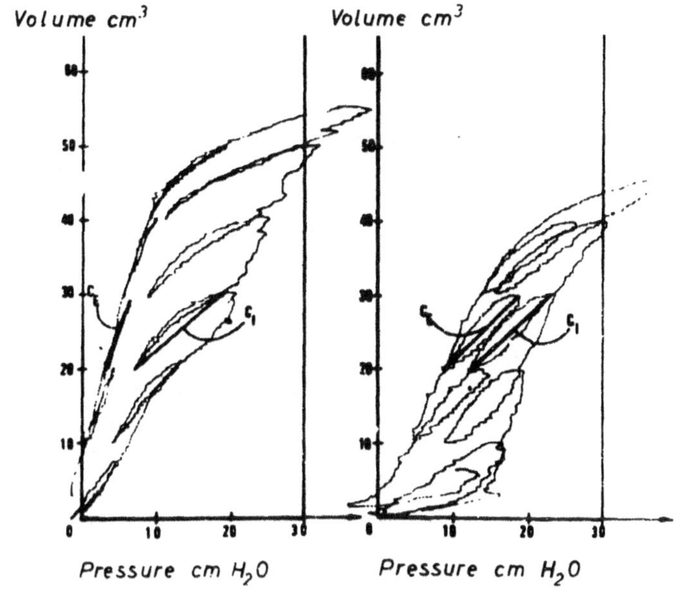

Fig. 4. Pneumoloop diagram for normal (left) and abnormal (right) surface activity

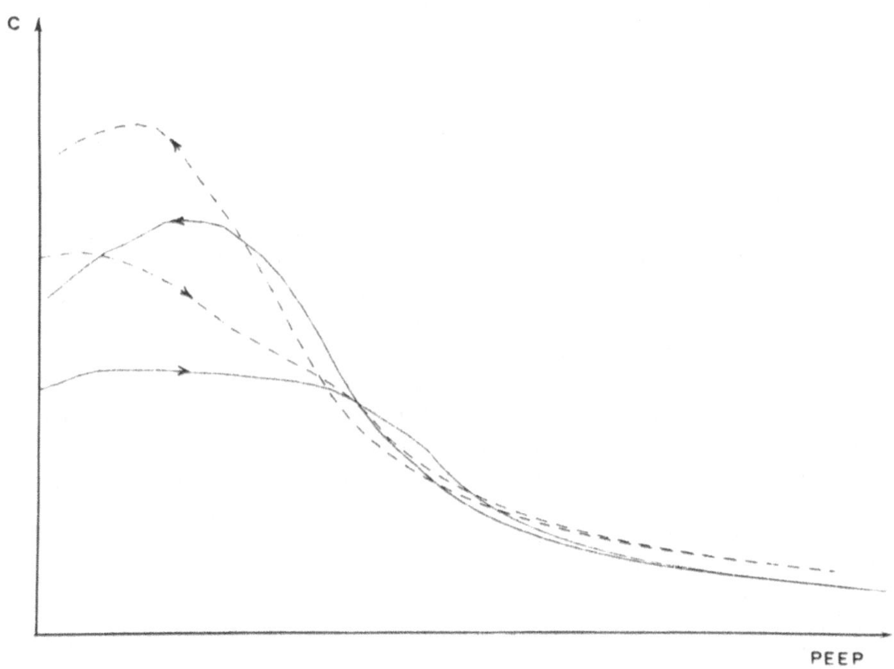

Fig. 5. Compliance-PEEP diagram calculated for pneumoloop data

decisions, and the rare (but regularly occuring) system breakdowns do not unduly distress the physicans and nurses.

Another area where we use computers routinely is for mechanical lung performance. On-line monitoring is not routinely practicable for this and we therefore developed some programs using a microcomputer that can be easily programmed and adjusted to immediate requirements to get more specific input to aid ventilatory therapy.

One of the main problems in monitoring critically ill patients is to have information about lung compliance to find the optimal positive end expiratory pressure (PEEP). For routine observations of lung compliance we developed a method that is easy to perfom and that is based on the so-called pneumoloop technique.

A step-wise increase as well as decrease of functional reserve capacity (FRC) will be caused by changes in PEEP during controlled mechanical ventilation. Electronically, compliance pressure (the difference between inspiratory hold and PEEP) will be calculated by an iterative computer program. This compliance pressure is adequate for the elastance of lungs, if tidal volume is constant. The duration of one cycle is ten to twenty minutes and includes an increase as well as decrease of PEEP, continuously controlled by computer from 0 to 20 cm H_2 0 and vice versa.

In Fig. 4 the registrations of PEEP is given on the *y*-axis and pressure difference on the *x*-axis. It will be observed in this "compliance" diagram that the slope in normal physiological conditions (left) differs markedly from the slope after infusion of olic acid (right) and therefore extremely damaged lungs. This race is converted into a compliance-PEEP diagram in Fig. 5. Here the point of best compliance is found at the highest point of the curve. And the best PEEP can be read directly. The injured lung (solid line) shows a right shift of maxima, suggesting some beneficial effects of higher PEEP levels.

Based on this experience of the bedside monitoring of compliance we developed another computer program, wich allows us to discover the status of compliance for different inflation levels of the lungs. Fig. 6 depicts volume-pressure (V/P) traces recorded at the bedside on different days; the reaction of inflation pressure influenced by the volume during inspiration as well expiration can be seen. The V/P curve differs according to the actual lung status; the curves are recorded daily and one can get an impression of the increase and decrease of restrictive pulmonary changes. This may be quite impressive but is not quantified and calculation and somewhat more definite decision aids may be necessary. The V/P curves traced at the bedside are therefore transfered via light pen or joystick to microcomputer memory; static compliance being marked by pressing the "fire" button (even a home computer could do some useful things besides playing games). Redrawing the curve on the screen results in Fig. 7, and once the static points are completed a print-out of compliance values and corresponding inflation volumes is given (Table 2).

All these data can be saved on floppy disks for later evaluation. Corresponding to more or less satisfactory results in computer controlled therapy, such as closed loop therapy with vasoactive substances, it seems to be possible to influence the respirator via a special interface using such a V/P diagram. So far it has not been possible to control the respirator using such a diagram because of the artifacts in the evaluation of patient's data.

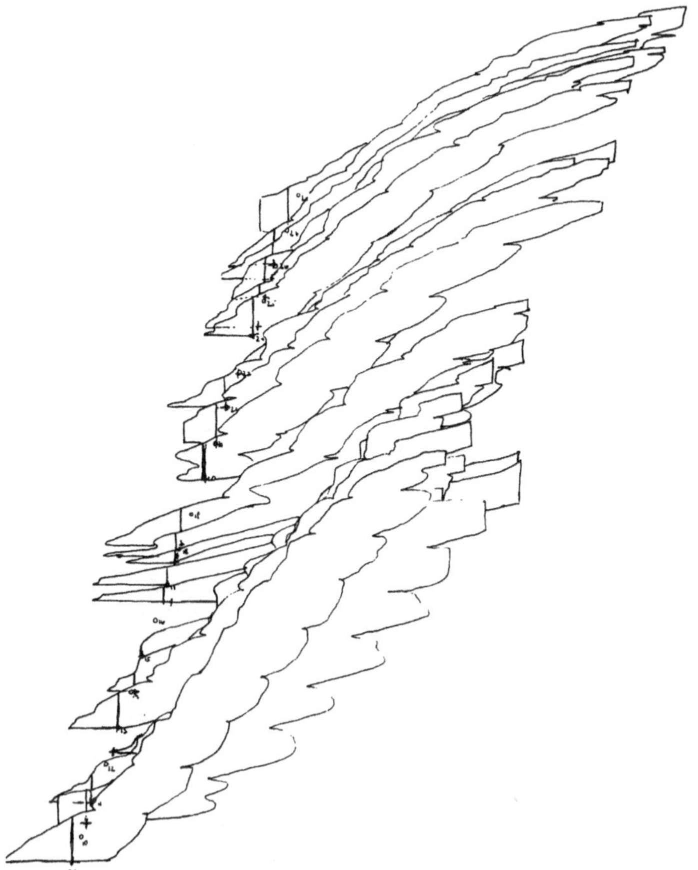

Fig. 6. Daily V/P diagrams of one patient drawn chronologically from front to back

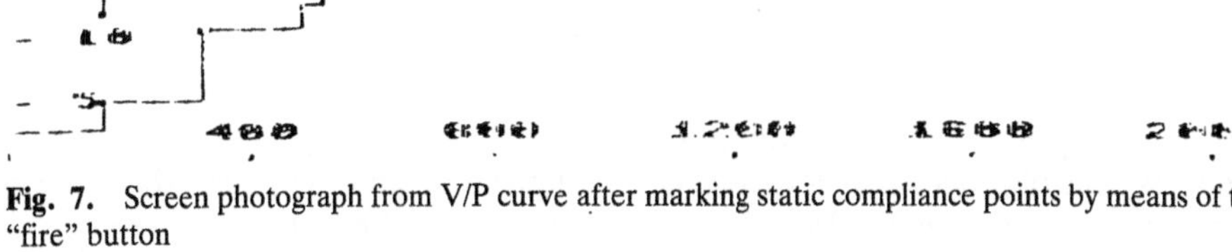

Fig. 7. Screen photograph from V/P curve after marking static compliance points by means of the "fire" button

Table 2. Printout of static compliance values for one V/P-curve (inspiration starts at bottom row)

82.13	ML/CM H20	BEI	275 ML	75.99	ML/CM H20	BEI	1512 ML	61.60	ML/CM H20	BEI	1065 ML
83.78	ML/CM H20	BEI	467 ML	67.07	ML/CM H20	BEI	1684 ML	55.67	ML/CM H20	BEI	838 ML
86.24	ML/CM H20	BEI	673 ML	67.07	ML/CM H20	BEI	1684 ML	51.30	ML/CM H20	BEI	639 ML
82.35	ML/CM H20	BEI	873 ML	61.18	ML/CM H20	BEI	1684 ML	42.43	ML/CM H20	BEI	426 ML
82.77	ML/CM H20	BEI	1093 ML	59.79	ML/CM H20	BEI	1512 ML	34.90	ML/CM H20	BEI	233 ML
81.66	ML/CM H20	BEI	1306 ML	64.50	ML/CM H20	BEI	1271 ML				

AUSDRUCK: ⟩ A ⟨ SPEICHERN: ⟩ S ⟨ NOCHEINMAL: ⟩ N ⟨ ENDE: ⟩ E ⟨ A

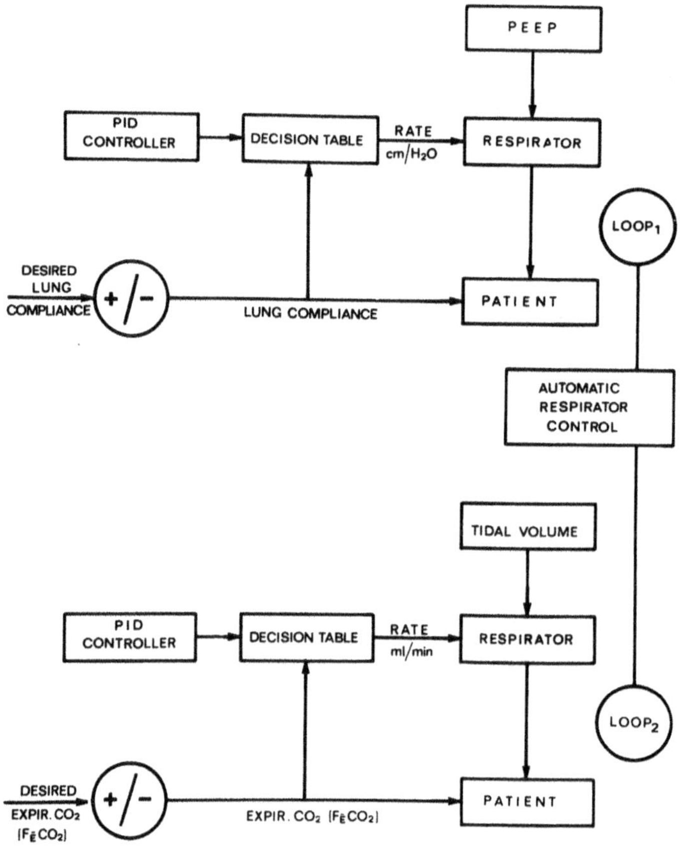

Fig. 8. Diagram depicting the closed loops which should assure adequate ventilation

One of the models which could be realized in the near future is introduced in Fig. 8. Two closed loops should maintain adequate ventilation; one is responsible for adjusting tidal volume according to expiratory CO_2 levels (lower half) and the other one for adjusting the PEEP level as indicated by volume-pressure calculations.

Therapy by means of a respirator has many components. It begins with pathological findings and observations, goes ahead making therapeutic decisions that lead to respirator settings, and then loops back to pathological findings etc., influenced by the

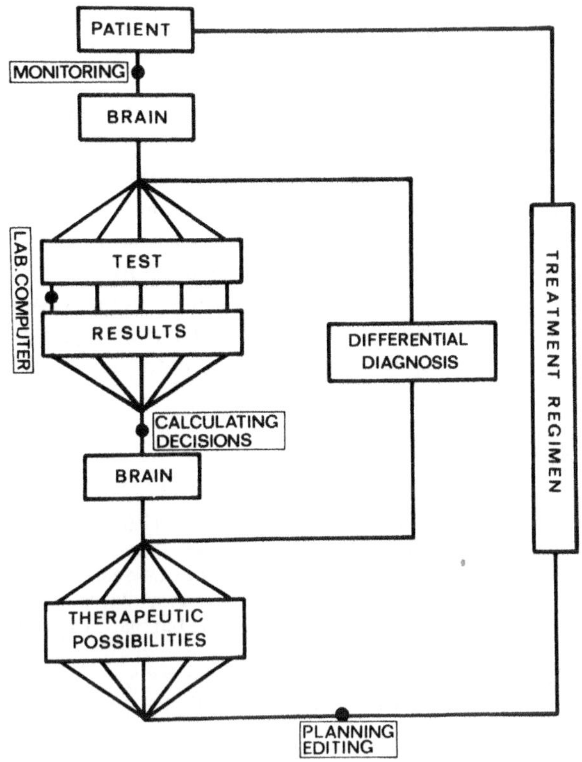

Fig. 9. Flow diagram of therapeutic concepts usually done routinely

therapy. Many steps and decision points have to be passed and it does not seem possible to develop algorithm for all of them (Fig. 9). One of the cycle's constituent parts is a biological system and minimal deviations may lead to strange and unexpected reactions that can result in life or death. Therefore although detailed parts of the system can be translated into machine language and controlled by an electronic processor, the synopsis between information, decision, and therapy cannot be made by a machine. Only a biological system can care for another biological system.

Computer controlled respirator setting is not possible today. The limiting factors to the satisfactory application of computers in this field are:

1. lack of sufficiently qualified basic data;
2. too many degrees of freedom;
3. using computers alone for therapy in a biological system means, even with high levels of technology, always failing; and
4. data obtained are never influenced by one factor and are therefore not suitable for controlling a single therapeutic loop.

A unique computerized treatment loop for any kind of patient will be certainly not be possible in the next decade, but technology can help in small problems, saving time and carrying out clear cut routines. Such routines could be (marked as dots in Fig. 9):

1. Early diagnosis of disturbances in lung mechanics as well as gas exchange.
2. Optimizing the respiratory therapy – friendly and adequate settings of the respirator for lung mechanics.
3. Monitoring results of therapeutic actions bringing improvements in the therapy itself.

Today, wide-spread discussion of jobs made redundant by the activities of electronic equipment suggests that both simple and complicated parts of working processes can be covered by machines. Decisions of principle, however, as well as any innovative actions are never carried out by computers. There is categorically a need for a well trained brain, which usually belongs to a member of a specified medical branch. We call them doctors, we have enough of them, and if they are well trained they will match the concept of computer-aided life-supporting therapy.

References

Baum M, Schmid D, Mendler N, Richter A (1975) Computerunterstützte Überwachung der Beatmung. In: Zindler M, Purske R (eds) Neue kontinuierliche Methoden zur Überwachung der Herz-Kreislauf-Funktion. Workshop Frankfurt Düsseldorf, June 1975

Mutz N, Pauser G, Schmid D (1981) Klinische Anwendung eines computerunterstützten Monitoringsystems an der Intensivstation. 10. Internat. Fortbildungskurs für klinische Anaesthesie, pp 137–141

Pauser G, Benzer H, Mutz N (1983) Computer documentation in critical care medicine. In: Computing in anaesthesia and intensive care, Rotterdam

Series Dead Space Volume Assessed as the Mean Value of a Distribution Function

G. Wolff and J.X. Brunner

Theory

The lung may be regarded as a gas-filled tree with an asymmetrical branching system, i.e. with both long and short pathways. During inspiration the transitional zone from convective to diffusive gas transport is localized in the respiratory units (acini). This transitional zone, the stationary interface (SI), was first described by Cumming et al. (1971) and has been set down mathematically by Paiva (1972).

If a patient is under controlled ventilation at a constant inspiratory flow rate (no end-inspiratory pause) each SI is established in its acinus at the end of inspiration. The volume which is contained in all pathways down the bronchial tree to the stationary interfaces is the series dead space (Vds). There is a mean pathway length down to the SIs with a distribution of shorter and longer pathways and analogous to that there is a mean dead space volume with a distribution of smaller and larger series dead spaces (Horsefield and Cumming 1968). The composition of gas distal to the stationary interfaces (alveolar gas) is determined by the amount of dead space gas and fresh gas received during inspiration and by the amount of CO_2 which is continuously released from the blood.

Our interest concerns the distribution of interfaces within the lung and the corresponding distribution of alveolar gas "behind" the interfaces. We therefore have to interpret the well-known CO_2 single breath diagram (CO_2 measured at the mouth of a patient as a function of the expired volume) as a cumulative distribution function. This distribution can be described with a mean value and a scatter without any assumption about its shape.

The contribution of a single interface is flow and concentration weighted and may be delayed due to sequential, emptying or long pathways. If a single interface is delayed so long that it is expired during phase III, it is impossible to separate the corresponding single series dead space from parallel (alveolar) dead spaces. We know of no solution to this problem because the CO_2 single breath diagram does not provide enough information. The approach to assessing series dead space at the mouth of a patient in terms of a distribution function therefore has to be a pragmatic one.

Established Methods

Two methods for assessing series dead space on a computer have been published. The THRESHOLD METHOD of Olson et al. (1980) is used in some commercially available set-ups. Series dead space is defined as the expired volume coinciding with the rise of CO_2 above the maximal expected noise of zero value (Vds threshold or Vds-T, see Fig. 1). This is achieved by setting the threshold for the CO_2 signal to a low percentage of the end-expiratory CO_2 value of the previous breath. Obviously with

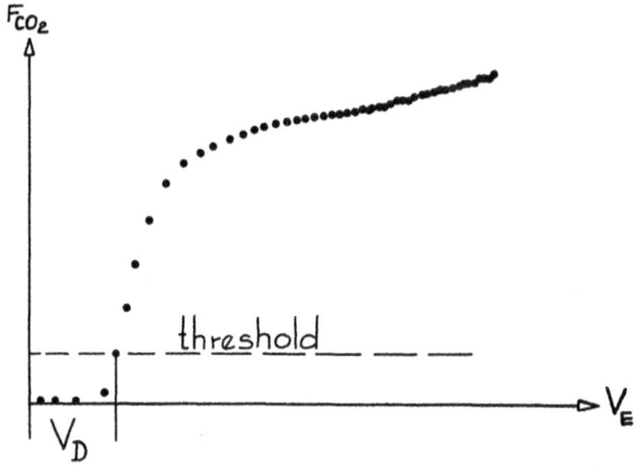

Fig. 1. Series dead space volume measured by the CO_2 concentration's crossing of a preset threshold (Langley method, giving Vds-L)

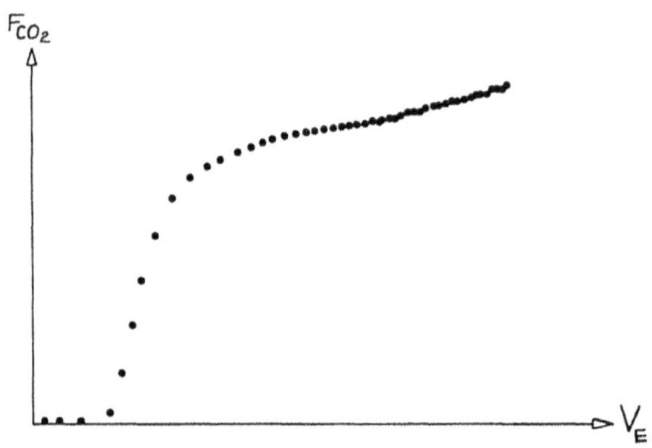

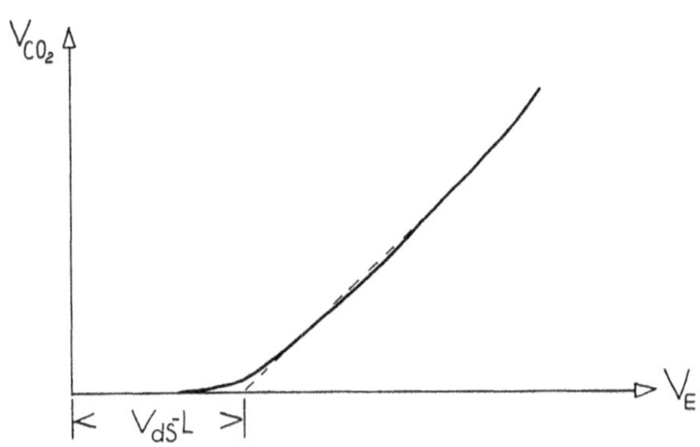

Fig. 2. Series dead space volume measured by integrating the CO_2 concentration to obtain the CO_2 volume, by fitting the CO_2 volume as a function of expired volume, and by reading the fit's intercept with the axis of expired volume (treshold method, giving Vds-T)

any such method series dead space is systematically underestimated, since it focusses on phase I and not on phase II. This error depends on many factors, varies according to the form of phase II, and cannot be corrected for.

The INTEGRATIVE METHOD, orginally published by Langley et al. (1975) and widely used by Fletcher et al. (1981) and by Fletcher and Jonson (1984), estimates series dead space by extrapolating phase III. This is achieved by integrating the CO_2 fraction to yield the CO_2 volume as a function of expired volume (Fig. 2). The curve is fitted with a straight line or a polynomial and the fit's intercept with the volume axis is read as the series dead space (Vds Langley or Vds-L). Our computer implementation of this method showed excellent applicability and reproducibility. However, since Vds-L focusses on phase III, series dead space is systematically overestimated and this systematic error depends on all the factors influencing phase III.

New Method

We therefore present a new method which concentrates on the analysis of phase II involving the following two steps:
Step 1: Focussing on phase II: the volume expired when the CO_2 concentration has reached half of the end-expiratory value is doubled, the rest of the points are excluded from further analysis (Fig. 3).

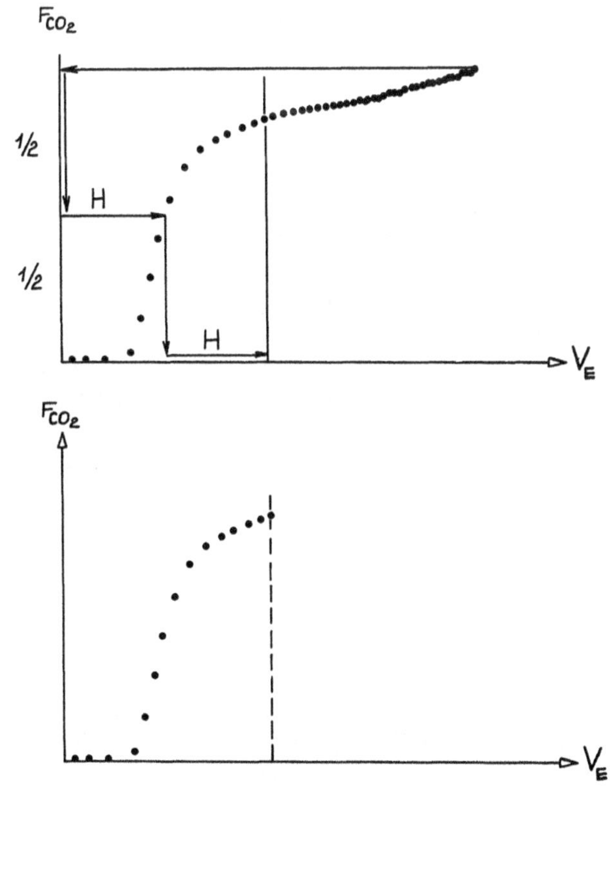

Fig. 3. New method, first step: focussing on phase II and excluding the rest of data from being processed

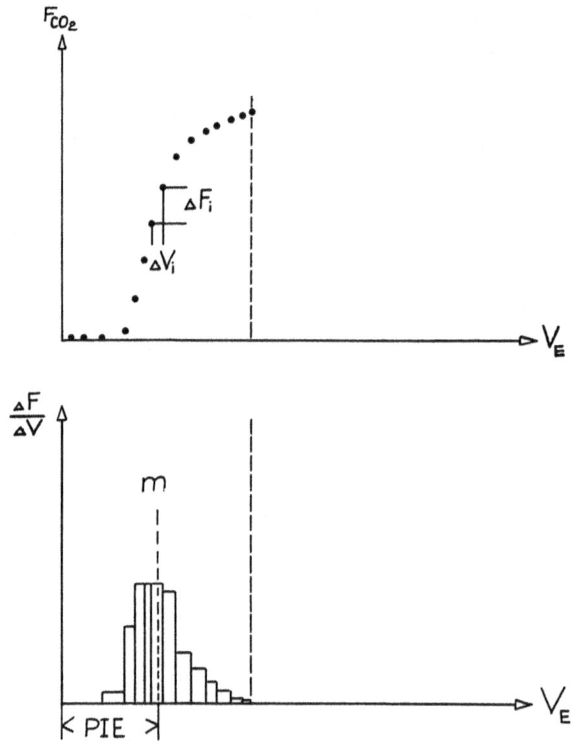

Fig. 4. New method, second step: analyzing dF/dV in the range focussed and regarding its mean value (first moment) as the smallest possible and largest determinable flow-, concentration-, and sequence-weighted mean series dead space volume (= pre-interface expirate = PIE)

Step 2: The volume expired up to the mean value of distribution of the change in concentration of CO_2 corresponds to the flow-, concentration-, and sequence-weighted minimal mean volume of the convective airways. We define this nonmixing volume as the measurable part of the series dead space and call it PRE-INTERFACE EXPIRATE or "PIE" [the change in concentration ($\Delta F/\Delta V$) is plotted against the expired volume (V) and the volume expired up to the mean value of this distribution is determined, see Fig. 4.

It follows that the sum of all series dead spaces cannot be smaller than the dead space volume deduced from the mean value of the distribution. Since, however, late interfaces are not included in the determination, the sum may be bigger. PIE therefore is to be defined as the smallest possible mean series dead space volume.

Investigation

To test the consistency of PIE and Vds-L with the described model we measured PIE under different conditions in ten stable patients under controlled mechanical ventilation. All investigations started out from the therapeutic situation as stabilized by the team in charge; this was referred to as standard situation (mean tidal volume: 1084 ml; mean inspiratory flow rate: 443 ml/s). In each situation 15 consecutive breaths were analyzed and mean values calculated.

Two different types of situation were investigated:

1. With standard inspiratory flow rate ($\dot{V}I$) and ZEEP, standard tidal volume was increased and decreased respectively (VT). As a consequence, end-inspiratory airway pressure (PAWI) was reduced by 3.6. cm H_2O and increased by 3.6 cm H_2O, respectively, compared with the standard situation.
2. With standard $\dot{V}I$ and standard VT we increased end-expiratory airway pressure (PEEP) by 7 cm H_2O, thus increasing PAWI by 7 cm H_2O.

Inspiratory flow rate within a breath was constant (square wave shaped flow rate), with no end-inspiratory pause. The end-tidal CO_2 concentration was kept constant by adjustment of the expiratory time. The inspired oxygen concentration was 40% in all patients who also had normal total compliance of around 80 ml/cm H_2O.

The measurements were carried out using the equipment described else-where Brunner and Wolff (1984), corrected and processed breath by breath (Brunner et al. 1983, 1984). All gas volumes are related to BTPS.

Results

Both PIE and Vds-L showed good reproducibility of ± 6% within 15 breaths. This allowed us to calculate mean values in each situation within ± 3% confidence limits. PIE increased proportional to PAWI, independent of the cause of pressure increase. Vds-L showed a pronounced dependence on VT, in contrast to only a slight dependence on PEEP (Fig. 5).

Discussion

Since series dead space (Vds) is contained within boundaries, given by anatomical walls and functional walls, any change of Vds must be explained by a change in function and/or a change in anatomy. Both may contribute to the dependence of series or "anatomical" dead space on airway pressure: Increased airway pressure distends the airways. This increases the volume of convective airways, i.e., Vds is increased.

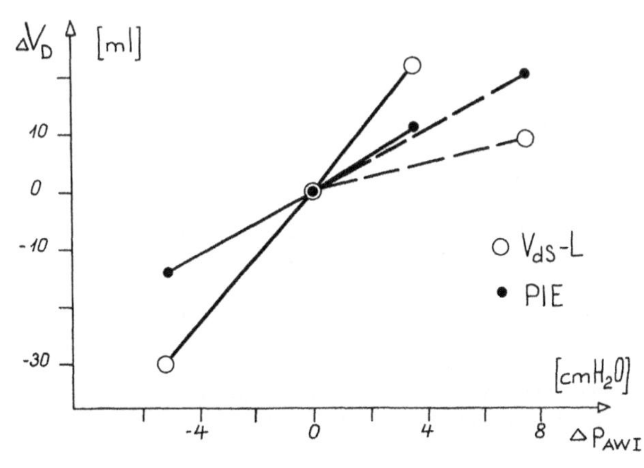

Fig. 5. ΔV_D, mean value of change in series dead space volume (ml); PAWI, end-inspiratory airway pressure; *continuous line*: PAWI depending on tidal volume; *broken line*, PAWI depending on end-expiratory airway pressure (PEEP)

However, due to airway distention total cross-sectional area within the acinus increases and therefore augments diffusion. Consequently the SIs move towards the entrance of the acinus, i.e., Vds is reduced. Paiva (1982) has shown in model calculations that the first effect dominates and Vds increases. These predictions of Paiva can be confirmed by our measurements.

The difference between increasing PAWI by VT or by PEEP must be discussed in the context of the time course: an increase in VT results in a more pulsatile increase of lung volume, whereas PEEP has a constant effect. VT therefore will influence regions with short time constants, while PEEP will influence regions with short and long time constants. It follows that if the effect of PEEP should differ from the effect of increased VT, series dead space would be increased more by PEEP than by VT. However, Vds-L is smaller when PAWI is increased by PEEP. Since the Langley method assesses phase III rather than phase II, it is probably phase III which responds differently to a change in PEEP than to a change in VT.

Conclusion

In conclusion, we understand PIE as the smallest possible and the largest determinable mean series dead space volume. We consider PIE to be an adequate description of the convective airways, since it it the mean value of the flow-, sequence-, and concentration-weighted distribution of all stationary interfaces which can be identified. The method proved to be simple, computer feasible, reproducible, and model consistent. The real time implementation of this algorithm is part of our breath-by-breath monitoring system used for investigations on intensive care patients. It has been in use for 2 years now, and has been found to be reliable at the bedside as well as in the laboratory.

Acknowledgment. This work was supported by the Swiss National Fund for the Advancement of Scientific Research, Berne, application no. 3.831-0.79.

References

Brunner J, Wolff G (1984) Reliable estimation of series dead space in ventilated patients. Clin Physiol (in press)

Brunner J, Langenstein H, Wolff G (1983) Direct accurate gas flow measurement in the patient: Compensation for unavoidable error. Med Prog Technol 9: 233–238

Brunner J, Wolff G, Langenstein H, Cumming G (1984) Reliable detection of inspiration and expiration by computer. J Appl Physiol in press

Cumming G, Horsefield K, Preston SB (1971) Diffusion equilibrium of the lungs examined by nodal analysis. Respir Physiol 12: 329–345

Fletcher R, Jonson B (1984) Deadspace and the single breath test for carbon dioxide during anaesthesia and artificial ventilation. Br J anaesth 56: 109–119

Fletcher R, Jonson B, Cumming G, Brew J (1981) The concept of deadspace with special reference to the single breath test for carbon dioxide. Br J Anaesth 53: 77–94

Horsefield K, Cumming G (1968) Functional consequences of airway morphology. J Appl Physiol 24 (3): 384–390

Langley F, Even P, Duroux P, Nocolas RL, Cumming G (1975) Ventilatory consequences of unilateral pulmonary artery occlusion. Les Colloques de l'Institut National de la Sante et de la Recherche Medicale 51: 209–214

Olsson SG, Fletcher R, Jonson B, Nordstroem L, Prakash O (1980) Clinical studies of gas exchange during ventilatory support – a method using the Siemens-Elema CO_2 analyzer. Br J Anaesth 52: 491–498

Paiva M (1972) Computation of the boundary conditions for diffusion in the human lung. Comput Biomed Res 5: 585–595

Paiva M (1982) Model analysis of inert gas mixing in the lung. Bull Eur Physiopathol Respir 18: 189–201

Evaluation of Indices for Respiratory Mechanics from an Automated System

B. Friberg, M. Forssblad , S. Baehrendtz, J. Hulting, K. Ekenbäck, M. Johansson, and G. Matell

Introduction

The traditional monitoring of respiratory mechanics in patients treated with ventilators includes airway pressure and expired volume minute by minute (Widemann et al. 1984). Semistatic compliance and resistance can be calculated from these parameters (Jonson et al. 1975). Automatic calculation and presentation of lung mechanics has become possible with the use of bedside monitors. Multipatient systems for automatic calculation of these parameters have been described (Matell et al. 1983; Baehrendtz et al. 1980; Brandt and Frank 1980). Reference values for lung mechanics calculated with the aid of such a system in anesthetized patients without pulmonary disease have been published (Carvalhas 1983). However, the influence of various diseases on monitored respiratory-mechanics parameters has, to our knowledge not been systematically studied. In order to establish the influence of common pulmonary disorders on mechanical variables of the lung, automatic respiratory monitoring was carried out in four well defined groups of patients who could be expected to have different lung-mechanical properties. Sampled variables were examined for intergroup differences. In addition, we wanted to test whether a more complex computer-calculated index gave better diagnostic seperation than conventional parameters.

Material

A total of 50 patients treated with ventilators at the Medical Intensive Care Unit (MICU), South Hospital, Stockholm during 1983 were included in the study. Twenty-three patients had no primary chest disease, common diagnoses were hypnotic drug poisoning and cerebrovascular disease. These patients were considered to be in good pulmonary health if they had a normal chest x-ray and normal blood gases (with forced inspiratory oxygen, FIO_2, < 0.3) and had no history of lung disease. The patients with diseased lungs comprised ten patients with pneumonia, eight with bronchial asthma and nine patients with pulmonary edema due to left ventricular failure. Patients with a mixture of pulmonary diseases, e.g., chronic obstructive lung disease with pneumonia, were excluded from the study. The study was approved by the local ethical committee, and there were no complications attributable to it.

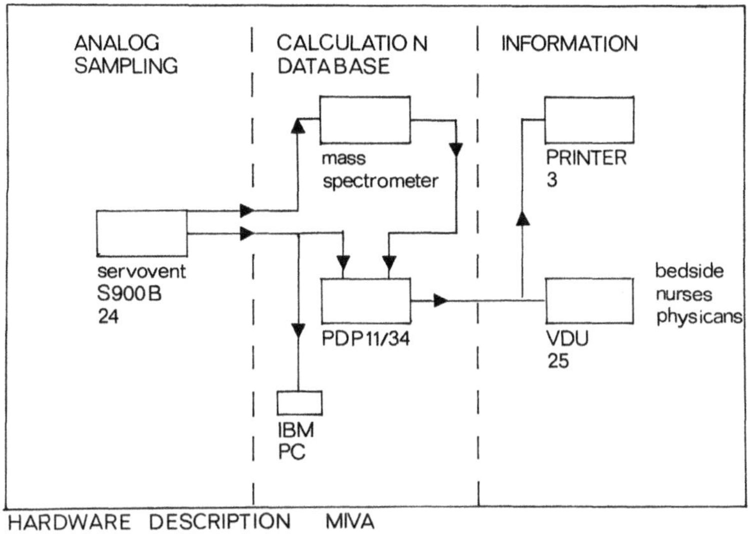

Fig. 1. A total of 24 ventilators can be connected to the system. A centrally positioned PDP 11/34 computer (Digital) calculates compliance and inspiratory resistance from analog signals representing flow and pressure from each ventilator. The parameters are recalculated once per minute. The results are stored in a data base and are available to the staff on 25 video display units (VDU) and 3 printers

Methods

The MICU has 24 beds, all of which are equipped with bedside connections to an automated cardiorespiratory monitoring and information system (Fig. 1) (Baehrendtz et al. 1980; Matell et al. 1983). Analog signals from electronic pressure and flow transducers are recorded once per minute from all running ventilators. A centrally positioned computer (PDP 11/34, Digital) is used to calculate semistatic compliance and inspiratory resistance. The information is stored in a data base and presented to the staff on video display units (VDU). The information can also be obtained as graphic on VDUs and as hard copy from printers.

The respiratory-mechanics variables from each patient in the present study were sampled once per minute for one hour starting one hour after the commencement of the ventilator treatment. Means were calculated after exclusion of artifacts (e.g., patient coughing) had been performed. At the end of inspiration peak pressure (P_{Peak}) and end-inspiratory flow ($\dot{V}_{EI}$) were recorded (Fig. 2). During the study an end-inspiratory pause of 10% of the respiratory cycle was used. The end-pause pressure (P_{Pause}) was recorded at the end of the end-inspiratory pause. The early expiratory flow ($\dot{V}_{EE}$) was measured 80 ms after onset of an expiration. This delay was included to compensate for the compressed volume of gas in the ventilator tubings. The end-expiratory pressure (P_{EE}) was measured at the end of an expiration. Compliance and inspiratory-resistance calculations were performed according to Jonson et al. (1975) as follows:

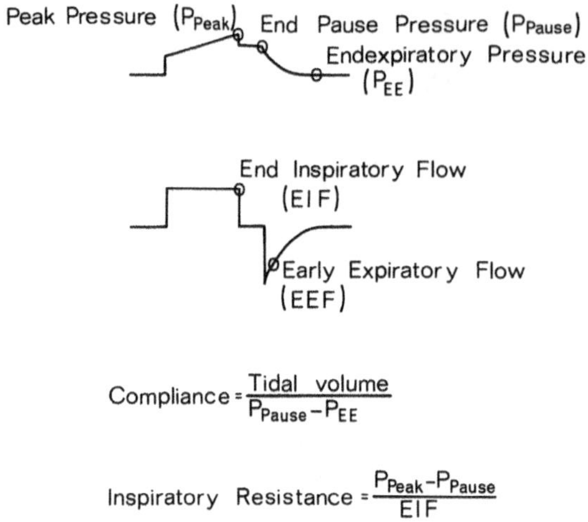

Fig. 2. Pressure and flow signals during one respiratory cycle. Peak pressure and end-inspiratory flow are recorded at end-inspiration. The end pause pressure (P_{Pause}) is recorded at the end of the inspiratory pause. End-expiratory pressure (P_{EE}) and end-expiratory flow ($\dot{V}_{EE}$) are recorded at end expiration

$$\text{Compliance } (C) = V_T / (P_{Pause} - (P_{EE} + \dot{V}_{EE} \times R_E))$$

$$\text{Inspiratory resistance } (R_I) = (P_{Peak} - P_{Pause}) / \dot{V}_{EI}$$

$$\text{Expiratory resistance } (R_E) = (P_{Pause} - P_{EE}) / \dot{V}_{EE}$$

where $\dot{V}_T$ = tidal volume, P_{Peak} = peak pressure, P_{Pause} = end pause pressure, $\dot{V}_{EE}$ = end expiratory flow, R_E = expiratory resistance, $\dot{V}_{EI}$ = end inspiratory flow, and P_{EE} = end expiratory pressure.

The product of end-expiratory flow ($\dot{V}_{EE}$) and expiratory resistance (R_E) is added to the end-expiratory pressure (P_{EE}). Compensation is thus made for low end-expiratory flow, such as occurs in highly obstructed patients. Tidal volume is obtained by integrating the expiratory flow with a delay of 80 ms. Linear regression and comparison of means and variances between groups have been used as statistical methods. A p-value > 0.05 was considered not significant.

Results

The results are summarized in Fig. 3–7. In the pulmonary healthy patients compliance averaged 0.461 $*$ kPa^{-1} and increased as expected with increasing tidal volume (Fig. 3). The inspiratory resistance was within the range 1.5–2.0 kPa $*$ l^{-1} $*$ s^{-1} and did not correlate with tidal volume. Patients with pulmonary edema (Fig. 4) had lower compliance (0.30 ± 0.07 l $*$ kPa^{-1}) than the pulmonary healthy patients ($p < 0.001$). However, the inspiratory resistance was within the same range as that of the pulmonary healthy group.

In the patients suffering from pneumonia (Fig. 5) compliance averaged 0.30 l $*$ kPa^{-1}, which was well below the pulmonary healthy group ($p < 0.001$). Inspiratory resistance (1.94 ± 0.46 kPa $*$ l^{-1} $*$ s^{-1}) was within the upper range of pulmonary healthy patients.

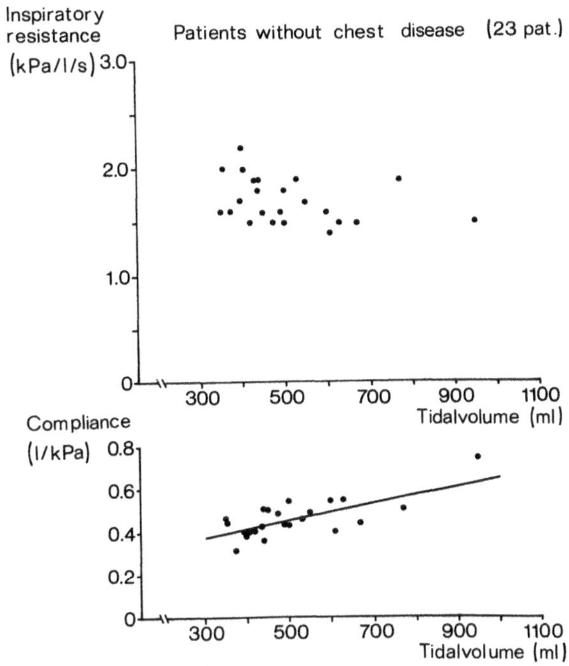

Fig. 3. Compliance and inspiratory resistance for the pulmonary healthy group. Compliance increases with tidal volume. Inpiratory resistance is within the range of 1.5–2.0 kPa $*\,l^{-1} * s^{-1}$ and displayed no correlation with tidal volume

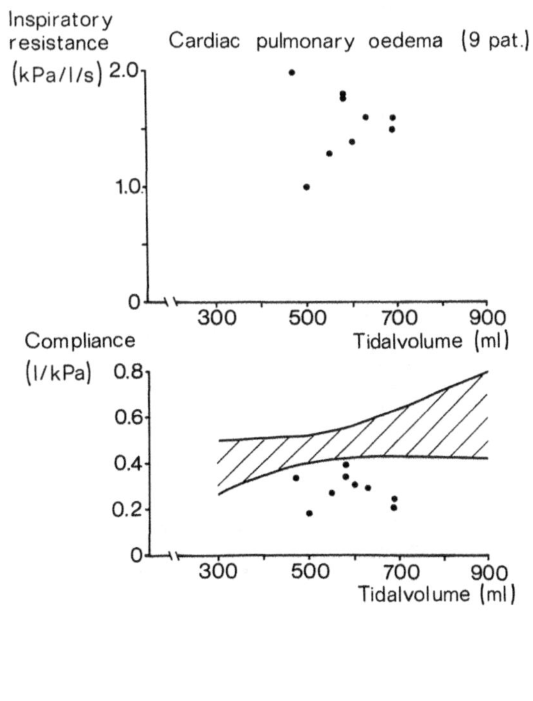

Fig. 4. Compliance and inspiratory resistance for nine patients with pulmonary edema. The hatched area represents the 95% confidence interval for the group with no lung disease. Inspiratory resistance did not differ from that of patients without chest disease

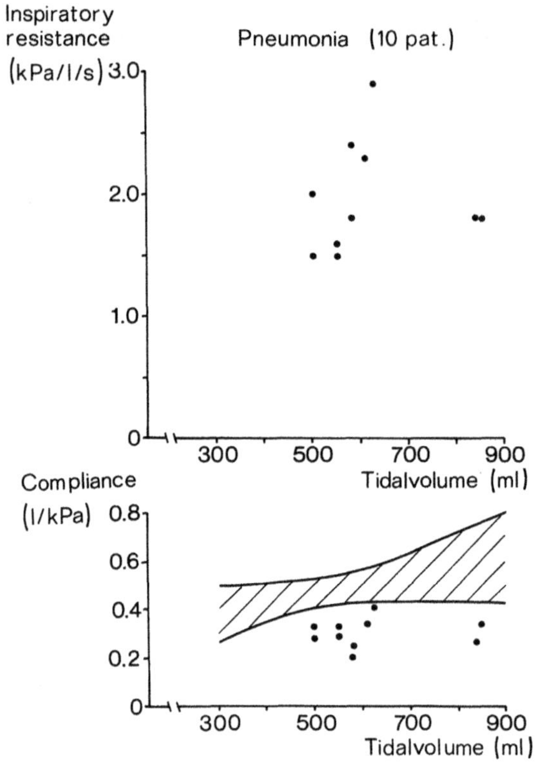

Fig. 5. Compliance and inspiratory resistance for ten patients with pneumonia. All individual compliance recordings are lower than for the patients without chest disease. The hatched area represents the 95% confidence interval for the group with no lung disease. Inspiratory resistance is within the same range as for the pulmonary healthy patients

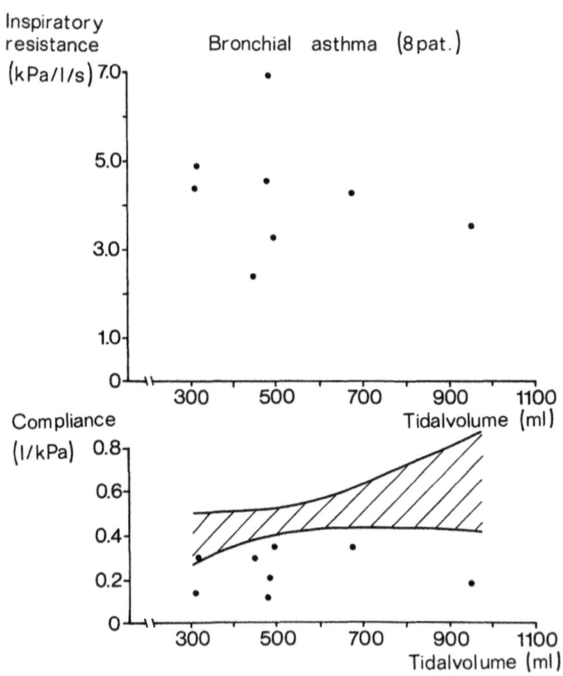

Fig. 6. Compliance for eight patients with bronchial asthma is lower than for the pulmonary healthy, while inspiratory resistance is higher. The hatched area represents the 95% confidence interval for the group with no lung disease

In patients with acute bronchial asthma (Fig. 6) compliance was 0.23 ± 0.08 l ∗ kPa^{-1} which was lower than for the pulmonary healthy group ($p < 0.001$) but not different from the patients with pneumonia or pulmonary edema. Inspiratory resistance displayed a mean of 4.24 kPa ∗ l^{-1} ∗ s^{-1} and was generally higher than in the other groups of patients.

Discussion

The system with automated sampling, computation, storing and presentation of lung-mechanics data provides a potential tool in the monitoring of patients treated on ventilators, especially in following the progression or regression of a pathological process. As expected, patients with pulmonary diseases (i.e., bronchial asthma, pneumonia and pulmonary edema) had lower compliance in comparison with the pulmonary healthy patients. However, inspiratory resistance was increased in acute bronchial asthma alone. It was not possible to differentiate between different groups of diseases by studying compliance or inspiratory resistance alone. The results emerging from the present study have provided us with a rough gauge for the evaluation of monitored respiratory parameters. However, it must be emphasized that these results are generated by one of many such systems in use around the world and that each and every system has to be evaluated on its own because of discrepancies in hard- and software set-up and different sampling techniques.

In an attempt to find a better discriminator we defined an index by dividing inspiratory resistance and compliance (R_I/C index). The R_I/C indices for the four groups of patients are displayed in Fig. 7. There is a difference ($p < 0.001$) between the pulmonary healthy patients and the three other patient categories. A difference also exists between bronchial asthma and pulmonary edema ($p < 0.01$) and also between bronchial asthma and pneumonia ($p < 0.01$). The index did not permit discrimination between the pulmonary edema and pneumonia groups. Consequently,

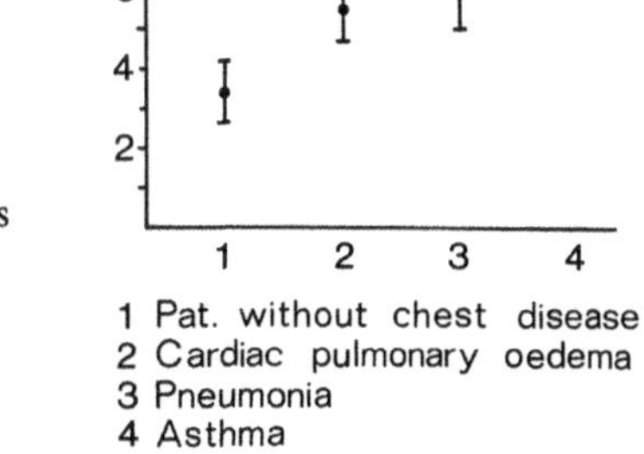

Fig. 7. By dividing inspiratory resistance by compliance an index (R_I/C) was constructed. Mean ± SD for this index is displayed for each patient category. There is a significant difference between patients without chest disease in comparison with the other groups. Patients with bronchial asthma had a significantly higher R_I/C index than those with pulmonary edeme or pneumonia

the R_I/C index failed to increase the discrimination rate between the different pathological processes studied. However, since increases and/or decreases of compliance *and* resistance will have greater impact on the constructed index than on the respective variables alone, it is probable that the R_I/C index will provide more obvious and possibly more prompt information regarding the progression or regression of a specific lung disease. If so, automatic monitoring of the index could be of additional help in the process of medical decision making and alarm signals can alert the staff when limits are first exceeded. In more favourable cases the patient can be weaned off the ventilator at an earlier stage than otherwise, or in the worse circumstances, e.g., due to increased obstruction, the staff have the opportunity of undertaking appropriate medical intervention at an earlier time. The R_I/C index may also be included in artificial intelligence programs for respiratory care.

Finally, we want to emphasize that in everyday intensive care we are not only dealing with patients with "pure" pneumonia, pulmonary edema or bronchial asthma but most frequently, with patients suffering from lung diseases involving several factors and this probably lessens the diagnostic usefulness of the R_I/C index. However, we suggest that the concept of the R_I/C index should be further evaluated.

We conclude that the range of inspiratory resistance and compliance obtained by an automated system can be fairly well defined for common groups of pulmonary disorders and that the ratio inspiratory resistance to compliance (R_I/C index) can be of help in differential diagnosis between bronchial asthma and pulmonary edema and pneumonia. The index is most probably more sensitive to variations in lung pathology than compliance or resistance alone and might therefore give faster and more prompt information as to whether a patient is deteriorating or improving.

References

Baehrendtz S, Hulting J, Matell G, Nygards ME (1980) Clinical evaluation of automated arrhythmia monitoring and its integration with respiratory monitoring in a general computerized information system. In: Nair S (ed) Computers in critical care and pulmonary medicine. Plenum, New York, pp 269–277

Brandt HJ, Frank W (1980) Automatisierte Kontinuierliche Überwachung der Respiration. Intensivmedizin 17: 220–6

Carvalhas AJB (1983) Relacoes de Ventilacao-Perfusao Pulmonar E Mecanica Respiratoria SOB Anaestesia. Thesis, University of Coimbra, Lisaboa, Portugal

Jonson B, Nordström L, Olsson SG, Åkerbäck D (1975) Monitoring of ventilation and lung mechanics during automatic ventilation. A new device. Bull Physiopathol Respir 11: 729–743

Matell G, Hulting J, Johansson M, Lindelöf B (1983) Computerized monitoring and information processing in the ICU – Attempts at an evaluation. In: Bemmel, Ball, Wigertz (eds) North Holland, Amsterdam, pp 84–87

Widemann HP, Matthay MA, Matthay RA (1984) Cardiovascularpulmonary monitoring in the intensive care unit. Chest 4: 537–549

Mathematical Modelling for Prediction of Optimal Ventilator Settings

R. RUDOWSKI, G. MATELL, K. EKENBÄCK, C. SPANNE, and B. OSSMER

Introduction

The goal of artificial ventilation is to stabilize CO_2 and O_2 concentrations in arterial blood at a desired level. This stabilization can be achieved at different combinations of ventilator settings. The question can therefore be raised as to which combination is optimal for the patient. The answer to this question depends on the chosen optimization criterion.

Some different factors to be optimized in intermittent positive pressure ventilation (IPPV) treatment can be mentioned:

- Cardiac output $\dot{Q}_T$
- Shunt fraction $\dot{Q}_S/\dot{Q}_T$
- Physiological dead space V_{DPhys}
- Functional residual capacity FRC
- Barotrauma risk

Reynolds (1978) proposed peak inspiratory pressure (PIP) and mean airway pressure (MAP) as performance indices and suggested reversed phases of ventilation (inspiratory time higher than expiratory time) to lower mean airway pressure.

Suter et al. (1975) chose lung compliance as the optimization performance index stating that maximum O_2 transport (arterial O_2 content × cardiac output) was achieved within the steepest part of the individual pressure-volume curve of the lungs.

Several authors (Darowski 1981; Rudowski et al. 1983) have proposed mean respiratory power (inspiratory work divided by the respiratory cycle time) as the performance index. The approach originated from Rohrer (1925) and Otis (1950). Their studies dealt with spontaneous breathing and suggested that man breathes with the frequency at which the mean respiratory power is minimum. Darowski (1981) and Rudowski et al. (1983) applied that concept to mechanical ventilation.

Jain and Guha (1972) proposed as the performance index the mean difference of alveolar pressure in the lungs of a healthy subject represented by a model of constant parameters and in the lungs of a patient represented by a model of variable parameters. The optimization goal is to minimize that difference. The index proposed by Jain and Guha can be used for estimation of the depressive influence of mechanical ventilation on the cardiovascular system.

Maffeo and Anné (1978) accepted physiological dead space and shunt as optimization performance indices. These indices reflect efficiency of the lungs as a gas exchanger.

Engström and Norlander (1962) took into consideration peak respiratory power (the maximum product of flow and pressure at the mouth level) (PRP) from the ventilator design point of view. A certain power reserve should be available during inspiration to meet patient demands.

Some of the indices mentioned can be used for prediction of the barotrauma risk. The definition of barotrauma according to Cullen and Caldera (1979) is the development of pneumothorax, pneumomediastinum, or subcutaneous emphysema in patients receiving respiratory therapy. The barotrauma problem is particularly important in the case of artificially ventilated children.

The reported incidence of barotrauma varies between 0.5% and 22%. Cullen and Caldera (1979) reported the lowest incidence – 0.5%. Other reported incidences are as follows: Kumar et al. (1973) – 10% in an IPPV group without PEEP (positive end expiratory pressure) and 11% in an IPPV + PEEP group; Mathru et al. (1983) – 22% in an CMV + PEEP group and 7% in an IMV + CPAP (intermittent mandatory ventilation plus continuous positive airway pressure) group; Petersen and Baier (1983) – 8% in an IMV + PEEP group of patients.

Several ways of barotrauma prevention and treatment have been proposed by Hillman (1984).

In view of the reported incidence of barotrauma, the barotrauma risk was accepted in our study as one primary optimization criterion. The prediction of the ventilator settings minimizing barotrauma risk can be based on the mathematical model of artificial ventilation combined with an optimization performance index. The mechanisms behind barotrauma are certainly not solely related to the peak power applied, since the condition to the pulmonary tissue must also be an important factor.

The purpose of this study was to define the mathematical model of artificial ventilation for predictions of the optimal ventilator settings, to use this model for simulation trials, and to verify it clinically. The computer-aided ventilator setting in clinical practice is the planned final stage of the work.

Mathematical Model of Artificial Ventilation and the Optimization Performance Index

Development of a computer program for prediction of the optimal ventilator settings requires firstly the definition of all equations describing the process. This set of equations is called the mathematical model. Its structure is shown in Fig. 1.

The first component of the model is the CO_2 elimination equation – metabolic hyperbola:

$$\dot{V}_A \cdot C_{ETCO_2} = \dot{V}_{CO_2} \quad (1)$$

It allows calculation of alveolar ventilation ($\dot{V}_A$) when CO_2 production of the patient ($\dot{V}_{CO_2}$) and desired end-tidal CO_2 concentration (C_{ETCO_2}) (equal to mean alveolar CO_2 concentration) are given. It is assumed that C_{ETCO_2} is equal to CO_2 concentration in arterial blood.

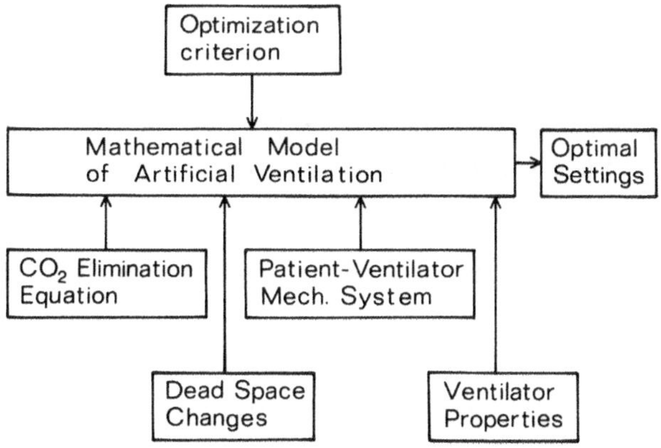

Fig. 1. The mathematical model structure of artificial ventilation

Equation (2) in turn defines alveolar ventilation

$$\dot{V}_A = V_A \cdot f \tag{2}$$

It can be seen from Eq (2) that a certain alveolar ventilation can be reached at many combinations of alveolar volume and the frequency of breathing. The choice of the best combination represents the optimization problem which is solved after defining an optimization performance index. The performance index will be discussed later.

The second component of our artificial ventilation mathematical model is a model of the patient-ventilator mechanical system (Fig. 2). It is a one-compartment model with R representing inspiratory resistance and C lung/chest complicance of the patient. The values of R and C are assumed to be constant, i. e., not dependent on the flow or pressure in the lung. The ventilator is represented by the constant flow source $\dot{V}$. This assumption is certainly true in the case of the Servoventilator (Siemens-Elema) or any device maintaining a constant flow to the patient. This simple model of a patient-ventilator mechanical system does not take into account the internal compliance of the ventilator, which usually is much smaller than the lung/chest compliance of an adult person.

The third component of the model is the equation describing the anatomical dead space changes with the change in tidal volume. It is necessary to consider this if the performance index is to be calculated for a certain range to tidal volumes or frequencies of breathing.

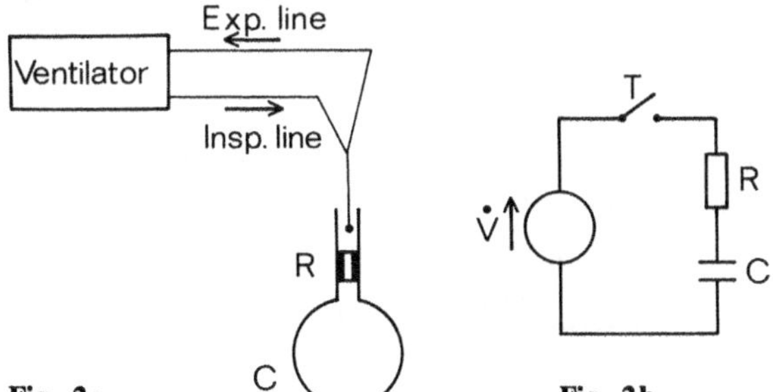

Fig. 2a, b. The accepted model of the patient-ventilator mechanical system. **a** the physical model; **b** the electrical analog of the model

Fig. 2a **Fig. 2b**

Tidal volume is described by the equation

$$V_T = V_A + V_D \tag{3}$$

where V_A = alveolar volume and V_D = anatomical dead space.

The simple model of the anatomical dead space changes is the equation

$$V_D = k \cdot V_T \tag{4}$$

where k = constant, found experimentally by Hedenstierna and McCarthy (1975) in healthy subjects.

Another model

$$\begin{aligned} V_D &= \text{const} = 150 \text{ ml for } V_T \geqq 500 \text{ ml} \\ V_D &= k \cdot V_T \text{ for } V_T > 500 \text{ ml} \end{aligned} \tag{5}$$

where k = constant can also be considered.

The fourth component of the mathematical model of artificial ventilation is the characteristic properties of the ventilator. For example the constant proportions of inspiratory, pause, and expiratory time in the respiratory cycle of some ventilators can be given.

The above-formulated model of artificial ventilation allows the construction of an algorithm for the ventilator settings calculation. The various setting combinations stabilizing C_{ETCO_2} at the desired level can be obtained in this way, and that combination chosen which minimizes the performance index.

The problem is finding a synthetic index which would be dependent on all ventilator settings and respiratory system parameters. This index should reflect both static (pressure) and dynamic (rate of pressure change) loads applied to the alveoli.

The peak respiratory power may be such an index. Power is defined as the amount of work performed in a unit of time. In pneumatic systems, such as a patient-ventilator system, the power is described by the formula:

$$P = \dot{V} \cdot p \tag{6}$$

where $\dot{V}$ = gas flow and p = gas pressure.

It is most convenient to consider power at the mouth level, where both flow and pressure can easily be measured. The highest risk of barotrauma accompanies the peak power marked PRP. The ventilator settings should be chosen to maintain correct gas exchange and at the same time to minimize PRP. The equation describing PRP for a constant flow ventilator is

$$PRP = \dot{V} \cdot p_{m\,max} = \dot{V}(p_{A\,max} + p_R) \tag{7}$$

where $P_{A\,max}$ = max alveolar (transthoracic) pressure and p_R = pressure drop across the resistance of the airways.

Substituting to (7)

$$\begin{aligned} p_{A\,max} &= PEEP + V_T/C \\ p_R &= \dot{V} \cdot R \end{aligned} \tag{8}$$

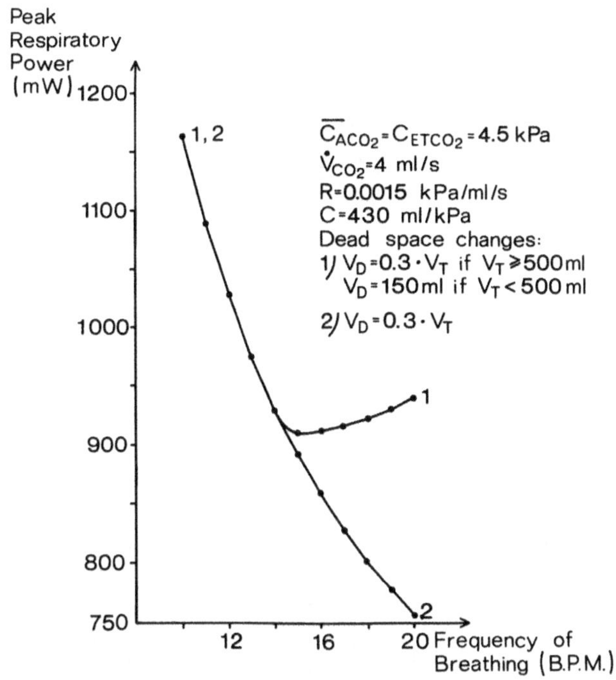

Fig. 3. The results of the model prediction

we finally obtain for PRP

$$PRP = \dot{V}(PEEP + V_T/C + \dot{V} \cdot R) \tag{9}$$

The results of the model prediction for different dead space changes are shown in Fig. 3. The PRP minimum was obtained within the frequency range normally used in IPPV when model (5) of the dead space changes was applied (Fig. 3, curve 1). When model (4) was tested the PRP minimum was found at the highest frequency (Fig. 3, curve 2). The results obtained in the simulation trials guided the clinical verification of the model performed in seven patients.

Clinical Verification of the Mathematical Model

Patients

Seven patients undergoing ventilator treatment were chosen for the study. The patients are listed in Table 1.

Methods

The technical arrangement is shown in Fig. 4. Its wider description is given by Matell et al. (1983). Three different computer systems were employed in the study.

Table 1. The patient material

No.	Age (years)	Sex	Diagnosis
1	66	F	Poisoning
2	70	M	Myocardial infarction, pulmonary edema, cardiogenic shock
3	80	M	Myocardial infarction. Died
4	42	F	Haemorrhagia cerebri NUD cum hypertonia. Died
5	77	F	Myasthenia gravis
6	71	F	Pulmonary edema
7	77	M	Statuspost-resuscitation, pulmonary edema

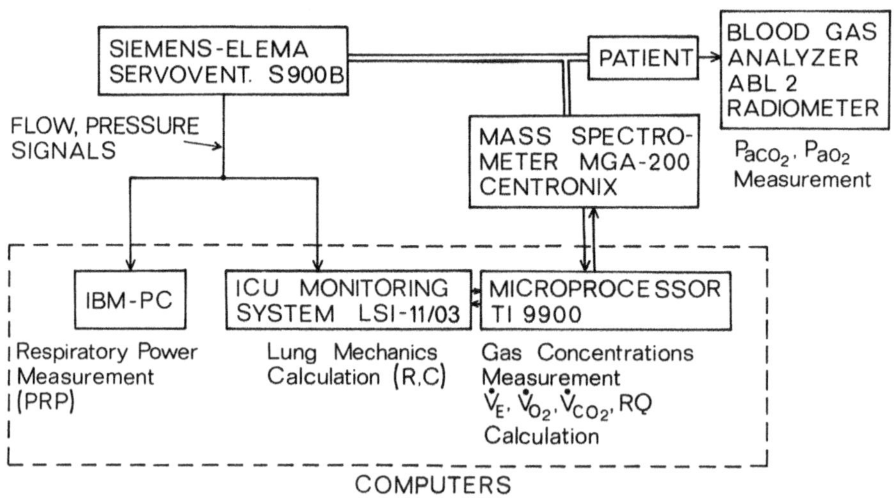

Fig. 4. The technical arrangement

The first, the ICU patient monitoring computer system (LSI 11/03 and PDP 11/34), was used to store information such as respiratory, blood gas, and cardiovascular system data.

The second computer was a microcomputer system (TI 9900) built into a mass spectrometer (MGA-200 Centronic) for displaying gas concentration [end-tidal CO_2 concentration (C_{ETCO_2}) and mixed expired CO_2 concentration (C_{ECO_2})] and calculations of expired volume ($\dot{V}_E$), CO_2 elimination ($\dot{V}_{CO_2}$), and O_2 consumption ($\dot{V}_{O_2}$).

The third computer system employed in the study was the IBM-PC for peak respiratory power measurement.

The respiratory mechanics – lung/chest compliance and inspiratory resistance – were calculated by the monitoring system from flow and pressure signals sampled form the Servoventilator. The formulas used for the calculation were the same as those applied in the Siemens-Elema Lung Mechanics Calculator.

All patients were ventilated with the Siemens-Elema Servoventilator S-900 B at a constant flow setting.

The blood gas concentrations were measured electrometrically (ABL-2 Radiometer, Copenhagen). The $(V_D/V_T)_{Anat}$ and the $(V_D/V_T)_{Phys}$ were calculated from Bohr equations:

$$(V_D/V_T)_{Anat} = \frac{p_{ETCO_2} - p_{ECO_2}}{p_{ETCO_2}} \tag{10}$$

$$(V_D/V_T)_{Phys} = \frac{p_{aCO_2} - p_{ECO_2}}{p_{aCO_2}} \tag{11}$$

Procedure

The goal of the clinical study was to investigate whether the peak respiratory power minimum occurs within the range of normally used ventilation frequencies for arterial CO_2 partial pressure (P_{aCO_2}) kept constant at all frequencies. The most frequent ventilator setting was no PEEP, inspiratory time/respiratory cycle ratio (T_I/T) = 25%, and pause time/respiratory cycle ratio (T_p/T) = 10%. In two patients the influence of 1 kPa PEEP and T_I/T = 15%, T_p/T = 20% on peak respiratory power was studied separately. After setting the frequency, at least 10 min was allowed for the patient to reach equilibrium before blood samples were taken and all measurements made. If p_{aCO_2} was not equal to the desired value, then a correction of the minute volume was performed at the same frequency in order to obtain a p_{aCO_2} value as close as possible to the desired value. Usually the measurements were done at four or five different frequencies ranging from 10 to 21 b.p.m.

The following parameters were measured at a given frequency after stabilization of the patient:

– Peak respiratory power	PRP (mW)
– Inspiratory resistance	R (kPa/ml/s)
– Lung/chest compliance	C (ml/kPa)
– End-tidal CO_2 concentration	C_{ETCO_2} (%)
– Mixed-expired CO_2 concentration	C_{ECO_2} (%)
– Arterial CO_2 partial pressure	P_{aCO_2} (kPa)

Results

The results of the study are presented in Figs. 5 and 6 and in Tables 2–5.

Peak Respiratory Power

Figure 5 illustrates the respiratory power change during inspiration for two different ventilator settings. The peak power for a constant flow setting is reached at the end of inspiration; this is different from spontaneous breathing, where the peak power occurs at mid-inspiration (Engström and Norlander 1962). Figure 5 shows how the ventilator setting affects the peak power.

The peak respiratory power as a function of frequency of breathing for all patients in the study is shown in Fig. 6. In five patients the PRP minimum was reached within the frequency range, in one patient at the highest frequency set, and in one patient at

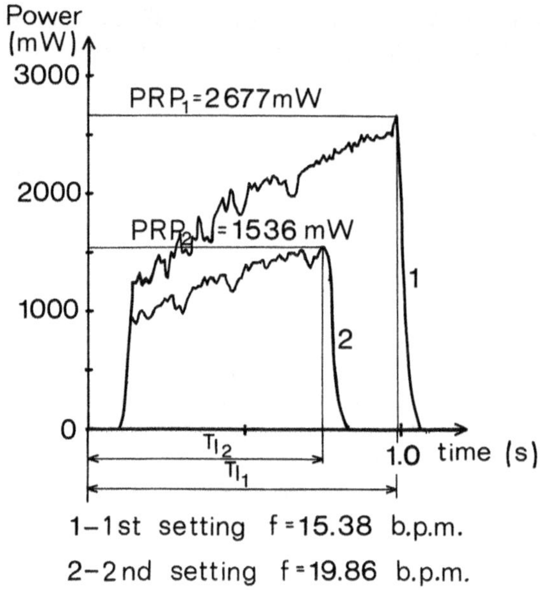

Fig. 5. The respiratory power change during inspiration for two different ventilator settings (patient 4)

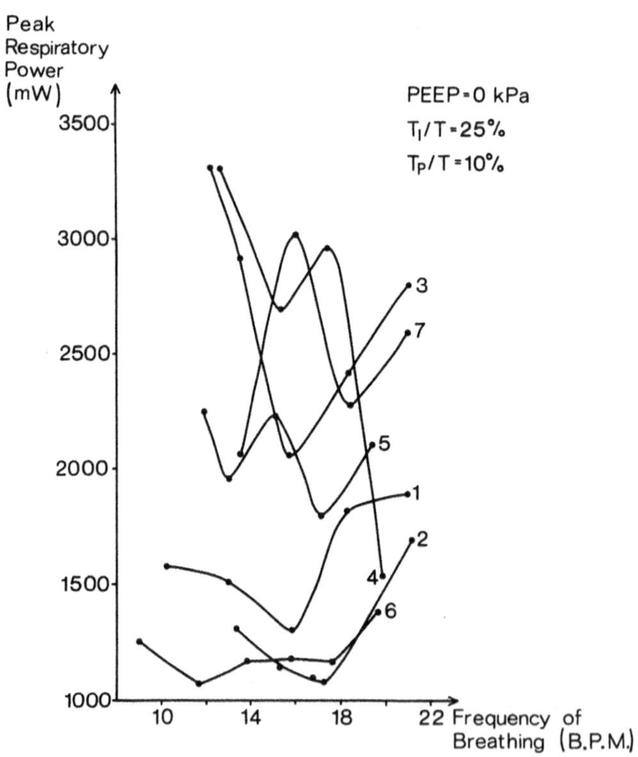

Fig. 6. The peak respiratory power curves for seven patients investigated in the study. For each patient P_{aCO_2} was kept approximately constant at all frequencies

the lowest frequency set. Thus the result of the model prediction was confirmed qualitatively in a clinical study. The mean frequency of breathing at which the PRP minimum occurred was $\overline{f^*} = 15.885 \pm 2.672$ (1 SD).

When adding a PEEP a moderate increase in PRP minimum was found (Table 2). However, in both cases PEEP improved the oxygenation of the patient. The result of the settings $T_I/T = 15\%$, $T_p/T = 20\%$ was a significant increase in PRP minimum (Table 2).

Table 2. The influence of PEEP and $T_I/T = 15\%$

Patient	3	4
Minimum PRP (mW), no PEEP, $T_I/T = 25\%$, $T_p/T = 10\%$	2050	1508
Minimum PRP (mW), 1 kPa PEEP, $T_I/T = 25\%$, $T_p/T = 10\%$	2569	2128
Minimum PRP (mW), no PEEP, $T_I/T = 15\%$, $T_p/T = 20\%$	5500	6428

Table 3. The effect of P_{aCO_2} on PRP minimum

Patient	1	2	3	4	5	6	7
P_{aCO_2} (kPa)	4.182	4.992	4.52	3.125	3.894	4.9	4.175
Min. PRP (mW)	1293	1080	2050	1508	1786	1073	2030

Table 4. Accuracy of the mathematical model

Patient	1	2	3	4	5	6	7
Min. PRP measured	1293	1080	2050	1508	1786	1073	2030
Min. PRP calculated	1303.6	944	1884.8	1443.5	1799.6	921.0	1729.0
Error (%)	0.8	12.6	8.1	4.3	0.8	14.2	14.8

Table 5. Mean values and SD of compliance and dead spaces at different frequencies.

	C (ml/kPa)	$(V_D/V_T)_{Anat}$	$(V_D/V_T)_{Phys}$
f = 13.5	410.0 ± 113.4	0.362 ± 0.026	0.457 ± 0.023
f = 16.0	395.8 ± 87.9	0.383 ± 0.052	0.483 ± 0.017
f = 18.5	381.6 ± 99.9	0.402 ± 0.035	0.500 ± 0.012
f = 21.0	386.4 ± 91.2	0.408 ± 0.046	0.515 ± 0.025
P	< 0.05	> 0.05	< 0.05

The effect of P_{aCO_2} on PRP minimum was studied (Table 3), and there was an obvious relation between higher P_{aCO_2} (= lower alveolar ventilation) and PRP minimum.

The accuracy of the mathematical model in predicting the value of PRP was tested. The test was performed for the PRP minimum in every patient and the following results were obtained (Table 4).

Lung/Chest Compliance, Anatomical and Physiological Dead Space

Paired differences were statistically evaluated (t-test) in five patients between f_1 = 13.5 b.p.m. and f_2 = 21 b.p.m. for lung/chest compliance C, $(V_D/V_T)_{Anat}$, and $(V_D/V_T)_{Phys}$. Statistically significant differences were found for C and $(V_D/V_T)_{Phys}$ (Table 5). No statistically significant difference was found for $(V_D/V_T)_{Anat}$.

The compliance of the patients ranged from 250 ml/kPa to 575 ml/kPa. The values of $(V_D/V_T)_{Anat}$ ranged from 0.318 to 0.45 and those of $(V_D/V_T)_{Phys}$ from 0.42 to 0.54.

Discussion

The purpose of the study was achieved by defining the mathematical model of artificial ventilation, using it for simulation trials, and verifying it clinically. The clinical studies showed that some modifications of the assumptions were needed. This applied mainly to the frequency-dependent lung/chest compliance.

A fall in compliance with the frequency of breathing was reported by Hedenstierna and Löfström (1972). They explained it by an altered, presumably less uniform gas distribution.

The constant $(V_D/V_T)_{Anat}$ (no statistically significant difference – Table 5) is in agreement with the results of Hedenstierna and McCarthy (1975), but contradicts those of Fletcher and Jonson (1982). The $(V_D/V_T)_{Phys}$ increment with the frequency of breathing (Table 5) is in agreement with the results of Fletcher and Jonson (1982). However, the values of $(V_D/V_T)_{Anat}$ and $(V_D/V_T)_{Phys}$ in our study are higher. The explanation is the different method of (V_D/V_T) calculation i.e., the Bohr equation in our study and the Fowler method in Fletcher and Jonson (1982).

The accuracy of the model (Table 4) (the difference between PRP values measured and those calculated from the model) depends on the accuracy of all the measurements involved, i.e., inspiratory resistance, lung/chest compliance, flow, and volume, as well as on the accuracy of the model itself. The possible explanation for the errors is that flow oscillations produced by the servosystem of the ventilator were not included in the model.

The other important question beyond the model itself is the choice of the optimization performance index. We believe that the choice of the peak respiratory power for the estimation of barotrauma risk is correct. Such a choice is based on the linkage of trauma with the amount of energy applied to the patient's lungs. Our clinical studies showed that PRP is very sensitive to the ventilator settings and that its minimum can be found within the ventilator frequencies normally used. However, a long-term clinical study of the ventilation of patients at minimum PRP is suggested to compare the incidence of barotrauma in such a condition with the present incidence.

Our results regarding peak respiratory power contradict those obtained by Hedenstierna and Löfström (1972), where minimum PRP within a frequency range was not found. A possible explanation for this is the different organization of the studies (p_{aCO_2} = constant in our study and MV = constant in theirs). A parabolic PRP curve depends on the combination of all the factors involved [see Eq. (9)]. The PRP increase at higher frequencies, however, can be explained by the deteriorating gas exchange manifesting itself by a higher $(V_D/V_T)_{Phys}$ ration and then by more ventilation being needed to keep p_{aCO_2} constant. The decrease of the lung/chest compliance at higher frequencies also contributes to the PRP increase.

In a way our results confirm those of McIlroy et al. (1954), i. e., a minimum of work is performed at around 15 breaths/min in healthy subjects during spontaneous breathing.

The results with regard to a PRP minimum increase in the case of PEEP (Table 2) can be explained by the fact that PEEP, which causes an increase in PRP failed to produce the compliance increase which would bring into effect a PRP decrease.

The higher flow values at the same tidal volume were the cause of a significant PRP increase when the T_I/T = 15% setting was applied (Table 2).

It can be generally noticed that hyperventilation of the patient (lower P_{aCO_2} values) requires more power (Table 3). The lowest values of PRP minimum correspond to the highest P_{aCO_2} values (Table 3).

Our preliminary study confirms the theoretical possibility of using the PRP index to estimate barotrauma risk. We envisage, however, a possible broader application of that index in optimizing the other factors encountered in ventilator treatment, such as physiological dead space, shunt fraction, and cardiac output. Combined monitoring of PRP with the other index – pulmonary blood flow – can also be foreseen. Simple methods of noninvasive measurement of the latter index have been reported recently (Linnarsson and Larsson 1984; Gedeon 1984). This will probably be helpful for selection of those PEEP and I_I/T_E settings which keep FRC sufficiently high to avoid airway collapse.

Conclusions

1. It is theoretically possible that peak respiratory power (PRP) is an index of barotrauma risk.
2. Our preliminary clinical study has confirmed this possibility.
3. Some assumptions underlying our mathematical model for prediction of optimal ventilator settings should be modified.
4. Optimization of ventilator settings has to take into consideration several different factors.

Acknowledgment. This study was performed with the support of grants from the Count Potocki Foundation, Warsaw, Poland.

References

Cullen DJ, Caldera DL (1979) The incidence of ventilator-induced pulmonary barotrauma in critically III patients. Anaesthesiology 50: 185

Darowski M (1981) The choice of a set of some respiration parameters for optimization of their settings. Biocyb Biomed Eng 1: 3/4, 33

Engström CG, Norlander EP (1962) A new method for analysis of respiratory work by measurements of the actual power as a function of gas flow, pressure and time. Acta Anaesth Scand 6: 49

Fletcher R, Jonson B (1982) Dead space analysis during different ventilator setting: use of the single breath test for CO_2. In: Prakash O (ed) Computers in critical care and pulmonary medicine. 2nd Int. Symp. vol 2 Plenum, New York, pp 179–181

Gedeon A (1984) Noninvasive pulmonary blood flow for optimal PEEP. In Abstracts: gas exchange symposium. Lund 1984

Hedenstierna G, Löfström B (1972) Breathing mechanics and gas exchange in normal subjects during artificial ventilation: influence of respiratory frequency and minute volume. Scand J Respir Dis 53: 135–148

Hedenstierna G, McCarthy G (1975) The effect of anaesthesia and intermittent positive pressure ventilation with different frequency on the anatomical and alveolar dead space. Br J Anaesth 47: 847

Hillman K (1984) Barotrauma. In: Vincent JL (ed) Intensive care and emergency medicine. 4th Inf. Symposium. Springer, Berlin, pp 52–55

Jain VK, Guha SK (1972) A control system for long term ventilation of the lungs. IEEE Trans Biomed Eng 19: 47

Kumar A, Pontoppidan H, Falke KJ, Wilson RS, Laver MB (1973) Pulmonary barotrauma during mechanical ventilation. Crit Care Med 1: 4, 181

Linnarsson D, Larsson H (1984) Pulmonary blood flow determination with selective rebreathing. In: Abstracts: gas exchange symposium, Lund 1984

Maffeo CJ, Anné A (1978) Optimal ventilation of critically ill patients, In: Klir GJ (ed) Applied general systems research. Plenum, New York

Matell G, Hulting J, Johansson M, Lindelöw B (1983) Computerized monitoring and information processing in the ICU – attempts at an evaluation. In: van Bemmell, Wigertz (eds) Medinfo 83, Proc. of 4th World Conference on Medical Informatics, North Holland, pp 84–87

Mathru M, Rao TLK, Venus B (1983) Ventilator induced barotrauma in controlled mechanical ventilation versus intermittent mandatory ventilation. Crit Care Med 11: 5, 359

McIlroy MB, Marshall R, Christie RV (1954) Work of breathing in normal subjects. Clin Sci 13: 127–136

Otis AB (1950) Mechanics of breathing in man. J Phys 2: 592

Petersen GW, Baier H (1983) Incidence of pulmonary barotrauma in a medical ICU. Crit Care Med 2: 67

Reynolds O (1978) Ventilator therap. In: Thibeault DW, Gregory GA (eds) Neonatal pulmonary care. Addison-Wesley, p 217

Rohrer F (1925) Physiologie der Atembewegung. Handb. d. norm. u. path. Physiol. vol 2, p 70

Rudowski R, Darowski M, Rondio Z, Rawicz M (1983) The computer program for ventilator settings calculation. In: Prakash O (ed) Proc Symp. on Computers in Anaesthesia and Intensive Care. Rotterdam, Sept 1983

Suter P, Fairley MB, Isenberg MD (1975) Optimum end-expiratory airway pressure in patients with acute pulmonary failure. N Engl J Med 232: 284

Indications for the Application of Closed Loop Systems in Perioperative Medicine

R. D. WESTENSKOW

Introduction

A closed-loop system compares a feedback signal with a control input, the difference signal drives an actuator which reduces the difference (Eveleigh 1972). The actuating signal continually changes so that the feedback signal tends to become equal to the control input, regardless of the external disturbance (Raven 1961). Everyday examples of control systems are thermostatic temperature control in our homes, power steering in our cars, and trajectory control during space flight.

Critical care medicine often deals with control: mechanical ventilators are set to control Pa_{CO_2}; fluids are given to control blood volume; sodium nitroprusside is given to control blood pressure. It would seem that the inclusion of closed-loop control in ICU equipment design would improve the equipment's function.

Control Theory

Classical closed-loop controllers incorporate one or more of the simple control effects called proportional, integral, and derivative (PID) (Ziegler and Nichols 1942). Proportional response, found in practically all controllers, gives an actuator signal proportional to the error (difference between the control input and the feedback signal). The proportional term is adjusted so that stability is achieved under the most difficult load condition.

The second response is the integral or automatic reset term. Its purpose is to eliminate offset or error. In action, it detects any disparity between the control input and the feedback signal and gives a slow and continuous actuator movement in the proper direction to correct the offset. It gives the actuator velocity proportional to the error signal.

The last control effect, derivative, gives an actuator movement proportional to the rate of change in the error. It is used only in conjunction with proportional response and provides the anticipatory control.

Three major methods are used to find the controller gains that give good controller performance:

1. Parameter optimization by minimizing a performance criteria using a process model and numerical methods.

2. Tuning rules using step responses or oscillation tests.
3. Trial and error starting with low gain for the parameters.

During closed loop operation the control parameters are systematically increased until the damping becomes too small. The parameters are then decreased by some fraction (Isermann 1981).

Although conventional PID regulation is remarkably effective, its initial tuning, and the maintenance of good tuning, can be a time consuming activity (Clarke 1981). Self-tuning control theory is one approach to the problem of tuning. This theory can be applied to the automatic tuning of the PID parameters, or control can be based on predictive control directly (Isermann 1981). Though most medical applications have used PID control, there are a few reports of success with self tuning control. Specific examples in anesthesia delivery, ventilation control, and blood pressure regulation will show how control theory has been applied to medical equipment design.

Anesthesia Delivery

In 1950 Bickford used the EEG to control the automatic intravenous injection of sodium thiopental. He used neither input nor error signal, the anesthetic was continuously administered as long as there was any EEG activity. His system required unacceptably deep levels of anesthesia. Later modification by Bellville allowed input of a reference EEG signal which was compared with the measured EEG level to produce an error signal (Bellville and Altura 1957). The intravenous infusion was controlled in proportion to the error signal. This improvement allowed a more controllable adjustment of depth of anesthesia as the system became a true proportional controller.

Halothane delivery has been controlled using mean arterial blood pressure (Coles et al. 1973). Coles et al. found that PI action was sufficient for controlling the end-tidal CO_2 and the anesthetic gas mixture, but blood pressure required adaptive control. PI action interacting with the log time delay in the blood pressure loop set up a severe limit cycle in the system. These authors state that biological systems are non-linear, multivariable, and interacting and exhibit significant variations from subject-to-subject and that the pressure control needed to be adaptive.

Enflurane delivery has been automatically controlled using end-tidal enflurane concentration and PID control (Westenskow et al. 1983a). The end-tidal concentration was held within 0.037 vol% ± 0.067 SD over a 4 h period in dogs (Westenskow et al. 1983b). In a study of 23 patients the controller kept the end-tidal enflurane concentration to within 0.1 vol% of the desired level (Westenskow et al. 1983c). In this system PID control also adjusted the oxygen concentration and circuit volume. Proportional control done has been used to keep the average of an anesthesia spirometer constant through the addition of oxygen (Pearce 1971). The end-tidal PCO_2 was maintained within 0.17 mmHg (SEM) of the desired value.

A self-adaptive algorithm applied to halothane delivery in a non-rebreathing system resulted in a much faster system. The desired end-tidal halothane concentration was achieved in 1–2 min (Morris et al. 1983).

The results obtained in 80 patients demonstrated the system was accurate, stable, robust, and able to adapt for variability between patients.

Ventilation Control

In 1957 Frumin described the first automatic artificial respirator (Frumin and Lee 1957; Frumin et al. 1957). His system increased or decreased lung inflation pressure by 0.1 mmHg per breath until the patient's end-tidal CO_2 concentration matched the desired value. The Frumin controller fits in a special category of integral controllers which give a constant velocity, the direction depending upon whether the input is above or below the setpoint. (Zierler and Nichols 1942). His controller performed well in a study of twelve patients, the difference between the desired and attained end-tidal PCO_2 was less than 3 mmHG (Frumin et al. 1959).

Both proportional and integral action were later used by Holloman to regulate CO_2 (Holloman et al. 1968). PI gains were adjusted by trial and error with step changes in the ventilatory stimulus. Their controller maintained a constant alveolar CO_2 during reduced oxygen breathing.

End-tidal PCO_2 has also been controlled using three term PID controllers. Ohlson kept $PaCO_2$ within 1.2 mmHg of the desired value even when CO_2 production increased by 44% (Ohlson et al. 1982). With an intraarterial sensor to measure $PaCO_2$ directly, a PID controller kept the average $PaCO_2$ within 2.4 mmHg of the desired level (East et al. 1982).

Coon evaluated a three term controller for the control of arterial pH (Coon et al. 1978). PI control produced the most stable system with a steady-state error less than 0.01 pH.

Blood Pressure Regulation

Sheppard et al. have considerable experience using PID control of blood pressure by the infusion of sodium nitroprusside (Sheppard 1980). Their non-linear PID controllers have been successfully integrated in a large ICU. In 10–15 min pressures are brought within 5 mmHg of the desired value. During anesthesia adaptive controllers may be needed to provide more rapid onset of control. These can bring the pressure down rapidly, within 2–10 min (Koivo et al. 1981; Stern et al. 1981; Westenskow et al. 1984) without the need for occasional tuning (Wernick 1984).

Indications for Closed-loop Control

From these successful examples we find at least six indications for closed-loop control.

1. Closed-loop control is advantageous when a drug is difficult to deliver manually. The rapid onset of action and wide range of sensitivities of sodium nitroprusside make it difficult to controll manually. The development of at least a dozen controllers substantiates the need for automatic control of nitroprusside.
2. Control is advantageous when the requirements for a drug change over time and vary from patient to patient. Inhalation anesthesia delivery is an example. Work in this area extends back to 1950.
3. Control is of value if a penalty applies to administering a drug in excess of that amount specifically needed. A minimum dose of neuromuscular blocker and

intravenous anesthetic should be given so that recovery following anesthesia will be more rapid.

4. Control of multiple drugs or multiple parameters may help compensate for interaction between drugs and help smooth control. The simultaneous control of ventilation, anesthesia delivery, oxygen delivery, and anesthesia circuit volume is an example.
5. When rapid control is needed, closed systems may be of value. Breath-by-breath adjustment of CO_2 is such a case (Lambertsen and Wendel 1960).
6. Closed-loop control may help when facing a shortage of trained personnel. This was true in Alabama (Sheppard and Kouchoukos 1977) and probably true for systems which control ventilation, insulin, and oxytocin.

With a clear indication of need and the application of proper control theory many closed-loop systems have succeeded. Future applications have the potential for expanding even further the capability of critical care and anesthesia personnel by providing equipment which is designed for specific control functions.

References

Bellville JW, Attura GM (1957) Servo-control of general anesthesia. Science 126–827

Bickford RG (1950) Automatic electroencephalographic control of general anesthesia. EEG Clin Neurophysiol 2: 93–96

Clarke DW (1981) Introduction to self tuning controllers. Self tuning and adaptive control. Theory and applications. Harris and Billings IEEE, London

Coles JR, Brown WA, Lampard DG (1973) Computer control of respiration and anaesthesia. Med Bio Eng 262–267

Coon RL, Zuperku EJ, Kampine JP (1978) Systemic arterial blood pH servocontrol of mechanical ventilation. Anesthesiology 49: 201–204

East TD, Westenskow DR, Pace NL, Nelson LD (1982) A microcomputer-based differential lung ventilation system. IEEE Trans Bioeng 29: 736–740

Eveleigh VW (1972) Introduction to control systems design. McGraw Hill, New York

Frumin MJ, Lee ASJ (1957) A physiologically oriented artificial respirator which produces N_2O-O_2 anesthesia in man. J Lab Clin Med 49: 617

Frumin MJ, Lee ASJ, Belmar NJ (1957) J Lab Clin Med 617–622

Frumin MJ, Bergman NA, Holaday DA (1959) Carbon dioxide and oxygen blood levels with a carbon dioxide controlled artificial respirator. Anesthesiology 20: 313–320

Holloman GH, Milhorn HT, Coleman TG (1968) A sampled-data regulator for maintaining a constant alveolar CO_2. J Appl Physiol 25: 463–468

Iserman R (1981) Digital control systems. Springer, Berlin Heidelberg New York

Koivo AJ, Larnard D, Gray R (1981) Digital control of mean arterial blood pressure in dogs by injecting a vasodilator drug. Ann Biomed Eng 9: 185–197

Lambertsen CJ, Wendel H (1960) An alveolar PCO_2 control system: Its use to magnify respiratory depression by meperidine. J Appl Physiol 15: 43–48

Morris P, Tatnall ML, Montgomery FJ (1983) Controlled anaesthesia: A clinical evaluation of an approach using patient characteristics identified during uptake. Br J Anaesth 55: 1065–1075

Ohlson KB, Westenskow DR, Jordan WS (1982) A microprocessor based feedback controller for mechanical ventilation. Ann Biomed Eng 10: 35–48

Pearce DH (1971) A system for measurement of oxygen consumption and control of inspired carbon dioxide. IEEE Trans Biomed Eng: 235–237

Raven FH (1961) Automatic control engineering. McGraw Hill, New York

Sheppard LC (1980) Computer control of the infusion of vasoactive drugs. Ann Biomed Eng 8: 431–444

Sheppard LC, Kouchoukos NT (1977) Automation of measurements and interventions in the systematic care of postoperative cardiac surgical patients. Med Instrum 11: 296–301

Stern KS, Walkter BK, Katona PG (1981) Automated blood pressure control using a self-tuning regulator. IEEE Frontiers of Eng in Health Care

Wernick R (1984) Evaluation of an adaptive blood pressure controller: medical teamwork by machine. Proceedings, AAMI 19th Annual Meeting, Washington, D.C., April 1984

Westenskow DR, Jordan WS, Hayes JK, East TD (1983a) Computer control of anesthesia delivery. In: Prakash O (ed) Computing in anesthesia and intensive care. Martinus Nijhoff, The Hague, pp 269–278

Westenskow DR, Jordan WS, Hayes JK (1983b) Feedback control of enflurane delivery in dogs-inspired compared to end-tidal control. Anesth Analg 62: 836–840

Westenskow DR, Jordan WS, Hayes JK (1983) Uptake of enflurane: A study of the variability between patients. Br J Anaesth 55: 595–601

Westenskow DR, Meline LJ, Pace NL, Bodily NM (1984) Sodium nitroprusside induced hypotension with computer adjustment for varying drug sensitivity. Anesth Analg 63: 281

Ziegler JG, Nichols NB (1942) Optimum settings for automatic controllers. Transactions of the ASME 759–768

Glucose-Insulin-Potassium Therapy Guided by a Glucose-Controlled Insulin Infusion System in Acute Myocardial Infarction

G. Müller-Esch, P. Ball, U. Bekemeyer, H. Djonlagic, A. Hauptmann, K. Heidbüchel, A. Peters, R. Tybussek, W. G. Wood, and P. C. Scriba

A number of hormonal and metabolic alterations have been observed during acute myocardial infarction (AMI): There is a rapid increase of catecholamine and cortisol secretion; free fatty acid (FFA) serum levels are markedly elevated (Gupta et al. 1969; Januszewicz et al. 1971; Vetter et al. 1974); and insulin secretion may be inappropiately low. These alterations result in a disturbance of glucose utilization, so-called stress hyperglycemia. Moreover, under these conditions and due to the accumulation of free fatty acids in the ischemic myocardium, severe ventricular arrhythmias as well as a progression of myocardial cell damage are likely to occur (Kurien and Oliver 1970; Kurien et al. 1971; Oliver et al. 1968).

Glucose-insulin-potassium infusions (GIK) in AMI have been used in a number of clinical trials in order to overcome these deleterious effects (Mantle et al. 1981; Rogers et al. 1976, 1979; Sodi-Palleres et al. (1962)). Some of the postulated benefits of GIK treatment in AMI are: a decrease of FFA, a reduction of potassium efflux, a repletion of intracellular potassium stores, an enhancement of myocardial glucose utilization, a reduction of myocardial oxygen consumption, and an improvement in coronary perfusion. These changes should reduce severe life-threatening arrhythmias, limit infarct size, improve left ventricular function, and reduce hospital mortality (von Arnim and Bolte 1980; Brachfeld 1973; Kurien et al. 1971; Manke et al. 1981; Oliver 1973). With an "open loop" fixed GIK regime as in the studies mentioned above, severe hyperglycemia as well as hypoglycemia were not infrequently seen, because the degree of impairment of the insulin sensitivity could not be predicted. We therefore decided to use a glucose – controlled insulin infusion system (GCIIS); this involves applying "closed-loop" control during treatment with GIK according to the individual insulin sensitivity and thereby studying hormonal and metabolic patterns in AMI.

Methods

Nine patients (eight male, one female; age 61.8 ± 8.8 years) with AMI admitted to our intensive care unit within 12 h after onset of chest pain received GIK for 24 h. The solution contained 430 g glucose, 166 U porcine regular insulin, and 133 mEq KCl per liter. The infusion rate was 0.9 ml/kg/h. Additional feedback – controlled insulin and/or glucose was given by the GCIIS (Biostator-Controller). The following constants were chosen: Mode 3:1, Var 100, BI 80, BD 60, and FI 500–1000. Insulin concentra-

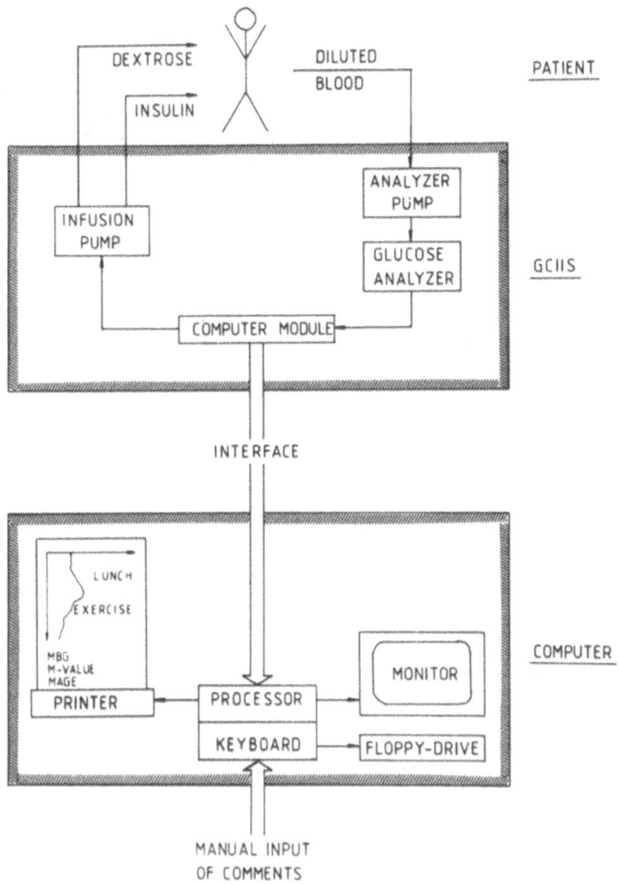

Fig. 1. Schematic diagram of device used for processing of GCIIS data

tion of the GIK solution was increased when blood glucose could not be kept below 250 mg/dl. Insulin, C-peptide, cortisol, GH, prolactin, and lactate were determined at 6-h intervals. FFAs were measured by gas-liquid chromatography (Tserng et al. 1981). Figure 1 shows a schematic diagram of the technical equipment. The patient is connected to the GCIIS. By means of an interface all data for blood glucose (BG), insulin infusion rate (IR), and dextrose infusion rate (DR) are transferred directly from the Biostator to a microcomputer for further processing (Muller-Esch et al. 1984). The microcomputer fulfils several functions:

1. *Monitoring:* BG, IR, and DR are plotted continuously
2. *Manual input:* comments concerning, for example, the actual therapy can be entered via the keyboard
3. *Calculations:* a BASIC computer program has been developed for the calculation of the glycemic indices mean blood glucose (MBG), M-value, and MAGE (Muller-Esch et al. 1984)
4. *Printer and floppy disks:* all values for BG, IR, and DR, as well as comments which appear in their time – related positions, and calculated parameters are plotted and documented on 5-in. floppy disks.

Results

The insulin sensitivity – as measured by blood glucose concentrations and total insulin requirements during GIK – varied markedly. Figure 2a is an example from a patient with high insulin requirements. Initial BG is about 110 mg/dl, rising to more than 250 mg/dl after starting GIK infusion. Despite submaximal additional feedback-controlled insulin by the GCIIS, BG did not fall below 200 mg/dl. In contrast, in the patient shown in Fig. 2b, euglycemia during GIK could be obtained with only minor additional feedback-controlled insulin administration. And in another patient, additional feedback-controlled dextrose had to be given to prevent hypoglycemia during GIK, MBG being in the range of about 80 mg/dl (Fig. 2c).

According to these data we can divide our patients into two groups: in five patients (group A), a total of 309 ± 52 U insulin/24 h was sufficient to maintain fair glycemic control (Table 1, top). In four patients, however (group B), insulin concentration of GIK had to be partially multiplied because of marked hyperglycemia: insulin requirements were 1193 ± 258 U/24 h; despite this, we did not achieve nearly normal BG values or nearly normal glycemic indices (Table 1, bottom).

When compared to the "low insulin" group, the "high insulin" group presented with higher serum insulin levels *before* GIK treatment. *During* therapy, this group had higher values for C-peptide, cortisol, prolactin, and lactate. GH and glucagon did not differ significantly (Table 1).

Table 1. Insulin, C-peptide, glucagon, cortisol, GH, prolactin, and lactate serum levels during GCIIS-guided GIK therapy in patients with low insulin requirements (group A) and high insulin requirements (group B). The glycemic indices MBG, MAGE, and M-value are also shown. ($P < 0.05$ vs. group A)

Group A (309 ± 52 U insulin/24 h, n = 5)

	0 h	6 h	12 h	18 h	24 h
Insulin (mU/l)	11.3 ± 7.5	191 ± 48	227 ± 181	289 ± 198	316 ± 219
C-peptide (µg/l)	2.6 ± 1.8	1.0 ± 0.7	0.6 ± 0.5	2.5 ± 4.1	2.1 ± 2.5
Glucagon (ng/l)	140 ± 25	158 ± 53	160 ± 84	176 ± 82	164 ± 74
Cortisol (ng/ml)	233 ± 131	172 ± 98	196 ± 95	212 ± 112	188 ± 92
GH (ng/ml)	2.1 ± 1.5	4.4 ± 2.9	4.2 ± 2.0	3.5 ± 2.5	2.1 ± 1.6
Prolactin (µU/ml)	398 ± 131	258 ± 64	242 ± 72	225 ± 79	248 ± 51
Lactate (mmol/l)	1.4 ± 0.5	2.0 ± 1.0	1.6 ± 0.8	1.3 ± 0.6	1.1 ± 0.3

MBG: 94 ± 28 MAGE: 51 ± 8 M-value: 17 ± 7

Group B (1193 ± 258 U insulin/24 h, n = 4)

	0 h	6 h	12 h	18 h	24 h
Insulin (mU/l)	● 43 ± 22	● > 500	● > 500	● > 500	● > 500
C-peptide (µg/l)	8.0 ± 7.5	● 13.4 ± 12.9	● 15.0 ± 14.3	21.6 ± 22.9	12.3 ± 15.6
Glucagon (ng/l)	152 ± 77	87 ± 62	90 ± 73	124 ± 140	15.1 ± 169
Cortisol (ng/ml)	301 ± 224	● 418 ± 135	● 418 ± 174	● 412 ± 203	● 418 ± 186
GH (ng/ml)	3.1 ± 2.4	6.1 ± 2.4	3.0 ± 1.8	1.7 ± 1.4	1.5 ± 1.2
Prolactin (µU/ml)	590 ± 281	● 549 ± 182	● 489 ± 150	● 532 ± 135	● 681 ± 191
Lactate (mmol/l)	● 2.7 ± 1.3	● 3.5 ± 0.8	2.7 ± 0.9	● 2.7 ± 1.2	● 3.5 ± 1.4

● MBG: 234 ± 42 ● MAGE: 159 ± 57 ● M-value: 46 ± 15

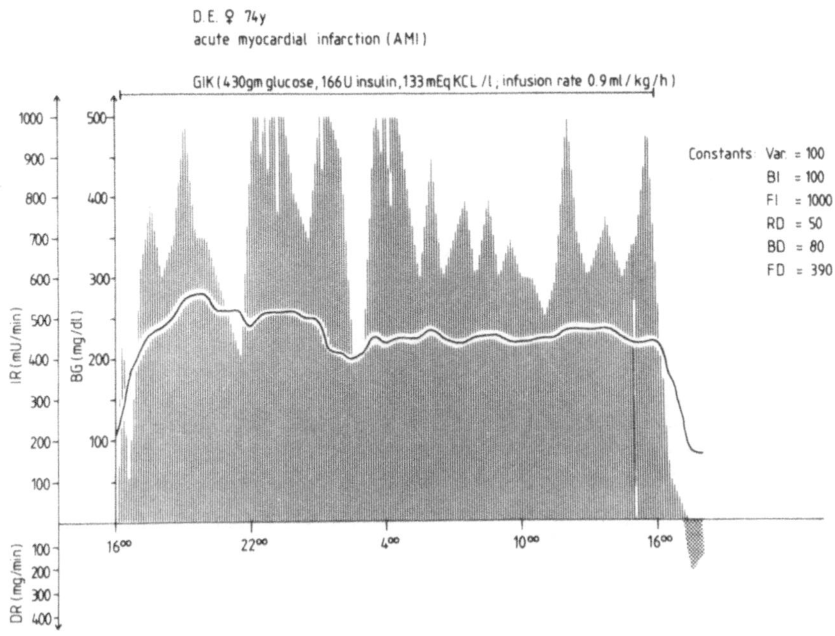

Fig. 2a

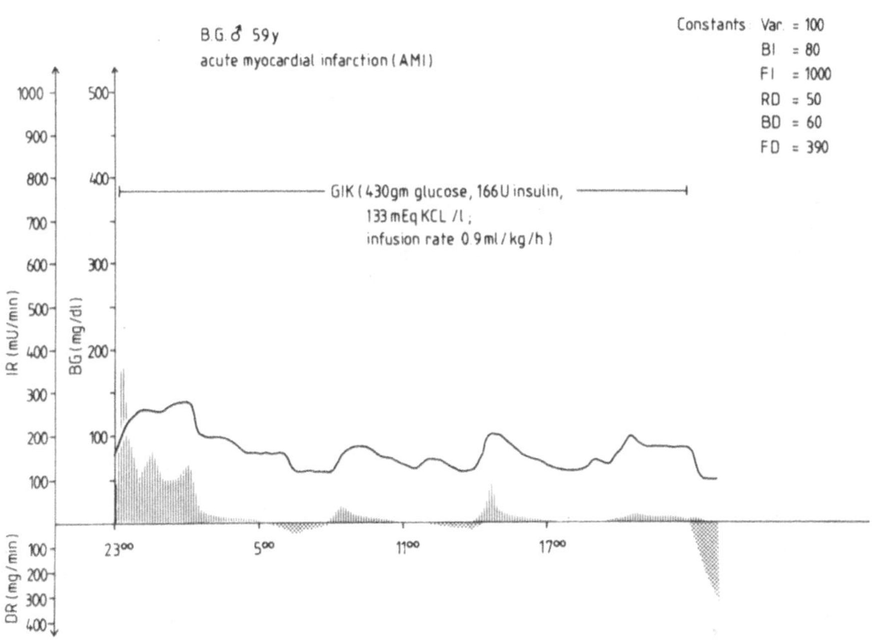

Fig. 2a–c. Blood glucose (BG), insulin infusion rate (IR), and dextrose infusion rate (DR) during GCIIS-guided GIK therapy in three patients with AMI

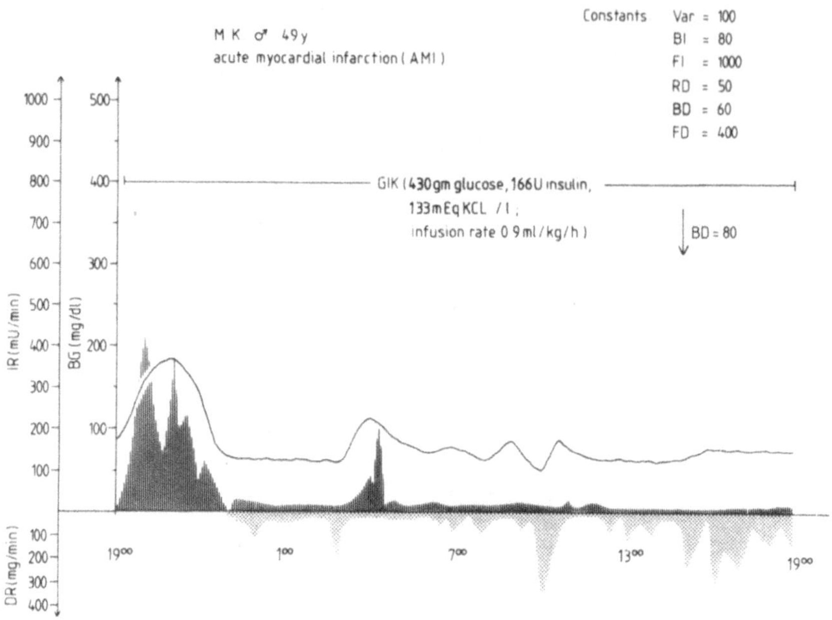

Fig. 2c

Table 2. Insulin, C-peptide, glucagon, cortisol, GH, prolactin, lactate, and blood glucose (BG) levels in seven conventionally treated patients with AMI as compared to four patients under GCIIS-guided GIK therapy (group B). ● $P < 0.05$ vs. controls)

Controls (n = 7)	0 h	6 h	12 h	18 h	24 h
Insulin (mU/l)	35 ± 17	18 ± 11	26 ± 24	26 ± 24	39 ± 34
C-peptide (μg/l)	5.4 ± 2.9	4.9 ± 3.3	4.7 ± 3.2	6.4 ± 3.3	8.6 ± 6.2
Glucagon (ng/l)	323 ± 446	373 ± 537	348 ± 412	431 ± 497	443 ± 407
Cortisol (ng/ml)	239 ± 145	266 ± 192	218 ± 108	247 ± 171	229 ± 163
GH (ng/ml)	2.1 ± 3.1	2.9 ± 3.8	2.4 ± 2.7	3.3 ± 6.5	2.6 ± 2.6
Prolactin (μU/ml)	834 ± 895	445 ± 256	273 ± 106	228 ± 50	306 ± 74
Lactate (mmol/l)	2.1 ± 2.1	2.1 ± 1.8	1.7 ± 1.1	1.4 ± 0.5	1.4 ± 0.4
BG (mg/dl)	147 ± 38	157 ± 49	122 ± 23	144 ± 48	162 ± 72

Group B (1193 ± 258 U insulin/24 h, n = 4)	0 h	6 h	12 h	18 h	24 h
Insulin (mU/l)	43 ± 22	> 500	> 500	> 500	> 500
C-peptide (μg/l)	8.0 ± 7.5	13.4 ± 12.9	● 15.0 ± 14.3	21.6 ± 22.9	12.3 ± 15.6
Glucagon (ng/l)	152 ± 77	87 ± 62	90 ± 73	124 ± 140	151 ± 169
Cortisol (ng/ml)	301 ± 224	418 ± 135	● 418 ± 174	412 ± 203	418 ± 186
GH (ng/ml)	3.1 ± 2.4	6.1 ± 2.4	3.0 ± 1.8	1.7 ± 1.4	1.5 ± 1.2
Prolactin (μU/ml)	590 ± 281	549 ± 182	● 489 ± 150	● 532 ± 135	● 681 ± 191
Lactate (mmol/l)	2.7 ± 1.3	3.5 ± 0.8	2.7 ± 0.9	● 2.7 ± 1.2	● 3.5 ± 1.4

MBG: 234 ± 42 MAGE: 159 ± 57 M-value: 46 ± 15

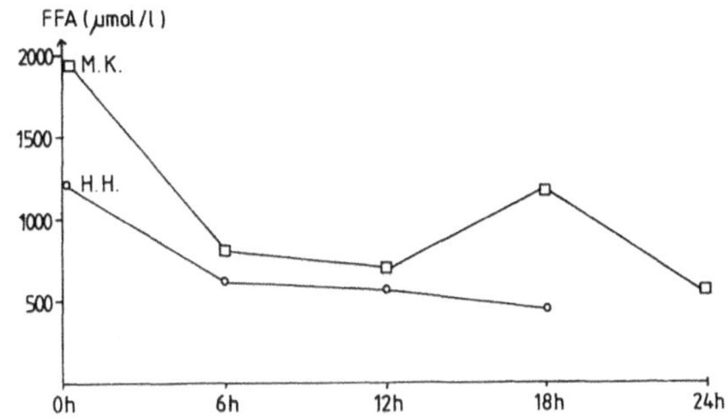

Fig. 3. Free fatty acids (FFA) during GCIIS-guided GIK therapy in two patients with AMI

Seven conventionally, treated patients with AMI served as controls (Table 2). In comparison with these patients without GIK, group B had higher serum levels for C-peptide, cortisol, prolactin, and lactate.

Serial FFA measurements in two patients show a decrease of FFA under GIK below the arrhythmia threshold (Oliver et al. 1968) of 1200 μmol/l (Fig. 3).

Discussion

Because of the small number of patients we are not yet able to decide whether the observed hormonal-metabolic differences between the groups are directly correlated to the infarct size or wheter they reflect different systemic reactions, different hormonal-metabolic patterns, during AMI.

In conclusion, these preliminary data indicate that the impairment of insulin sensitivity and glucose utilization during AMI varies markedly. FFA can be reduced below the arrhythmia threshold. Further studies should compare metabolic, hemodynamic, and antiarrhythmogenic effects of GCIIS-guided GIK support in patients with AMI.

References

Von Arnim T, Bolte HD (1980) Therapie mit Glukose-Insulin beim kardiogenen Schocksyndrom. In: Brückner JB (ed) Kreislaufschock. Springer, Berlin Heidelberg New York, pp 500–505

Brachfeld N (1973) The glucose-insulin-potassium (GIK) regimen in the treatment of myocardial ischemia. Circulation 47: 459–462

Gupta DK, Jewitt DE, Young R, Hartog M, Opie LM (1969) Increased plasma-free-fatty-acid concentrations and their significance in patients with acute myocardial infarction. Lancet 2: 1209–1213

Januszewicz W, Sznajdermann M, Ciświcka-Sznajdermann M, Wocial B, Rymaszewski Z (1971) Plasma free fatty acid and catecholamine levels in patients with acute myocardial infarction. Br Heart J 33: 716–718

Kurien VA, Oliver MF (1970) A metabolic cause for arrhythmias during acute myocardial hypoxia. Lancet 1: 813–815

Kurien VA, Yates PA, Oliver MF (1971) The role of free fatty acids in the production of ventricular arrhythmias after acute coronary artery occlusion. Eur J Clin Invest 1: 225–241

Mantle JA, Rogers WJ, Smith LR, McDaniel HG, Papapietro JE, Russell RO, Rackley CH (1981) Clinical effects of glucose-insulin-potassium on left ventricular function in acute myocardial infarction: results from a randomized clinical trial. Am Heart J 102: 313–324

Müller-Esch G, Peters A, Göhl M, Heidbüchel K, Scriba PC (1984) Simplified evaluation and documentation of data from glucose controlled insulin infusion systems (GCIIS). Biomed Technik 29: 62–66

Oliver MF (1973) Glucose, insulin, potassium in acute myocardial infarction. Acta Cardiol [Suppl] 17: 257–262

Oliver MF, Kurien VA, Greenwood TW (1968) Relation between serum-free-fatty acids and arrhythmias and death after acute myocardial infarction. Lancet 1: 710–715

Rogers WJ, Stanley AW, Breinig JB, Prather JW, McDaniel MG, Moraski RE, Mantle JA, Russell RO Jr, Rackley CÊ (1976) Reduction of hospital mortality rate of acute myocardial infarction with glucose-insulin-potassium infusion. Am Heart J 92: 441–454

Rogers WJ, Segall PH, McDaniel HG, Mantle JA, Russell RO Jr, Rackley CE (1979) Prospective randomized trial of glucose-insulin-potassium in acute myocardial infarction. Effects on myocardial hemodynamics, substrates and rhythm. Am J Cardiol 43: 801–809

Sodi-Pallares D, Testelli MK, Fishleder BL, Bisteni A, Medrano GA, Friedland C, DeMicheli A (1962) Effects of an intravenous infusion of a potassium-glucose-insulin solution on the electrocardiographic signs of myocardial infarction. Am J Cardiol 9: 166–181

Tserng KY, Kliegmann RM, Miettinen EL, Kalhan SC (1981) A rapid, simple, and sensitive procedure for the determination of free fatty acids in plasma using glass capillary columm gas-liquid chromatography. J Lipid Res 22: 852–858

Vetter NJ, Strange RC, Adams W, Oliver NF (1974) Initial metabolic and hormonal response to acute myocardial infarction. Lancet 1: 284–289

Changes in Monitoring Methods Caused by the Use of Intelligent Bedside Equipment

E. Epple, W. Bleicher, M. Kopp, and H. Junger

Introduction

The reduction in the real cost of computing power has caused bedside hardware monitors to be replaced by firmware or software systems (microprocessors). There has been some pioneering work, for example from C. Zeelenbergs group of the Thorax Center Cardiology Departments, Rotterdam. They developed the Unibox-Unibed System (Zeelenberg et al. 1977). In the meantime several commercial "intelligent bedside monitors" have been presented. With those monitors we have greater possibilities and there arises the necessity of a critical reexamination of appropriate clinical tasks for those units. Fortunately a lot of experience in the abilities of "intelligent" devices has been gained by applying minicomputers in patient monitoring (Epple et al. 1981, 1983a, c; Kopp et al. 1980; Sheppard et al. 1983; Shoemaker et al. 1979).

In contrast to centralized minicomputer systems a decentralized microcomputer monitor has two main advantages:

1. Expenses for data transmission are reduced.
2. Data security is improved, especially when a background computer is used for double storage. (Data storage at the bedside has to be provided for a limited time only, about one shift. After that time, reports may be generated and the long-term storage (legal reasons, scientific work, long-term reports) can be provided by the background computer.)

There are some other advantages, such as improved response time and reduced software overheads.

In contrast to hardware electronics a computerized system has the ability to store data over longer periods of time. We may differentiate the stored data as off-line and on-line data. In addition, the system may contain information that is not subject to change (default values, help frames and so on).

We will restrict ourselves to the on-line data, because in this area there are specific methodological strengths in comparison with conventional monitoring:

1. The amount of recorded data can be increased significantly in comparison with a handwritten chart. This holds for the number of recorded vital parameters as well as for the sampling rate of the individual parameter.
2. The collected data can be shown in different styles of presentation on various sorts of display devices.
3. Further algorithmic processing is possible (e.g., trend analysis, trend alarms, prognostic indices, hemodynamic values, fluid balance).

To record and process measured values has the aim of presenting significant information in an as impressive form as possible. The time constant for collecting and processing significant information is determined by several conditions:

(a) Physiological or pathophysiological changes in organ functions bearing relevant clinical information require an appropriate sampling rate.
(b) The most dangerous situations occur suddenly and have an intervention time of less than five minutes. Therefore a warning or sign has to be processed and presented in a fraction of this time span (e.g., at half-minute intervals) to allow a timely reaction by the medical staff.
(c) The processed data have to be presented in a manner acceptable to physicians and nurses during routine working. The amount of data presented has to be reduced as far as possible, without neglecting topics (a) and (b).

The conditions of topic (b) indicate a minimum of data required in patient monitoring, (a) represents conditions which help to get deeper insight and to improve therapy control. In practice we have to find an adequate compromise between the needs of detailed information, topic (a), and data reduction from the point of view of routine use, topics (b) and (c).

Data Collection and Storage

The specifications for topics (a, b and c) lead primarily to consequences for the measuring methods. It is helpful to differentiate between techniques suitable for detecting short-term emergency situations and those which allow control over the development of patient's situation over a longer period of time or which answer specific diagnostic questions. The first will be called "monitoring methods", the second "diagnostic methods".

The requirements for a monitoring method in respect of the sampling rate (respectively time constant) must at least match the conditions of topic (b). This means that the transducers have to work continuously with time constants of less then one minute.

A monitoring method can fulfill the needs of topic (a) in addition. Rapid changing signals – the ECG or blood pressure signals – have in this case to be sampled at a rate of more than 100 values per second (according to Shannon's theorem). For reasons of economy and because of condition (c) these signals are not usually stored over longer periods of time without data reduction. Therefore a first step in bedside data processing consists of feature extraction from the original signals. Thus we get vital parameters, e.g., heart frequency from the ECG or systolic and diastolic pressures from the original blood pressure signal. The highest time resolution of such sequences of repeated events is on an event-to-event basis. This means in the case of the ECG a beat-to-beat registration with time intervals of the order of one second. We thus get a remarkable data reduction from more than 100 samples per second to about one value per second.

As we know from perinatology (Hammacher 1967), information is produced in the courses of cardiotachograms which is clinically relevant (corresponding to topic (a)). In an intensive care ward even this sampling rate is felt to be too high. The procedure mostly applied for further data reduction is to calculate mean values from a series of consecutive values. Because this means low pass filtering, it suppresses or smoothes sudden changes in vital parameters. Besides providing data reduction it is thought to be helpful because it reduces artifacts.

At the same time, of course, real events of physiological origin in the plots of vital parameters are smoothed out. As we were able to show (Bleicher et al. 1980; Epple et al. 1983a; Kopp et al. 1980), this is not desirable, as relevant clinical information will be destroyed. The aspect of artifact suppression will be treated in detail in a separate contribution and therefore some statements only will be given:

(a) Artifact suppression has preferrably to be done at the place of origin.
(b) Artifact suppression by digital data processing has to be done by means of pattern recognition and not in an unspecific manner.
(c) Presentation of artifacts can be helpful in order to analyze the reason for their origin. They should not therefore be totally suppressed.

On the one hand, storage of all the data (on the level of original signals or even on the level of beat-to-beat feature sequences) is not practicable. On the other hand data reduction by low-pass filtering is problematic. The best solution would be to select features out of sequences with a resolution of the order of some 10 s (according to topics (b) and (c)). These reduced sequences will be called "vital parameter trends". For selected time intervals original signals and beat-to-beat feature sequences should be stored in addition, to allow interpretation of certain patterns in vital parameter trends.

These selected time intervals may be detected by suitable pattern recognition programs or the data recording may be started manually by a clinical observer. In the latter case it would be very helpful to use some kind of delayed registration (e.g., a ring buffer) for getting detailed data from the past. The content of the buffer can be saved by special request. In addition the content could be saved per time schedule in fixed time intervals.

It would be necessary to store the vital parameter trends in such a way that one is able to get some hints of any change in the character of the signals. One possibility is to sample with constant time intervals (e.g., 30 s) and to take the instantaneous feature value. In this case certain periodic changes could be missed (aliasing). A different method, avoiding this effect, would be to select one feature out of the appropriate time interval by a random process. In this way single short-term events will be missed, but long-term changes in the characteristics of the feature sequence can be observed. The best solution for that purpose, however, would be to store a minimum and a maximum value for every time interval, together with a corresponding mean value.

Data Presentation

As usual the most important original signals should be displayed on oscilloscopes. Vital parameter trends shown on a graphical display are very informative (Epple et al. 1981, 1983a, c; Smalhout and Zalenda 1975). They should be presented with an adequate time resolution to match the conditions of topic (b). The display form should also contain some hint of changes in variability. As discussed in the provious section, this could be provided in different ways.

Because variability and patterns in the vital parameter trends are very important there are some requirements for the graphical display:

(a) The most important monitoring parameters (arising from the monitoring methods) should be displayed simultaneously, because correlations and phase shifts between different parameters are very informative.
(b) To get an adequate dynamic range in ordinate direction it is helpful to use one ordinate scale for several parameters. The problem of crossing signals can be solved by different techniques (the optimal consists of color display).
(c) In a standard display the scale relationship between ordinate and abscissa should be fixed; otherwise significant patterns cannot be recognized. This means especially:

Auto-scaling is not a good solution.
Longer time intervals should be displayed on-screen, not by data compression, but by moving window, scrolling or paging techniques.

Of course these conditions may be neglected in non-standard displays, which are helpful in special cases. To these non-standard displays particularly, belong the presentation of original signals and beat-to-beat sequences collected intermittendly or on request. By these means we get improved possibilities in monitoring (Kopp et al. 1980; Smalhout and Kalenda 1975). Observation of short-term dynamic changes in vital parameters can be used for improved monitoring, for prognosis and therapy control.

Monitoring methods are needed to show that something is happening. In consequence they have to meet these conditions:

(a) They have to be applicable continuously over longer periods of time.
(b) They have to react fast (in a fraction of a minute).
(c) They need not to be very specific (e.g., end-expiratory CO_2 is influenced by many organ functions).
(d) They need not to be very precise; that means systematic errors can be tolerable. (Control of absolute values or recalibration can be performed from time to time.)

Diagnostic methods are applied to answer the question: "What happens?" Therefore they have to meet other conditions:

(a) They can be applied as instantaneous measurements (e.g., the measurement of hemodynamic values by the thermodilution method). This sort of diagnostic parameter has to be controlled by adequate monitoring methods, to make sure that the measured values are representative and not the result of a momentary instability in patient's situation.
(b) They should be specific.
(c) They should be as precise as necessary for the subsequent decision making.

This comparison of monitoring and diagnostic methods in connection with intelligent bedside monitors marks a certain monitoring philosophy. Depending on the disease and the situation of the patient, a selection of monitoring methods have to be applied; these have primarily to show the dynamic behaviour of organ functions. Characteristic patterns can occur spontaneously or when provoked (e.g., by therapeutic measures). Such events can be studied in more detail by recording data at a higher sampling rate. Spontaneous changes proved to be of prognostic value and can therefore be used as warnings. It should be emphasized, that some non-invasive methods are well suited to match those requirements (Bleicher et al. 1980, Epple et al. 1983b). In addition diagnostic methods can be applied. An indication for their application can often be taken from the dynamic behaviour of vital parameter trends.

Further Data Processing

There are some well established algorithms to be applied in an ICU. Whether they should be performed at the bedside or in a background computer depends to a large extent on economy. That is especially true for diagnostic methods which have to be applied with longer time intervals. Some of them may require large data bases and complicated algorithms (e.g., prognostic indices have been calculated on powerful background computers (Shoemaker et al. 1979)). These methods are, of course, not suitable for processing at the bedside.

Data processing at the bedside is preferable in those cases where there are large amounts of data which can be reduced with algorithms effective in small computers with a reasonable processing time. In our opinion controlled infusion could be such an example (Sheppard et al. 1983).

In the preceeding section we discussed characteristic patterns in the courses of vital parameters being perceived and analyzed by the visual system of an observer. For warnings and alarms it would be helpful to use pattern recognition algorithms to do that automatically and in that way to assist the medical staff. Research in this direction is in progress (Swoboda 1981). Of course it is possible to analyze patterns and to give warnings in some well known examples. At present, however, this does not solve the problem of routine application. Automatic pattern recognition will be useful in an ICU only when complete. That means that all the patterns and their clinical meaning have to be known. Otherwise there would be a lot of false and missing alarms. In fact we are in a learning period with a long way to go and we should not like to lose the consideration by physicians and nurses of this very helpful information.

Final Comments

This overview treats only a few special aspects of the tasks of intelligent bedside monitors. As an example of topics not treated: courses of vital parameters need comments to be understandable (clinical observations, therapeutic measures and so on). Techniques to input off-line data is therefore a special topic of great importance. Another example not discussed is: automatic generation of patient charts with the help of a plotter at every bedside would be desirable. It is rather expensive at present; therefore the best solution would be to employ a background computer or a special central processor.

The methodological changes discussed may be taken as examples for developments which will improve monitoring of patients in critical situations. Because of the experience gained with more powerful computers there will be some development of very new methods, but in general increased availibility of more complicated methods in routine, and a shifting of monitoring philosophy. Powerful local networks will lead to flexible and economical systems, which can be tailord to the needs of different clinical problems.

References

Bleicher W, Zahn S, Fiderer F, Frey R, Steil E, Faust U (1980) Automatic device for noninvasive monitoring of stroke volume, cardiac output, systolic time intervals, and derived hemodynamic parameters. In Computers in Cardiology, IEEE Catalog 80CH1606-3. IEEE Computer Society, Long Beach, CA

Bleicher W, Frey R, Zahn S, Steil E, Budwig G, Epple E (1980) Characteristic trend patterns in computerized intensive care monitoring In: Computers in Cardiology, IEEE Catalog 80CH1606-3. IEEE Computer Society, Long Beach, CA, pp 423–426

Epple E, Junger H, Bleicher W, Schorer R, Apitz J, Faust U (eds) (1981) Rechnergestützte Intensivpflege (Symposium in Tübingen). Thieme, Stuttgart (INA vol 26)

Epple E, Bleicher W, Faust U (1983a) Clinical importance of patterns in the courses of on-line recorded vital parameters. In: Lecture notes in medical decision-making, vol 22. Springer, Berlin Heidelberg New York Tokio, pp 202–208

Epple E, Bleicher W, Steil E, Kopp M, Junger H (1983b) Invasive versus noninvasive parameters – the influence of the use of a computerized monitoring system. Acta Anaest Scand [suppl 78] 27: 11

Epple E, Frey R, Bleicher W, Apitz J, Schorer R, Faust U (eds) (1983c) Rechnergestützte Intensivpflege II (2. Tübinger Symposium). Thieme, Stuttgart (INA vol 44)

Hammacher K (1967) Die kontinuierliche Elektronische Überwachung der fetalen Herztätigkeit vor und während der Geburt. In: Gynäkologie und Geburtshilfe, vol 2. Thieme Stuttgart, pp 793–803

Kopp M, Junger H, Bleicher WU, Heipertz W, Epple E (1980) Rapid dynamic changes of vital parameters shown in graphical presentation by a computerized intensive care system. In: Nair S (ed) Computers in critical care and pulmonary medicine Plenum, New York

Sheppard LC, Shotts JE, Wallace FD, Kouchoukos NT, Kirklin JW (1983) Computer based critical care system applied to post surgical cardiac patients In: Epple E (ed) Rechnergestützte Intensivpflege II. Thieme, Stuttgart, pp 156–162 (INA vol 44)

Shoemaker WC, Chang P, Bland R, Czer L, Clifton JF, Shabot MM (1979) Cardiorespiratory monitoring in postoperative patients: I. Prediction of outcome and severity of illness II. Quantitative indices as guides to therapy. Crit Care Med 7: 237–249

Smalhout B, Kalenda Z (1975) An atlas of capnography. Kerckebosch, Zeist, Netherlands

Swoboda A (1981) Trend Analysis in Medicine using the Box-Jenkins Method. In: Computers in Cardiology, IEEE Catalog 81CH1750-9, IEEE Computer Society, Long Beach, CA, pp 247–250

Zeelenberg C, Engels WAH, Deutsch LS (1977) A Hierarchical patient monitoring computer network. In: Computers in Cardiology, IEEE Catalog 77CH1254-2C. IEEE Computer Society, Long Beach, CA, pp 439–444

Automated Arrhythmia Detection in Intensive Care

C. Zeelenberg, S. H. Meij, M. R. Hoare, and P. G. Hugenholtz

Introduction

The field of arrhythmia monitoring, and more specifically automated arrhythmia monitoring, is a relatively new one which first became important with the introduction of the first coronary care units (CCU). In the late fifties it was shown that the majority of deaths from ischaemic heart disease (IHD) taking place in hospital–about 50% of the total IHD deaths–were due to ventricular fibrillation (VFIB). It was found that ventricular fibrillation itself was often subsequent to, or triggered by, certain other cardiac arrhythmias, notably ventricular tachycardia and runs of unifocal or multifocal premature ventricular contractions (PVC), while these arrhythmias in their turn were frequently preceded by other, less serious, cardiac irregularities, such as intermittent PVCs or the R on T phenomenon. Early detection, and hence treatment, of these nominally less serious rhythm disturbances was soon shown to reduce the incidence of potentially lethal arrhythmias and thus of sudden death among IHD patients (Lown et al. 1969). Even when it was subsequently shown that premonitory rhythm disturbances were of much less predictive value than was earlier assumed, the reasons for continuous monitoring were enhanced. For ventricular fibrillation and asystole both proved to be conditions which were readily amenable to emerging treatment, provided their occurence was instantly detected. Indeed a modern CCU would currently be expected rarely to encounter deaths due primarily to arrhythmia's of any kind. All these experiences have led by degrees to the present-day situation in which almost every major hospital, and many smaller ones, in the developed world has at least one CCU.

One of the major features of coronary care is the need for continual, or more often continuous, monitoring of the patient's electrocardiogram (ECG) in order to detect any signs of trouble and to determine the efficacy of any anti-arrhythmic drugs being administered. Continuous ECG monitoring is not confined to coronary care of course, as it is widely used in most types of intensive care, for instance after open heart surgery. Detailed arrhythmia analysis, however, tends to be largely confined to coronary care and it is for this reason that this paper will concentrate mostly on this particular area.

Fully continuous ECG monitoring round the clock, without any automated aids, requires considerable reserves of trained manpower. It is also extremely wearisome. Early monitoring "systems" consisted basically of oscilloscope screens showing a continuous ECG trace. These screens were positioned at the bedside or central nursing station or both. Monitoring consisted of visual observation of the screens by the clinical staff, who often, at times usually, had to combine this chore with their other duties. Only a few institutions could afford to dedicate staff to continuous ECG observation and even then a single observer would have to monitor several patients at once. Monitoring in this way was clearly in no way continuous; it was, in fact, intermittent sampling and in practice many premonitory signs of ventricular arrhythmias might be missed in this way (Lindsay and Bruchner 1975; Romhilt et al. 1973; Ryden et al. 1975).

From the earliest days of coronary care, therefore, attempts were made to automate ECG monitoring, whether partially or fully, using special purpose analog or digital devices or else general purpose digital computers. This paper will concentrate on the latter type of application since the greater part of true arrhythmia monitoring today uses some type of digital computer.

Although digital computers were used quite early in the history of coronary care, the first kind of monitor to become widely accepted was the analog heart-rate monitor. This is still probably the most popular variety of ECG monitor in intensive care. This type of device, which is usually coupled to an ECG display and often to a strip-chart recorder, triggers on each heartbeat and gives an alarm whenever the current rate exceeds preset limits. The introduction of these devices relieved some of the burden on the clinical staff as it was now possible to detect low heart-rates, high heart-rates and, at least in principle, their extreme forms namely, cardiac arrest and ventricular fibrillation. Unfortunately, this type of automatic device is far from problem free in practice. Briefly, the problems can be divided into those of a technical nature and those of a clinical nature. The technical problems all relate to the difficulty, or near impossibility, of detecting all heartbeats from any given patient under the conditions prevailing in intensive care without increasing the false positive rate (number of events incorrectly seen as heartbeats) to an unacceptable value. Signal artifact caused by muscle activity or poor electrode contact tends to be recognised as heartbeats or else masks true beats thus causing false alarms. As a result of this, the clinical staff may, or will, ignore alarms or else set the limits to extreme values, thus effectively nullifying much of the monitor's purpose. The clinical problem with a ratemeter is that the alarm, if genuine, is generated too late. That is, the event to be prevented has in fact already taken place in many cases and the device is not capable of detecting and indicating most of the precursory arrhythmias whose prompt treatment might have reduced the likelihood of the more serious ones occurring. Many attempts have been made to overcome the shortcomings of these devices. Beat detectors have been made less sensitive to artifact in an attempt to cure some of the technical problems. The clinical problem has been approached by going a step beyond the mere detection of a beat and calculation of a mean heart-rate to attempts to classify the beat within the context of its neighbours and hence say something about both the beat itself and the underlying rhythm. The increase in complexity of the logic required to make the step from error-prone, simple ratemeters to reliable arrhythmia monitors made analog logic less attractive and resulted in some researchers turning to the digital computer.

Several early monitoring systems were, in fact, already a combination of a ratemeter, used as preprocessor, with a digital computer for calculation. In some cases attempts were made to use the positions of the heartbeats as determined by the ratemeter to determine the type of rhythm. The problems previously described made this approach unsatisfactory and later work always omitted the analog preprocessor in favour of purely digital techniques. The one remaining analog feature to be found in many systems is a band-pass filter to remove some of the artifacts. Other systems use digital techniques which can be conveniently "tailored" to the application in hand but carry a heavy overhead in terms of computer time. The dramatic decrease in the price of microcomputers has made this a less objectionable consideration.

Although computer ECG monitoring for arrhythmia detection is itself largely confined to coronary care, it is only a small part of the much wider application of computerized ECG analysis which covers such fields as Holter tape analysis and diagnostic ECG. Holter tape analysis is, in fact, widely regarded as a branch of arrhythmia monitoring, as it makes use of similar algorithms and shares many techniques. Table 1 lists the main characteristics of monitoring, Holter, and diagnostic ECG analysis, and indicates the principal differences between the three. There is a certain amount of feedback between Holter analysis and ordinary monitoring in the sense that improvements in techniques for the one are often applied later to the other. The most important differences are probably that in the case of Holter analysis there may be multiple passes through the data and the whole tape (3, 6, 12 or 24 hours) can be considered as basically "stable" and is used to set the "context;" whereas in intensive care monitoring the basic rhythm may be changing rapidly, two or more passes are only possible in terms of very short lengths of data since alarms must be immediate and the "context" is usually set up during a short "initialisation" run and then continuously updated. Diagnostic ECG differs radically from either of the other two branches. Not only does it usually concentrate on the morphological features and analyze multiple leads but it can afford to use averaging techniques to produce a satisfactorily "clean" signal and a representative beat and does not suffer from any real-time constraints. There is one type of diagnostic ECG, however, which combines features from both diagnostic ECG proper and from monitoring. This is stress or exercise testing. Much of the analysis resembles diagnostic systems but the type of system, display and time-constraints are closer to monitoring systems, and while the section of ECG for diagnosis can be selected in order to be as artifact and arrhythmia free as possible this is not wholly true of exercise testing.

Table 1. Computer processed ECGs

Arrhythmia analysis		Diagnostic interpretation
Continuous real-time monitoring and Holter recording		Rest and exercise
Large number of complexes Order (100000)	⟷	Small number of complexes Order (10–100)
1–2 leads	⟷	Multiple leads (6–12)
Fast processing (1–120 times real-time)	⟷	Detailed analysis (0.1–0.01 times real-time)
Mainly oriented to measuring ventricular ectopic activity	⟷	Analysis of complete polarisation sequence to determine underlying pathology

Characteristics of Computer-based Systems

The majority of monitoring systems in clinical use today are essentially similar where data acquisition and analysis are concerned. Differences tend to be mainly in the methods of presentation of the results, in the front-end equipment and displays and in the interactions between system and user. The vast majority use more or less dedicated mini or microcomputers which may or may not handle other signals as well (pressures, cardiac output etc.). Systems range considerably in size from one microcomputer per bed to over 50 beds per computer. Current systems all work in real-time in order to ensure that nothing is lost and that alarms are generated soon after the initiating event. Some obsolete systems were forced to drop a number of beats if time constraints became too severe but this is not now considered acceptable. Virtually all production systems analyse a single ECG lead. This restriction is in part historical. Multiple leads require considerably more complex recognition algorithms and more computer resources. This is less of a consideration with today's microprocessors, and it would seem advisable to employ multiple leads.

System Structure

Figure 1 shows the "standard" elements of an automated arthythmia detector (AAD). Systems do not necessarily contain all these elements. The ECG is registered by the

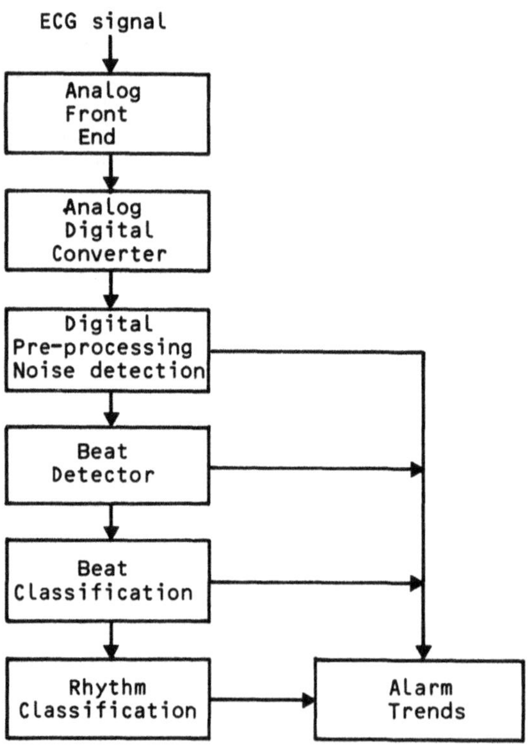

Fig. 1. Structure of an automated arrhythmia detector

electrodes and transmitted through the leads or by telemetry to the front-end which amplifies, filters, and displays it. The front-end also contains isolation amplifiers for patient safety, and logic to protect the apparatus from damage if the patient is defibrillated. Most front-ends also have a strip-chart recorder with a delay-memory to enable the nurse to check the cause of an alarm. Normally, the front-end will also contain a ratemeter with its own alarms, which can be used as back-up if the computer fails. In addition, the front-end often provides duplicate display and registration features at the nurse desk. The analog signal from the front-end is then transmitted through a cable to the computer, where it is sampled using an analog-digital converter (ADC). Sample rates vary considerably but are most commonly in the range 100–250 Hz. The sampled signal then normally undergoes a pre-processing stage which may include any or all of the following items: digital filtering, differentiation, noise detection, data compression. The next stage is beat detection and characterization. Note that the systems which make use of intervals alone could in theory use special purpose analog hardware in place of ADC, preprocessing and beat detection/characterization. Beat detection may be used merely to establish a fiducial point for systems using the raw data in later steps, it may be used to provide R-R intervals and detect noise, it may be used to determine a number of features (QRS width/duration, QRS height, R-R interval etc.), or it may be used to characterise the morphology by some measure of correlation to a template. The next stage is beat classification. Beat classification normally precedes, though it may include, rhythm classification and alarm generation. The final step is the presentation of the results to the clinical staff in a suitable format. Here systems using the same basic detection algorithms may vary greatly in methods of presentation and in ways of interacting with the clinician. As a general rule, systems provide a frequently updated review of the data of some or all patients with more detailed reports on demand. Time-trend, various types of graphic display and sometimes histograms or scatter diagrams are also commonly provided. Some systems provide much more complex facilities, often based on links to larger computers, but these fall outside the scope of this paper.

Algorithms for Arrhythmia Detection

Algorithms for automated arrhythmia monitoring have attracted a great deal of attention from cardiologists and signal analysts, among others, over the last two decades. Attempts have been made to apply most of the techniques of signal analysis and of pattern recognition to the problem. However in practice there are only a few algorithms in general use today outside development systems and the vast majority of systems use either ARGUS (Nolle 1972) or the WPI (Feldman et al. 1971) algorithm or some modification of one or other (Dillman et al. 1978; Sanders et al. 1977; Shah et al. 1977; Zeelenberg et al. 1977). This does not mean that methods not in current use should necessarily be forgotten. New advances in hardware (array processors, special purpose chips etc.) may well make techniques that in the past required a large mainframe become feasible on-line in the CCU. Algorithms for arrhythmia monitoring can be classified in various ways. Some authors divide them into groups depending on the number and type of ECG leads they require (single bipolar lead, orthogonal leads, subset of 12-lead, bipolar leads plus intra-atrial or esophageal). In practice, however, most AADs contain more or less the same elements regardless of lead system, although multiple leads naturally complicate the analysis. The majority of algorithms contain four main elements: a preprocessing stage in which the raw data is filtered, compressed etc., a beat detection and characterization stage, a beat classification stage and finally the rhythm classification. The remainder of this section will give a brief, and far from exhaustive, overview of the commoner techniques used at each stage. More extensive overviews can be found in several surveys (Hulting 1979; Oliver et al. 1977; Plokker 1978; Thomas et al. 1979; Willems and Peperstraete 1978).

Data Preprocessing and Reduction

Most AADs use a fairly high sampling frequency in order to retain the high-frequency details of the QRS. This results in a very large number of samples being available for processing. Most systems contain a preprocessing stage which precedes the beat detection and whose primary aims are usually the reduction of the raw data to more manageable proportions and/or the removal of some of the artifact and undesirable frequency components present by applying suitable digital filtering. The most widely used data compression algorithm for this purpose is AZTEC (Amplitude-Zone-Time-Epoch-Coding) (Cox et al. 1968) which reduces ADC samples to a set of slopes and horizontal lines (see Fig. 2). Many systems also retain the raw data, whether for display, research or further analysis. Other compression schemes have been applied to reduce the data for storage, the best known being Huffman coding (Cox and Ripley 1963). Digital filtering, with or without differentiation and second derivative, is almost always matched to the special requirements of the beat detector used. Orthogonal leads may be combined to give polar coordinates at this stage. In this preprocessing stage many AADs also check the signal for excessive noise level, and suppress further analysis if required.

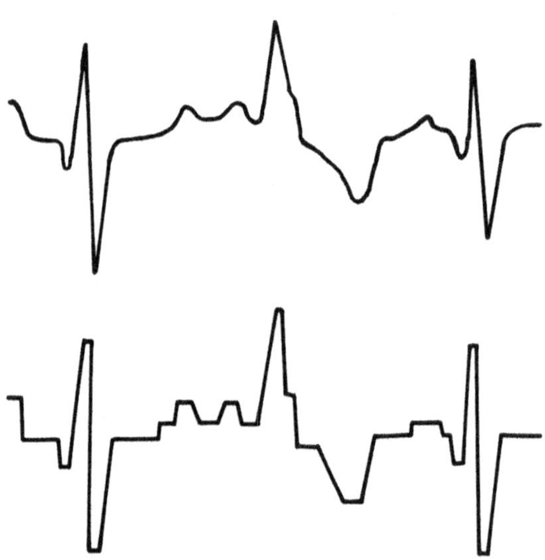

Fig. 2. Example of AZTEC transformation

Beat Detection and Characterization

This step, seemingly the simplest, is in practice often the most difficult, the more so as errors at this point propagate through succeeding stages and may ultimately lead to errors in rhythm classification. This stage aims to determine the existence of a beat, to locate it in time by defining a fiducial point and then to characterize the beat by extracting one or more measurements. Most systems use detection schemes based on a search for threshold crossings in the basic signal and/or its first derivative. Threshold values differ from scheme to scheme. They may be fixed values or may be derived (intermittently or continuously) from the ECG being monitored, with or without cut-off points. Once a potential QRS has been detected it must fulfil a further set of criteria with respect to shape and/or timing before it will be classified as a true QRS (Dillman et al. 1978; Engelse and Zeelenberg 1979; Hulting 1979; McClelland and Arnold 1976; Mead et al. 1979; Nolle 1972). In some schemes potential QRS complexes that do not fulfil these criteria may be tested against a separate set of criteria for classification as artifact. Once all conditions are met, a fiducial point is declared which locates the beat in time and hence enables comparison with other beats. Examples of commonly used fiducial points are: QRS-onset, R-peak and point of maximum slope. Each detection scheme has its own pecularities and weak points. None of them work perfectly and a lot of research work is still being devoted to the definition of more reliable fiducial points, particularly ones which are less sensitive to muscle noise and

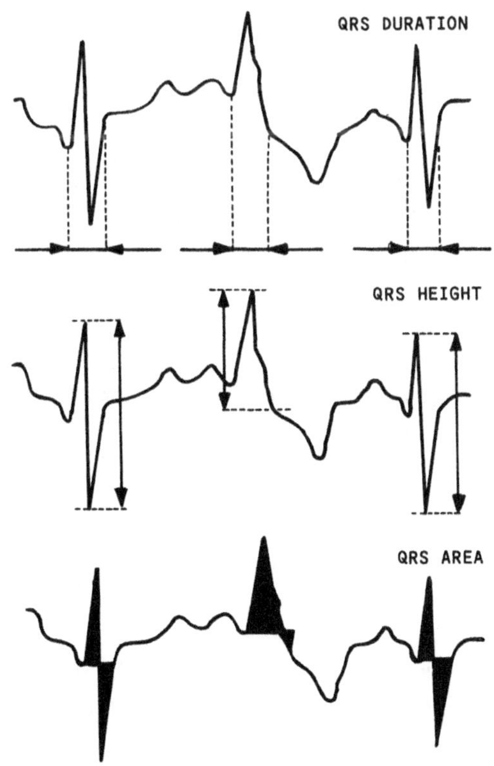

Fig. 3. Typical time domain QRS features

other artifact. The fiducial point provides the first and probably the most important single parameter in beat characterization, the interval length. A number of monitoring techniques have been based solely on this parameter, although most current systems do extract additional shape information from the QRS complex.

There are two main approaches to beat shape characterization and they form the basis of the two most widely-used AADs. The first approach requires a set of absolute measurements from the complex (Fig. 3), while the second derives one or more parameters by comparing the complex with one or more stored templates which, in their turn, may be either "standard" forms or beats derived from the ECG being monitored (Fig. 4). ARGUS (Nolle 1972), the best known example of the first approach, uses QRS height, duration, offset and area as measurements of QRS morphology. An example of the second approach is the use of a normalized cross-correlation coefficient to compare the test beat with a standard template (modified to allow for physiological variability) found in the WPI (Feldman et al. 1971) algorithm developed at Worcester Polytechnic Institute. Both approaches have certain drawbacks and tend to fail on certain specific types of beat morphology. Some users have modified the ARGUS approach at this point, for instance, in an attempt to increase its reliability. Some schemes tend to trigger on abnormally sharp or high P or T waves. The latter problem is often avoided by having a "dead-time" (typically 150–200 ms) after a QRS has been detected, although this does mean that some physiologically important phenomena (R on T) may be ignored.

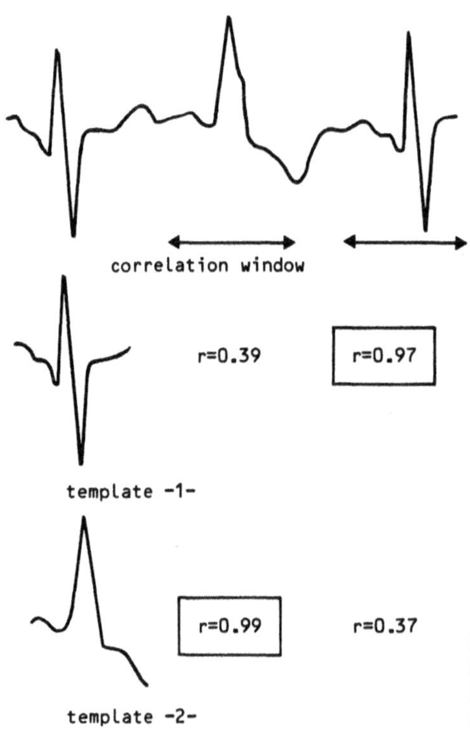

Fig. 4. Shape classification using multiple template correlation. The R-peak is used as the fiducial point for positioning the correlation window

The feature extraction approach usually requires less computation time than the cross-correlation method, particularly where multiple leads or multiple templates are concerned, but the latter method is potentially more satisfactory. A variant of the method whereby the fiducial point is determined by sliding the beat across the template, thus avoiding all pitfalls of precise determination of its location, was until recently too time-consuming for any practical application. These objections, however are rapidly disappearing with new advances in low-cost hardware.

It is perhaps worth mentioning at this point that systems analyzing multiple leads can use this fact during beat location, as well as during beat classification, in order to locate beats where one or more leads are noisy or where the amplitude in one of the leads is extremely low and hence not seen by the detector.

Beat Classification

At this point, most AADs attempt to classify the individual beat, based on the measurements obtained from the detection and beat shape characterization. Beat classification may take place in various ways, the two principal being based on either decision tables or on distance measurements in feature space (Fig. 5). Clearly either method can be applied to the outcome of either approach from the preceding stage. Classification is usually into a number of categories which normally correspond to beats of known morphology. An exception to this rule occurs, for instance, where time intervals only are considered. They are often merely categorised as, for instance, "standard", "short" and "long" without any decision being taken as to their normality in terms of, say, sinus rhythm (Gersch et al. 1972; Hoare and Arntzenius 1971; Jenkins et al. 1976; Vinke et al. 1979). Both decision table and distance measurement techniques can again be subdivided into methods depending on fixed criteria, methods depending on variable criteria (learning methods) and learning methods where a "normal" beat must be indicated by the operator. Decision table methods are usually based directly on the experience of one or more cardiologists together with data from the literature, while the second technique attempts to calculate the distance

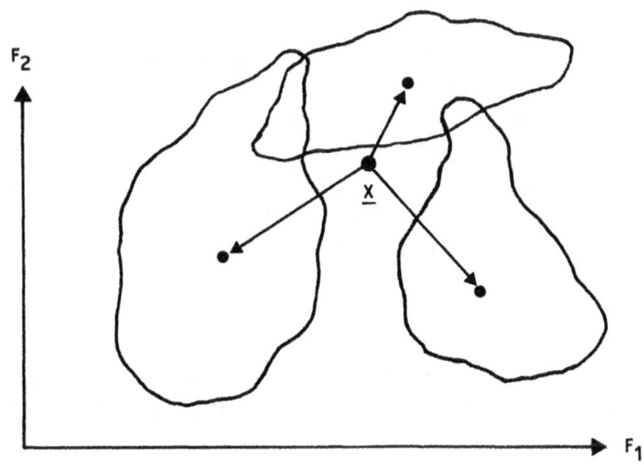

Fig. 5. Beat morphology clusters in feature space. Classification of unknown beat depends on "distance" to clusters of known morphology. Only two-dimensional case is shown, usually more features are used

of the vector of beat characteristics from a given predefined class and hence to assign the beat to that class or another one using some preset threshold distance. Thus beats may be classified into types or into degrees of abnormality. Some systems then update the class with the new beat thus compensating somewhat for physiological, variability over long periods of time.

Rhythm Classification

The techniques used at this stage are very similar to those used for beat classification but are now usually applied to multiple beats. There is, of course, a certain overlap here with beat classification in that the most commonly sought phenomenon, the PVC, can be classified either at this point or during beat classification (Spitz and Harrison 1978). In addition to the two methods mentioned earlier, decision table and distance measurements, rhythm classification may also make use of syntactic analysis (Hoare and Arntzenius 1971; Jenkins et al. 1976), Markov-chain analysis (Gersch et al. 1972; Vinke et al. 1979; Algra et al. 1982), Bayesian methods or other statistical techniques (Epple et al. 1975; Haisty et al. 1972; Knoebel and Lovelace 1978; Rompelman et al. 1977; Willems and Pipberger 1972). Most AADs are very limited in the range of arrhythmias they can detect. The emphasis has traditionally been on the detection of ventricular dysrhythmias: PVCs, ventricular tachycardia, ventricular fibrillation etc. and on bradycardia, tachycardia and asystole. The lack of a P-wave in most conventional (i.e., single-lead) systems makes even this limited set extremely difficult to detect with any degree of reliability. Special (multiple) lead systems, e.g., intra-atrial or esophageal, combined with surface leads or orthogonal leads may partially overcome this limitation (Bernard et al. 1974; Jenkins et al. 1976; Lorente et al. 1977; Mantle et al. 1978; Rey et al. 1971).

In practice most systems use at least two different types of logic, one for PVCs and one for other arrhythmias. For example, PVCs (single or multiple) might be detected using distance calculations, bradycardia and the like using decision-table logic and atrial fibrillation using spectral analysis.

Some AADs place less emphasis on single beat and more on the classification of a string of beats. This is particularly true of systems using only interval information. Syntactical techniques can be applied to R-R intervals only but do not give very satisfactory results due to insufficient data. They have also been applied to the combination of bipolar and esophageal leads, i.e., to P and R waves (Jenkins et al. 1976). Simple statistical techniques (standard deviation, autocorrelation applied to R-R intervals, dispersion) have been more satisfactory for giving additional information than for basic rhythm classification. Markov chain analysis seems et present to be better at detecting sinus rhythm than arrhythmias. Clustering techniques applied, for instance, to displays of R-R intervals (nth interval against n-1th) have been used in some systems but have not found general application.

Almost all forms of rhythm classification have problems with the detection of ventricular fibrillation (VFIB), since QRS detectors frequently classify it as artifact and must therefore use special logic. The most promising method to date compares the contribution of a narrow-band low-frequency component of the ECG to the total power in the signal (Kuo and Dillman 1978; Nygards and Hulting 1977). It remains, however, difficult to discriminate between VFIB and artifacts simulating as beats. Also, some isolated VFIB records can not be correctly classified by this method without excessive amounts of false-positives (Nolle et al. 1980).

Problems

None of the above algorithms are completely without problems. The main technical problem is still that of artifact. Signals are often "noisy" and, as with the simple ratemeters, this results in wrongly detected or ignored beats. The effect is even more serious in true arrhythmia monitoring as these artifacts are usually recognised as an arrhythmia, often generating an alarm, or else mask an actual arrhythmia. Systems with a short-term "memory" and/or automatic strip chart generation allow the nurse to check whether it was really a true alarm, but a high rate of false alarms will cause irritation and engender lack of faith in the computer system. It is not always sufficiently appreciated, however, what dramatic improvement in signal quality can be achieved by better electrode placement (Hugenholtz et al. 1974), by more care in applying electrodes, and even by the type of electrode itself (Feldman et al. 1979). Several systems now attempt to monitor the amount of artifact and include poor signal quality among the automatic alarms. Prompt action to improve signal quality and regular attention to this will greatly improve the performance of any arrhythmia monitoring system. Certain traditional problems due partly to human error, such as poor gain setting or loose electrodes which may be seen as cardiac arrest, have been eliminated in the newer systems where the front-end is incorporated in the system itself. Problems still occur, even in clean signals, with algorithms generating incorrect rhythm classification and alarms. The accuracy of the best known algorithms has been evaluated many times. Unfortunately, there is as yet no general agreement on a "best" algorithm, partly because these results are not identical when the same algorithm is used at different institutions. One very serious problem is found with ventricular fibrillation. This is a relatively rare occurrence nowadays but it is essential that the computer system should always generate a serious alarm if it does occur. No algorithm up to now has proved completely foolproof in general clinical use.

Evaluation

Formal evaluation of the performance of an analysis system is far from simple and interpretation of the results can be extremely difficult (Hulting et al. 1977). Even in the case of fully automated systems it is rarely possible to compare results directly, as until recently there was no standardised database to use as a yardstick and there is still little agreement as to the best methods of presenting the results, although several approaches have been proposed (Hermes and Cox 1980). In addition, most systems can be "tuned" to fit certain requirements, and institutions seldom specify identical system characteristics. The increasing use of receiver operator characteristics (ROC curves) is helping to clarify this and the existence of two standard (and reasonably compatible) arrhythmia databases should make it easier to compare results in future (Ripley and Oliver 1977; Schluter et al. 1980). In the case of interactive systems the evaluation becomes one of comparing system/operator combinations. There are as yet no satisfactory techniques for extracting the operator component of the total systems performance. Evaluation of an arrhythmia system, however, should not be confined to the technical accuracy of the detection algorithms. It cannot be emphasized strongly enough that user-acceptance of a system is governed by many factors, physical and psychological, which may have little to do with the theoretical performance of the system. A system which is inconvenient, arkward to use, complicated to understand or does not provide satisfactory, easily-read output is unlikely to be a success, whatever its technical advantages. Again, a system whose technical performance is not necessarily optimal may be well engineered for the particular environment and thus engender complete satisfaction among its users. On the other hand, a system is remembered for its failures and the occasion an algorithm failed to recognise a life threatening event will weigh very heavily. It is perhaps unnecessary to emphasize that the use to which the system is to be put is a very important part of the overall evaluation. A system to be used to record the number of PVCs for studies comparing two drugs is somewhat different in its requirements from one used, say, to take over as much as possible of the nurse's surveillance work in units with low staffing. The quality of technical support too, will make a considerable difference to acceptance or otherwise of a system. Signal quality is perhaps the most important single factor in reliable monitoring, and in some centers the technicians are completely responsible for this, starting with the electrode placement.

Recent Developments

The increasing use of microprocessors and microcomputers has led to a number of new developments in arrhythmia monitoring (Willems and Peperstraete 1978). The micro's cheapness means that more computing power can be devoted to each patient. One result of this is that systems are now being built which omit the conventional analog bedside equipment, replacing this by computer-controlled display and logic. The most elaborate of these systems has a microcomputer per patient which controls all signal handling; plugging the signal into the unit is sufficient to initiate appropriate conditioning, display and processing. The unit itself guides the user through complex procedures such as calibration or cardiac output measurements. Bedside micros are linked to another micro at the nurse station for strip chart alarms and displays (Deutsch et al. 1978). Other similar structures are being built whereby more or less of the bedside equipment is replaced (Augenstein et al. 1979; Sabean et al. 1977). This approach simplifies the user interface considerably, thus increasing user acceptance.

The Future

Much of the work of the past five years has been a question of consolidating existing work, improving the system design and equipment and "tuning" algorithms. It seems likely that this will continue for some time yet. On the other hand, the relative cheapness of computing power today makes it possible to reconsider techniques that were discarded in the past as too slow or too wasteful (Fourier analysis, autocorrelation). There is a new interest in techniques which do not rely on human-type pattern recognition (Markov chain etc.). Again, electrode improvements (such as the esophageal electrode) may enable recognition of P-waves and hence more sophisticated and reliable arrhythmia detection. Another development which is becoming increasingly popular in teaching and research hospitals is the coupling of the monitoring computer directly to the central database. This can in theory open up a wide range of possibilities – the ability to make suggestions for therapy based on previous experience of this type of case, the provision of teaching material in the same way and, of course, ready access to past and present details of the patient, have all received much attention. However, it seems most probable that the greatest effort will be put into microprocessor-based applications and that over the next ten years the arrhythmia monitor will replace the ratemeter as the latter took over some of the drudgery of the clinical staff a decade ago. Certainly, as long as clinical heart disease shows no decline in its incidence, cheaper and better monitoring systems will remain a necessity.

References

Algra A, Vinke RVH, Zeelenberg C (1982) Prescanning 24 hour ECG recordings selecting normal sinus rhythm using the theory of Markov chains. In: Computers in cardiology. IEEE Computer Society, 82CH1814-3, Long Beach, CA, pp 49–55

Augenstein JS, Civetta JM, Lustig J, Konowalchuk T (1979) Clinical experience with a distributed intelligence intensive care data management system. In: Computers in cardiology. IEEE Computer Society, 79CH1462-1C, Long Beach, CA, pp 447–449

Bernard R, Rey W, Vainsel H, Boothroyd M, Demeester M (1974) Computerized dysrhythmia monitoring with an intra-auricular lead. In: Computers in cardiology. IEEE Computer Society, 74CH0879-7C, Long Beach, CA, pp 17–21

Cox JR, Ripley KL (1963) Compact digital coding of electrocardiographic data. In: Proc. 6th Hawaii Int. Conf. on System Sciences, Honolulu

Cox JR, Nolle FM, Fozzard HA, Oliver GC (1968) AZTEC a pre-processing program for real-time ECG rhythm analysis. IEEE Trans Biolmed Eng 15/2: 128–129

Deutsch LS, Engelse WAH, Zeelenberg C, Voorde F vd, Hugenholtz PG (1978) The Unibed patient monitoring system: a new approach for a new technology. Med instrum 11/5: 274–277

Dillman R. Judell N, Kuo S (1978) Replacement of AZTEC by correlation for more accurate VPB detection. In: Computers in Cardiology. IEEE Computer Society, 78CH1391-2C, Long Beach, CA, pp 29–33

Engelse WAH, Zeelenberg C (1979) A single scan algorithm for QRS-detection and feature extraction. In: Computers in Cardiology. IEEE Computer Society, 79CH1462-1C, Long Beach, CA, pp 37–43

Epple E, Bleicher W, Decker W, Faust U (1975) Analysis of time intervals in the ECG by statistical methods. In: Computers in Cardiology. IEEE Computer Society, 75CH1017-1C, Long Beach, CA, pp 189–193

Feldman CL, Amazeen PG, Klein MD, Lown B (1971) Computer detection of ventricular ectopic beats. Comput Biomed Res 3: 666–674

Feldman CL, Hubelbank M, Haffajee CI, Kotilainen P (1979) A new electrode system for automated ECG monitoring. In: Computers in Cardiology. IEEE Computer Society, 79CH1462-1C, Long Beach, CA, pp 285–289

Gersch W, Eddy DM, Dong E (1972) Cardiac arrhythmia classification: A heart-beat interval-Markov chain approach. Comput Biomed Res 4: 383–392

Haisty WK, Batchlor C, Cornfield J, Pipberger HV (1972) Discriminant function analysis of RR intervals: an algorithm for online arrhythmia diagnosis. Comput Biomed Res 5: 247–255

Hermes RE, Cox JR (1980) A methodology and performance evaluation of ventricular arrhythmia detectors. In: Computers in Cardiology. IEEE Computer Society, 80CH1606-3, Long Beach, CA, pp 3–9
Hoare MR, Arntzenius AC (1971) First steps in real-time arrhythmia screening. In: Snellen HA, Hemker HC, Bemmel JH v (eds) Quantitation in cardiology. Leiden University Press, Leiden
Hugenholtz PG, Lubse J, Miller AC, Immink A, Hagemeijer F (1974) Selection and placement of electrodes in computer monitoring of arrhythmias. In: Miller, Harrison (eds) Biomed Elect Technol. Academic, New York
Hulting J (1979) Application and evaluation of automated arrhythmia monitoring in the coronary care unit. Acta Med Scand [Suppl] 630
Hulting I, Nygards ME, Wigertz O (1977) Problems in the evaluation of arrhythmia monitoring systems. In: Bemmel JH v, Willems JL (eds) Trends in computer-processed electrocardiograms. North-Holland, Amsterdam
Jenkins JM, Wu D, Arzbaecher RC (1976) Computer-based arrhythmia classification utilizing the PR interval. In: Computers in cardiology. IEEE Computer Society, 76CH1160-1C, Long Beach, CA, pp 149–157
Knoebel SB, Lovelace DE (1978) A two-dimensional clustering technique for identification of multiform ventricular complexes. Med Instrum 12/6: 332–333
Kuo S, Dillman R (1978) Computer detection of ventricular fibrillation. In: Computers in cardiology. IEEE Computer Society, 78CH1391-2C, Long Beach, CA, pp 347–350
Lindsay J, Bruchner NV (1975) Conventional coronary care unit monitoring: non-detection of transient rhythm disturbances. JAMA 232/1: 51–53
Lorente P, Henzel D, Bardon A, Lesignie C, Levy B (1977) A hardware device for recognition of P and QRS waves. Med Prog Technol 4: 177
Lown B, Klein MD, Hershberg PI (1969) Coronary and precoronary care. Am J Med 46: 705–724
McClelland KM, Arnold JM (1976) A QRS detection algorithm for computerised ECG monitoring. In: Computers in cardiology. IEEE Computer Society, 76CH1160-1C, Long Beach, CA, pp 447–451
Mantle JA, Strand EM, Wixson SE (1978) Atrial electrogram monitoring in a cardiac care unit. Med Instrum 12/5: 289–292
Mead CN, Clark KW, Potter SJ, Moore SM, Thomas LJ (1979) Development and evaluation of a new QRS-detector-delineator. In: Computers in cardiology. IEEE Computer Society, 79CH1462-1C, Long Beach, CA, pp 251–255
Nolle FM (1972) Argus, a clinical computer system for monitoring electrocardiographic rhythms. D. Sc. dissertation, Washington University, St. Louis, MO
Nolle FM, Ryschon KL, Zencka AE (1980) Power spectrum analysis of ventricular fibrillation and imitative artifacts. In: Computers in cardiology. IEEE Computer Society, 80CH1606-3, Long Beach, CA, pp 209–213
Nygards ME, Hulting J (1977) Recognition of ventricular fibrillation utilizing the power spectrum of the ECG. In: Computers in cardiology. IEEE Computer Society, 77CH1254-2C, Long Beach, CA, pp 393–398
Oliver GC, Ripley KL, Miller JP, Martin TF (1977) A critical review of computer arrhythmia detection. In: Pordy L (ed) Computer electrocardiography: Current status and criteria. Futura, New York
Plokker HWM (1978) Cardiac rhythm diagnosis by digital computer. Dissertation, Institute of Medical Physics TNO, Utrecht
Rey W, Laird JD, Hugenholtz PG (1971) P-wave detection by digital computer. Comput Biomed Res 4: 509–522
Ripley KL, Oliver GC (1977) Development of an ECG database for arrhythmia detector evaluation. In: Computers in cardiology. IEEE Computer Society, 77CH1254-2C, Long Beach, CA, pp 203–210
Romhilt DW, Bloomfield SS, Chou T-C, Fowler NO (1973) Unreliability of conventional electrocardiographic monitoring for arrhythmia detection in coronary care units. Am J Cardiol 31: 457–461
Rompelman O, Coenen AJRM, Saat RG (1977) A special purpose computer for on-line statistical analysis of the heart rate. Med Prog Technol 5: 149–156
Ryden L, Walderstrom A, Holmberg S (1975) The reliability of intermittent ECG sampling in arrhythmia detection. Circulation 52 no 4: 540–545

Sabean R, Scharnberg B, Schillings H, Ehlers CTh (1977) Gottingen information system for intensive care. In: Computers in cardiology. IEEE Computer Society, 77CH1254-2C, Long Beach, CA, pp 431–439
Sanders WJ, Alderman EL, Harrison DC (1977) The development of a second generation; ECG monitoring system. In: Bemmel JH v, Willems JL (eds) Trends in computer processed electrocardiograms. North-Holland, Amsterdam
Schluter P, Mark R, Moody G, Olson W, Peterson W (1980) Performance measures for arrhythmia detectors. In: Computers in cardiology. IEEE Computer Society, 80CH1606-3, Long Beach, CA, pp 267–271
Shah PM, Arnold JM, Bliss DT, McClelland KM, Clarke WB (1977) Automatic real-time arrhythmia monitoring in the intensive coronary care unit. Am J Cardiol 39: 276–283
Spitz AL, Harrison DC (1978) Automated family classification in ambulatory arrhythmia monitoring. Med Instrum 12/6: 322–323
Thomas J, Clark KW, Mead CN, Ripley KL, Spenner BF, Oliver GC (1979) Automated cardiac dysrhythmia analysis. Proc IEEE 67/9: 1322–1337
Vinke RVH, Algra A, Ros J, Zeelenberg C (1979) Classification of cardiac rhythms using the theory of Markov chains. In: Computers in cardiology. IEEE Computer Society, 79CH1462-1C, Long Beach, CA, pp 255–259
Willems J, Peperstraete J (1978) Survey report on cardiac arrhythmia monitoring based on special purpose analog and microprocessors within the ECG. Contract 338–77-ECI B, Leuven
Willems J, Pipberger H (1972) Arrhythmia detection by digital computer. Comput Biomed Res 5: 263–278
Zeelenberg C, Deutsch LS, Engelse WAH, Corbeij HMA (1977) Experiences with implementing Argus in a cardiac surveillance unit. In: Bemmel JH v, Willems JL (eds) Trends in computer processed electrocardiograms. North-Holland, Amsterdam

Monitoring Intracranial Pressure – Nuisance to, or Advantage for, Ward Personnel?

K. Wiedemann, G. Schmidt, and M. Müller

Introduction

Over the past two decades clinical application of intracranial pressure measurement has developed into an almost routine procedure in larger intensive care units, and there is an abundance of papers on this issue. Few studies, however, have addressed the fact that intracranial pressure is the only parameter monitored in intensive care that is immediately and regularly influenced by routine nursing care. Moreover it may demonstrate to nurses and physicians the presence of acute danger to patients with increased intracranial volume, at the very moment the staff are caring for the bedfast and comatose.

There is rather limited space for accommodating volume increases in any of the components of the intracranial contents, arterial blood volume, venous blood volume, brain tissue and cerebrospinal fluid (csf), especially if the spinal dural sac has been extended to its maximum capacity or is inaccessible to cerebrospinal fluid due to herniation. It is common knowledge that a volume increase in any one component will lead to a different increase in intracranial pressure, depending on the preexisting brain and csf volumes. This is expressed in the exponential nature of the intracranial pressure/volume curve (Langfitt et al. 1965). Nursing procedures may therefore produce rather different reactions in intracranial pressure due to different states of the intracranial compliance or elastance.

Table 1. Causes of raised intracranial pressure related to nursing procedures

1. Increased cerebral blood volume:	
(a) Arterial inflow:	Coughing
	Straining
	Isometric muscular contraction
	Emotional arousal
	Painful stimuli
	Respiratory disturbances: $PCO_2 \uparrow$, $PO_2 \downarrow$
(b) Venous outflow:	Head flexion-extension
	Head rotation
	Valsalva maneuvre
	(PEEP)
2. CSF increase:	Head rotation, flexion

Miller and Leech (1975) have shown that any change in mean intracranial pressure exceeding 2 mmHg with a volume challenge of 1,0 ml, i.e., a volume-pressure response of 2 or more, will represent a state of high elastance or low compliance.

Apart from common causes of increased brain mass, such as edema, tumor, or hemorrhage, increased blood volume as in posttraumatic hyperperfusion syndrome, or in the use of certain volatile anesthetics, and increased amounts of spinal fluid due to increased production, decreased absorption, or obstructed spinal fluid pathways, there are many nursing procedures that will significantly alter the volume of the intracranial contents (Table 1).

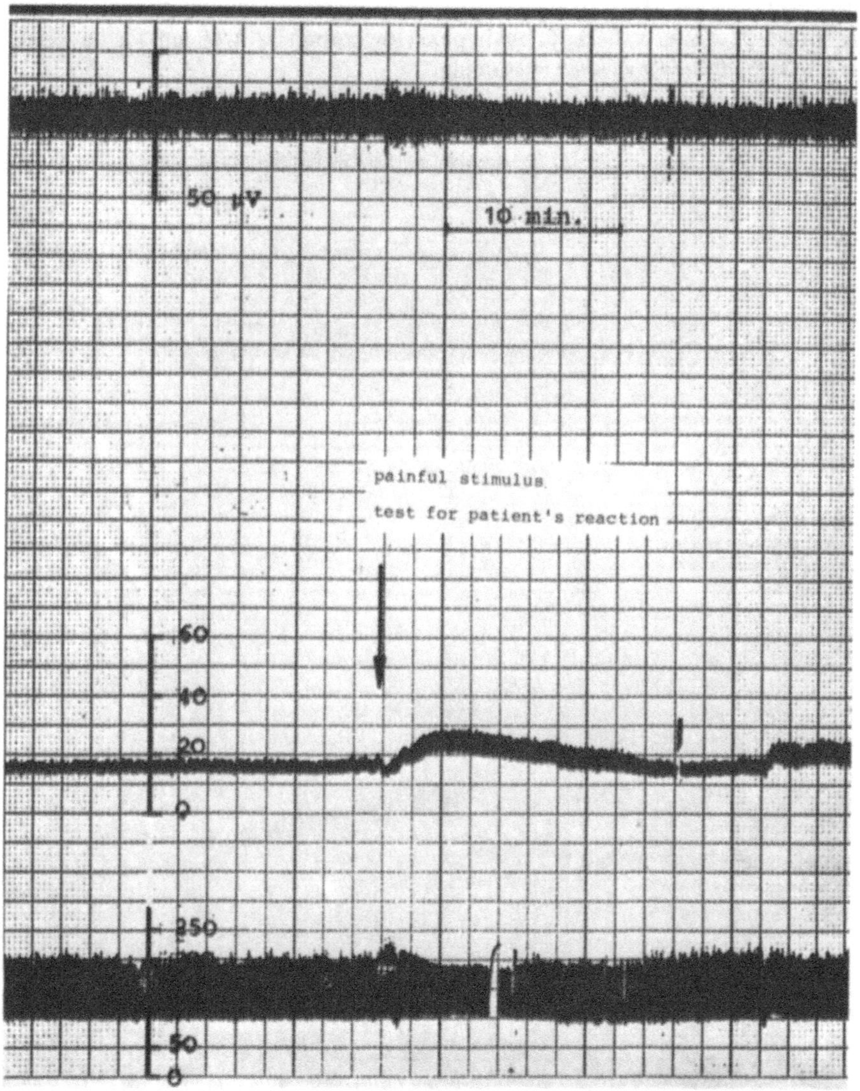

Fig. 1. Intracranial pressure (ICP) increase upon testing response to pain in a 41-year-old male with frontotemporal contusion. Traces from top to bottom: EEG, ICP, arterial pressure. Note independence of ICP increase from arterial pressure

Conditions and Nursing Procedures

Increases in Arterial Inflow. These will occur consequent to rises in systemic arterial pressure, whenever autoregulation of cerebral blood flow is disturbed. This has been shown to occur in focal or global damage to the brain, as with contusions, and in moderate to marked levels of preexistent intracranial hypertension, i.e., when cerebral perfusion pressure is decreased below 50–60 mmHg in the normal adult.

Special attention should be called to arterial vasodilation on account of emotional or pain-induced arousal, which will increase cerebral blood flow according to acutely increased demand (Fig. 1). Respiratory disturbances are mainly thought to occur in insufficient respirator therapy, but hypoxia lower than PaO_2 60 mm Hg has also been demonstrated during routine suctioning.

Venous Outflow from the Cranial Vault. This may be impeded by occlusions of the jugular veins (Mitchell 1980) and even the vertebrobasilar drainage systems on rotation of the head (Fig. 2) or flexion-deflexion of the neck. Hulme and Cooper

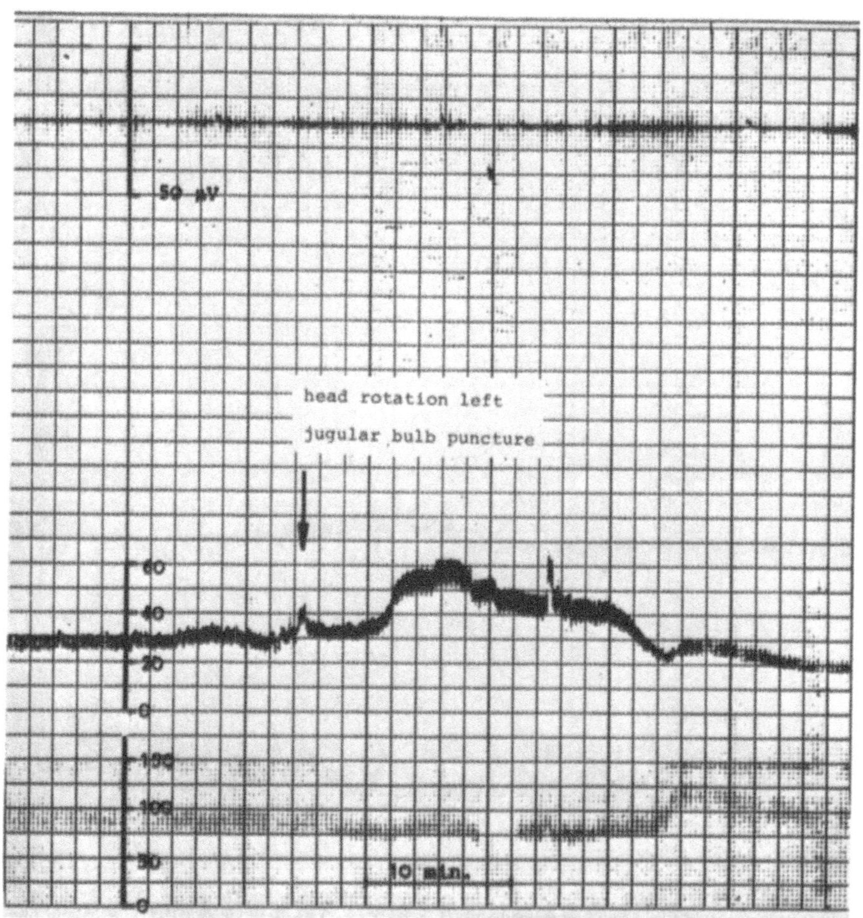

Fig. 2. ICP increase due to head turn for jugular bulb catheterisation. Patient and traces as in Fig. 1

(1976), in 18 patients with diverse intracranial pathology, demonstrated abrupt rises and falls of intracranial pressure (ICP) with head positioning or jugular vein compression. In some of their patients with high ICP, increases resembling plateau waves were seen, and the increments were most pronounced in subjects with increased opening pressures.

Turning patients to lateral recumbent positions (Mitchell et al. 1980) also caused intracranial pressure to rise, irrespective of whether the patient's head was being kept from additional rotation or not, in 88% at least during half the turns performed.

Any event resembling a Valsalva maneuvre, such as coughing or straining at stool, will cause a rise in arterial pressure after the event due to intrathoracic pressure increases, and in addition will impede cranial venous outflow and thus will augment intracranial volume. Shalit and Umansky (1977) entertain the idea, that intracranial pressure increases consequent on head positioning are caused by temporary entrapment of cerebrospinal fluid in the cranial vault due to occlusion at the craniovertebral junction.

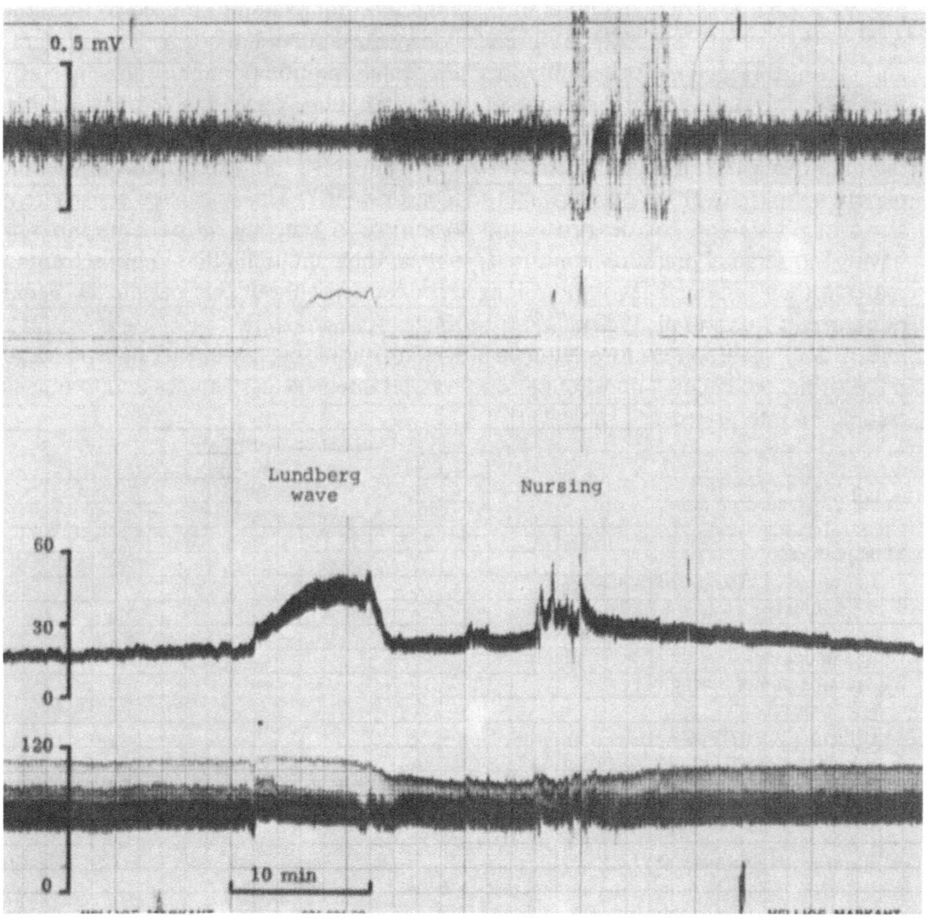

Fig. 3. Lundberg wave and pronounced ICP increase upon nursing procedures in an 11-year-old boy with temporobasal contusion. Note protracted return to baseline of ICP. Traces as in Fig. 1

In a more recent series of 33 cases Tsementzis et al. (1982) showed in 14 of these a transient rise of intracranial pressure upon routine nursing procedures, such as suctioning with or without chest physiotherapy, testing the pupillary light reflex, taking the blood pressure by sphygmomanometry, inserting a nasogastric tube, giving IM injections and performing oral or skin hygiene. In most cases this could be traced to increased intrathoracic and thus increased jugular venous pressure. In five patients, however, dangerous rises in intracranial pressure were seen, unexplained by venous outflow mechanics; pressure waves were accompanied by pressure increases, intractable by conservative means in one case, and were thought to be due to primary cerebral arterial vasodilation.

Staff Reactions. The nursing staff are thus faced with the puzzling and at times rather distressing situation, that nursing duties (Fig. 3) expected to be carried out regularly and to the best of their knowledge and skill, may cause acute, and sometimes irreversible danger to the cerebral perfusion in their patients.

Under conditions of high intracranial compliance, for example induced by barbiturate coma, the same procedures will cause only transient and minor rises of intracranial pressure (Fig. 4). Conceivably this additional emotional load on nursing staff, i.e., probably harming the patient by caring for him, might cause considerable reluctance in dealing with patients thus monitored, or might lead to simply ignoring the data displayed, not unlike Sir Robert Macintosh's reported attitude towards a patient's dropping blood pressure: "Stop measuring it!". This may even constitute a trend in physicians, for despite claims to improved outcome in patients through having intracranial pressure monitored, some authors maintain that in brain trauma patients they obtained favourable long term results without this parameter being monitored (Stuart et al. 1983).

In order to gain some information on nurses' attitudes towards intracranial pressure monitoring, we issued a questionnaire to trained intensive care nurses and to nurses training in intensive care (Table 2).

Table 2. Questionnaire

Main features:

1. Experience in recognizing raised ICP
   < 15 mmHg < 30 mmHg
2. Experience in nursing with ICP monitored
   < 5 patients > 5 patients
3. Training in monitoring ICP:
   (a) Bedside only
   (b) Additional lessons
4. Influence of ICP monitoring on nursing preparation:
   (a) Better
   (b) Usual
   (c) Less
5. Intimidation or assurance by ICP information?
6. Preference for ICP monitoring in comatose patients
   Yes / No
7. Transfer of nursing considerations to non-monitored comatose patients possible
   Yes / No

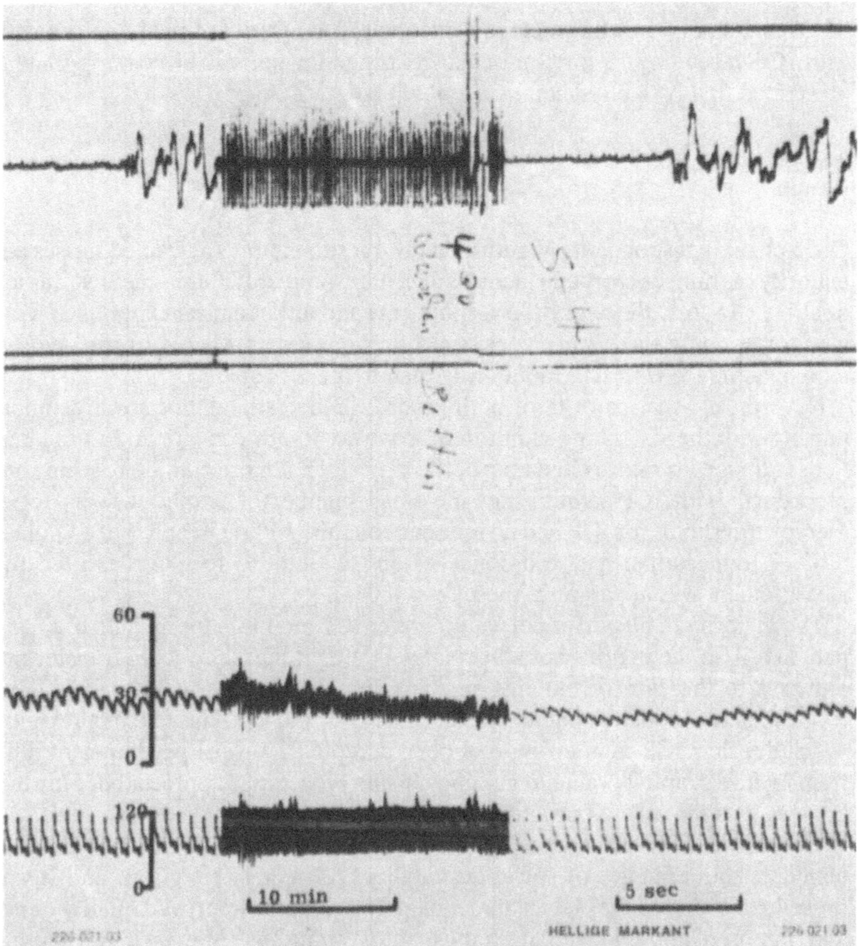

Fig. 4. Amelioration of ICP reactions to nursing due to increased intracranial compliance following institution of barbiturate coma (thiopentone 4 mg-kg-h) Patient as in Fig. 3, traces as in Fig. 1

Fisher's exact test was used on the results. All staff were accustomed to ICP being monitored in their patients epidurally, either by a Statham device (Gobiet et al. 1975) or by a Gaeltec manometer (Gaab et al. 1979). The epidural intracranial pressure was displayed constantly on a slow speed chart recorder together with arterial pressure and electroencephalogram (see Figs. 1 to 4). Interpretation of major events had been explained to all nurses and trainees at the bedside; an additional lesson had been offered.

Brain-oriented intensive care in these patients consisted of hyperventilation to $PaCO_2$ 30 torr, administration of steroids, infusion of mannitol 0,3 g kg^{-1}, if ICP was consistently higher than 15 torr and institution of thiopentone coma with ICP higher than 25 torr. Muscle relaxants were added if posturing occured either spontaneously or upon stimulation.

All personnel were allowed to inject fentanyl 0,1 mg prior to suctioning and nursing with ICP exceeding 15 torr; muscular relaxants for periods of posturing had to be prescribed first by a physician.

Results

Of 53 possible respondents 36 returned the questionnaire. All trained nurses and the majority of trainees correctly identified the threshold of ICP treatment at our institution, i.e., 15 torr. Since only 33 respondents had any practical experience with ICP monitoring, only these were considered further. As a probable truism, nurses had more experience with ICP monitoring than trainees (Table 3).

Nevertheless the majority of both groups claimed stimulation towards improved nursing with the ICP being monitored. Contrary to our concern and to the implications from the literature cited above, the majority felt more confident during nursing procedures with ICP monitoring; the small number of wrong answers regarding therapy thresholds for ICP had no influence on this. Although only 4 of 14 nurses and 5 of 19 trainees had had additional lessons, a trend to feeling reassured by ICP measurement was apparent in these ($p = 0{,}054$).

The majority of all personnel would prefer ICP monitors for nursing brain trauma patients. Also the majority of all personnel thought that they could transfer nursing attitudes to the care of patients similarly injured but not monitored. Additional lessons tended to yield a higher transfer rate ($p = 0{,}04!$). Thus one might cautiously conclude, that ICP monitoring had been accepted by ward personnel of different training levels, and its value in guiding nursing procedures appreciated. However we are aware of the severe limitations in interpreting these results.

Only 33 out of 53 candidates could be evaluated fully, no provisions were made to eliminate the influence of social desirability on the answers given, and it was not possible to evaluate the claims made, namely as regards improved quality of nursing and transfer of improved nursing habits. Since the author's interest in ICP monitoring was known to all nurses, further influences on the choice of answers cannot be ruled out. Nevertheless it is possible to state that monitoring ICP, despite all the considerations cited in the beginning, would not present such a conflict to ward personnel as seriously to endanger acceptance of the method.

However, in order to augment the yield of information to nurses, especially as regards prognosticating the incidence as well as the severity and duration of dangerous pressure increases in any given patient, several provisions have to be made:

1. Intracranial pressure, arterial pressure, and cerebral perfusion pressure should be displayed on a slow speed chart recorder or trend oscilloscope as usual, to facilitate interpretation of past noxious events and for teaching purposes.
2. Data processing at the bedside should provide the nurse with a very simple display of information on the impending development of the ICP, the degree of risk from nursing procedures for a given patient, and of deliberations concerning postponement or modifications of those procedures. As already shown by Kullberg (1972), this may be accomplished by observing the skewness of frequency histograms of intracranial pressure (Fig. 5). Widening of the histogram basis, skewing to the right, differences between arithmetic mean, median and mode all point to

Table 3. Results. TN, trained nurses; NIT, nurses in training

Lowest limit for treatment of ICP

	15 mmHg	30 mmHg	Total
TN	16	0	16
NIT	15	5	20
	31	5	36

Experience in nursing patients with ICP monitoring

	Patients		
	< 5	> 5	Total
TN	3	11	14
NIT	16*	3	19
	19	14	33

* $p = 0.05$

Influence of ICP monitoring on nursing preparations (analgetics, timing)

	Better	Usual	Less	Total
TN	12	2	0	14
NIT	14	4	1	19
	26	6	1	33

Intimidation or assurance by ICP monitoring?

	Intimidated	Assured	Total
TN	3	11	14
NIT	4	15	19
	7	26	33

Preference for ICP monitoring in brain trauma patients

	Preference		
	Yes	No	Total
TN	12	2	14
NIT	17	2	19
	29	4	33

Transfer of nursing attitudes to brain trauma patients without ICP monitoring

	Transfer		
	Yes	No	Total
TN	11	3	14
NIT	14	5	19
	25	8	33

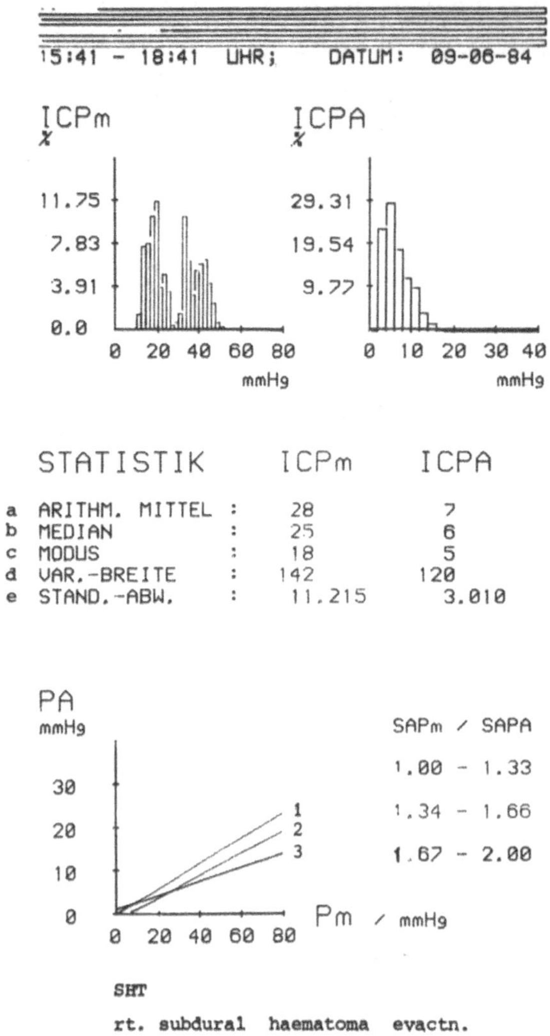

(Lower panel) Regression lines of intracranial pressure amplitude (PA) plotted against intracranial mean pressure (PM), corrected for influence of high *(1)*, intermediate *(2)* and low *(3)* systemic pulse pressure. Correction ratios shown on the right: Systemic arterial pressure mean (SAPm) by systemic pulse pressure (SAPA). All three regression lines indicate acceptable intracranial compliance

Fig. 5. Frequency distribution of mean ICP (ICPm) and ICP amplitude (ICPA) during 3 h sampling time *(upper panel)*. Display of arithmetic mean *(a)*, median *(b)*, mode *(c)*, variation *(d)* and standard deviation of the mean *(e)* of ICPm and ICPA. The double-humped frequency distribution reflects effective reduction of raised ICP by starting thiopentone infusion 6 mg-kg-h at 16.50

increased incidence of pressure waves. This in turn indicates danger to the patient from further pressure increases by common nursing procedures, due to reduced intracranial compliance. Turner et al. (1976) maintained that nurses, even regardless of their experience, were able to interpret ICP histograms and, with a tendency to overestimate the skewness of the histograms, would render the system fail-safe. Any bedside computer in neurosurgical wards can be expected to be capable of producing histograms and indicating arithmetic mean, median, and mode.

3. Work from many authors (Szewszykowski et al. 1977; Avezaat et al. 1976) has shown that the ratio of intracranial pulse pressure to intracranial mean pressure closely reflects pressure-volume tests in yielding information on intracranial compliance. This feature is highly desirable in a bedside computer for neurological intensive care. With increasing experience it will be possible to make the resulting diagrams (Fig. 5) interpretable not only by individual dedicated physicians, but also by trained nurses. With the latter group the one and only purpose is, of course, to aid in decisions regarding nursing procedures and alterting the intensive care physician.

Computers capable of displaying data thus processed, fed from a conventional chart recorder preamplifier, have been developed during recent years, and may soon be available to a broader public.

Details of this development may be taken from the following contribution of Dr. Gaab and it is to be hoped, that computers of this type may help to convert routine monitoring of ICP from a nuisance into an advantage to nurses.

References

Avezaat CJJ, van Eijndhoven JHM, de Jong DA, Molenaar WCJ (1976) A new method of monitoring intracranial pressure/volume relationship. In: Beks JWF, Bosch DA, Brock M (eds) Intracranial pressure III. Springer, Berlin Heidelberg New York, pp 308–313

Gaab MR, Knoblich OE, Dietrich K (1979) Miniaturisierte Methoden zur Überwachung des intrakraniellen Druckes: Techniken und klinische Ergebnisse. Langenbecks Arch Chir 350: 13–31

Gobiet W (1977) Intensivtherapie nach Schädel-Hirn-Trauma. Springer, Berlin Heidelberg New York

Hulme A, Cooper R (1976) The effects of head position and jugular vein compression on intracranial pressure. In: Beks JWF, Bosch DA, Brock M (eds) Intracranial pressure III. Springer, Berlin Heidelberg New York, pp 259–263

Kullberg GA (1972) A method for statistical analysis of intracranial pressure recordings. In: Brock M, Dietz H (eds) Intracranial pressure. Springer, Berlin Heidelberg New York, pp 65–69

Langfitt TW, Weinstein JD, Kassell NF (1965) Cerebral vasomotor paralysis produced by intracranial hypertension. Neurology 15: 622–641

Miller JD, Leech P (1975) Effects of mannitol and steroid therapy on intracranial pressure-volume relationships in patients. J Neurosurg 42: 274–281

Mitchell PH (1980) Intracranial hypertension: implications of research for nursing care. J. Neurosurg Nurs 12: 145–154

Mitchell PH, Mauss NK, Ozuna J, Lipe H (1980) Relationship of nurse/patient activity and ICP variation. In: Shulman K, Marmarou A, Miller JD, Becker DP, Hochwald GM, Brock M (eds) Intracranial pressure IV. Springer, Berlin Heidelberg New York, pp 565–568

Shalit MN, Umansky F (1977) Effect of routine bedside procedures on intracranial pressure. Isr J Med Sci 13: 881–886

Stuart GC, Merry GS, Smith JA, Yelland JDN (1983) Severe head injury managed without intracranial pressure monitoring. J Neurosurg 59: 601–605

Szewszykowski J, Sliwka S, Kunicki A, Dytko P, Korsak-Sliwka J (1977) A fast method of estimating the elastance of the intracranial system. J Neurosurg 47: 19–26

Turner JM, McDowall DG, Gibson RM, Khalili H (1976) Computer analysis of intracranial pressure Measurements: Clinical value and nursing response. In: Beks JWF, Bosch DA, Brock M (eds) Intracranial pressure III. Springer, Berlin Heidelberg New York, pp 283–287

Tsementzis SA, Harris P, Loizou LA (1982) The effect of routine nursing care procedures on the ICP in severe head injuries. Acta Neurochir 65: 153–166

Computerized Neuromonitoring*

M. R. Gaab

Introduction

The results presented at this symposium make it clear that the computer has finally found its way into the intensive care unit (ICU). It helps us to accumulate, select and examine the value of data; it records and improves biosignals and eliminates artifacts (Wiener et al. 1982).

So far, however, only peripheral service systems – if I may so designate the vital functions of heart, lungs, and kidneys – have been monitored with the support of a computer. It is not only in neurological and neurosurgical cases, however, that the brain is the organ that determines the prognosis, but also in all cases of vital function disorder and intoxication (Brierley and Meldrum 1971; Gaab 1981). After all, the whole purpose of intensive therapy is to maintain the brain's supply. Yet the current methods of brain monitoring still hardly differ from those used 100 years ago – we check motor systems and reaction to pain and tap reflexes (Gaab 1984). This is regrettable as there are, in fact, technical methods available which make reliable continuous control of the brain function and of any risks possible.

Useful Biosignals for Cerebral Monitoring

The functional activity and metabolism of the brain are shown by the EEG (Prior 1979); the utility of a trace of this spontaneous cerebral autorhythm is increased by a

List of Abbreviations and Units Used

ARM = arithmetic mean value, CBF = cerebral blood flow (ml min^{-1} per 100g, CPP = cerebral perfusion pressure (mmHg), CVP = central venous pressure (mmHg), EEG = electroencephalogram (Hz, μV), EMG = electromyogram, EVP = evoked potentials, FFT = fast Fourier transformation, ICP = intracranial pressure (mmHg), ICU = intensive care unit, IFT = interval Fourier transformation (power spectrum), MAP = mean arterial pressure (mmHg), MED = median, MOD = modus (mode, modal, value), p = partial gas pressure (mmHg), P/V diagram = pressure-volume diagram (intracranial), PVI = pressure-volume index (ml), SAH = subarachnoid hemorrhage, SAP = systemic arterial pressure (mmHg), TIA = cerebral transitory ischemic attack

* supported by grants from DFG (Ga 273) and BMFT (MMT 19)

recording of different (up to "multimodal", Chiappa and Yiannikas 1983) stimulus-related EEG responses, or evoked potentials (EVP), which allow an in vivo investigation of the conduction paths and a definition of neuronal failure (Chiappa and Yiannikas 1983).

The most significant danger parameter for the brain, on the other hand, is the intracranial pressure (ICP) (Gaab 1981; Marshall et al. 1979;) intracranial hemorrhages, disturbances of the CSF circulation and brain swelling increase the ICP and will finally decrease the cerebral blood flow (CBF). After only a few minutes, however, a critical decrease of the CBF will produce irreversible cerebral damage (Toole 1984); a complete arrest of the CBF is followed by brain death. Therefore the earliest possible recognition and immediate treatment of an ICP disturbance is of the utmost importance (Bramm et al. 1982; Gaab and Haubitz 1983); here the computer can play a decisive role (Gaab 1981; Gaab and Heissler 1984).

In the near future, direct measurement of the cerebral oxygen supply, of its CO_2 tension, of the cerebral pH and of ional cerebral homeostasis will be possible. We are now developping and testing miniaturized sensors for monitoring PO_2, PCO_2, pH, the concentrations of K^+ and Ca^{++} directly on the brain surface (Heller et al. 1984) or within deep brain structures; the O_2 supply of the brain via the internal carotid artery can also be estimated from conjunctival PO_2 monitoring (described later).

A continuous, reliable evaluation of these three groups of signals for complete neuromonitoring requires computerized data processing at the patient's bedside. We have therefore developed a special neuromonitor which is a now commercially available (Dr. Weiss Neuromonitor). The scope of the the monitor is indicated in Table 1.

Recording of Signals

The prerequisites for a computerized EEG, ICP and PO_2 analysis are reliable, artifact-free signals. In the EEG such signal is achieved by special stick-on electrodes and integrated preamplifiers (preamplification to over 100 mV, Gaab et al. 1982). As the recognition of focal EEG changes is not important in the ICU, a 2-channel EEG (F_1-P_3 / F_2-P_4, Gaab et al. 1982) is sufficient; this placement of the electrodes is also suitable for somatosensory evoked potentials (Chiappa and Yiannikas 1983). For the measurement of ICP, we use microtransducers, implanted epi- or subdurally. Initially developed by us, (Dietrich et al. 1977; Gaab 1981), such microtransducers are now commericially available (Gaeltec Ltd., Isle of Skye, Scotland). The epi- or sub-dural implantation is completely without risk except in cases of coagulatory disturbances (Gaab 1981; Gaab and Heissler 1984). We monitored the ICP over days and weeks in more than 900 patients and never encountered meningitis or any other serious infectious complication; this method of ICP monitoring with perfect signal quality (Gaab and Heissler 1984) is therefore less invasive than lumbar puncture or a subclavian catheter. It impedes neither the patient's freedom to move nor the nursing; at present we are working on a new sensor with telemetric pressure transmittance (Bramm et al. 1982).

For continuous registration of tissue PO_2 tension, we use platinum surface electrodes. A multiwire 8-channel electrode (Eschweiler, Kiel) allows a histographical

Table 1. Signals for neuromonitoring and methods of computerized evaluation. Intracranial "risk" parameters (A) and parameters of neuronal function/metabolism (B). The evaluations shown are provided by the Dr. Weiss Neuromonitor, or in preparation as software

A. "Risk" Parameters: ICP, (S)AP and CPP	
Scan rate	Sample AT ≥ 25 HZ
Graphics	Time-plot (with magnification) Histogram Amplitude mean pressure regression Fourier spectrum of Frequency
Statistics	Mean pressure, mode, median curtoisis, skewness Frequency and power of amplitudes Regression slope and R
Autoregulation and Complicance	Frequency transfer SAP and CVP to ICP

B. Neuronal function and metabolism		
EEG	FFT (Fourier/Berg)	PO_2, pH, PCO_2, ions
Scan:	≥ 70 Hz	Scan ≥ 2 min^{-1}
Graphics	IFT-Spectrum Chronospectra	time-plot histogram as for ICP
Statistics	Mean frequency Dominant frequency 95% frequency Total power % power	Mean, mode, median Curtoisis, skewness
EVP	Graphics and statistics Latency (interpeak) Amplitudes Form	

evaluation of the PO_2 distribution on the brain surface; a continuous PO_2 measurement is possible with specially sterilized microelectrodes from Orange (from Fresenius AG., Germany) which we use routinely for PO_2 registration at the conjunctiva. These microsensors have a sufficient stability for about 2–3 days of PO_2 registration on the brain surface after implantation.

The Computerized Neuromonitor

As a prototype we used a HP 9845 computer to monitor one patient at a time (Gaab 1981; Gaab et al. 1982). With this system, we developed programs now in an improved version in the Dr. Weiss Neuromonitor. We then attempted monitoring simultaneously up to six patients in our ICU by means of larger computer (Intertechnique IN 110, Gaab et al. 1982). Its usefullness lies in its qualities as a rapid analyzer of biosignals on a hardware basis. However, the complex system is easily disturbed by artifacts, and the installation of a central computer requires additional technical personnel. In the meantime, the microprocessors have reached such a high level of refinement that, given the low prices of the necessary high storage demand, we succeeded in packing the whole amount of functions into a small bedside neuromonitor (Fig. 1).

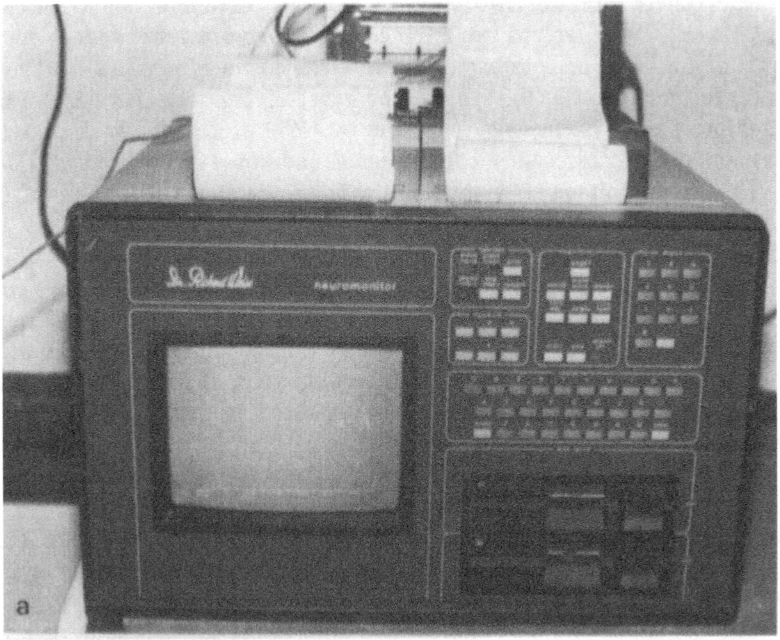

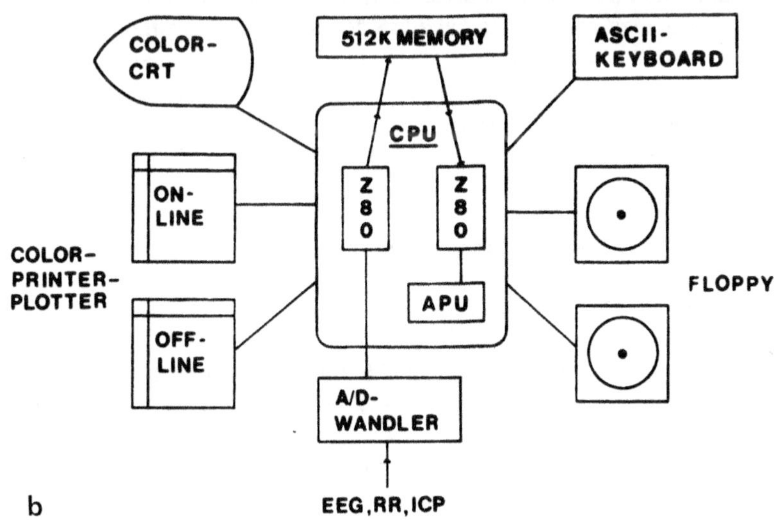

Fig. 1a, b. The Dr. Weiss Neuromonitor. **a** Compact bedside monitor with color display, two disc drives, two integrated color plotters and functional keyboard. **b** The multiprocessor system with 512 kb and devices for data presentation and storage

The system monitors two pressure channels, usually systemic arterial pressure, SAP, and ICP, as well as two EEG channels; one pressure channel can be used for PO_2 monitoring, and an expansion to eight channels is possible. The signals are recorded analogously (4–8 input channels) or digitally (RS 232). The core is a multiprocessor system (Fig. 1b). The two Z80 processors work in a "ping-pong" fashion, one processes the incoming signals and stores them after fast Fourier analysis (FFT), and simultaneously operates the first integrated 4-color plotter and the color display for on-line representation of the signals. The second processor turns to the files and analyzes the off-line values such as histogram statistics, pulse amplitude regression etc., and represents these independently on the second 4-color plotter. This constitutes also an on-line representation; for example a histogram measured over 30 min is put out without a perceptible time lag immediately after the recording, and without interrupting the further accumulation of data. All data are stored on floppy disc and may at any time be newly plotted, used for various computations, or transferred to a central computer.

The Neuromonitor requires no preliminary knowledge, in particular no experience in progamming; like any intensive care monitor it can be operated by physicians or nurses. The programs are stored on the system disc (Fig. 1), which makes a constant complementation and expansion of the programs possible. The monitor recalls all important values by itself, the questions are answered by the keys; wrong operation is practically impossible. First the configuration of the signal input is determined, then the alarm limits are set (intelligent alarms using size and duration of signals!) and the duration of measurement and analysis defined. The Neuromonitor processes not only biosignals but also clinical data input, thus administration and storage of anamnesis, diagnosis etc. are possible. Comments on the mesurement, for example, cause of alarm, therapy may be added at any time. A complete record of a coma scale (expanded Glasgow Scale, Gaab 1984) can also be kept.

Functions, Results, and Perspectives

Presentation of the Original Signal

A display of the original input signal (continuously or at least on demand in case of alarm) is indispensible in computerized monitoring. Only visual control of the signal allows a qualitative check and a safe decision between artifacts and a real danger signal in case of alarm. up to now, almost all algorithms for computerized biosignal processing have neglected the shape of single signal elements, e.g., of epileptic discharges in the EEG (spikes, waves, etc.), or the changes in the pulse wave of the ICP. A computerized monitor should therefore provide visual control and a graphical output of the unprocessed signal.

Trend Analysis of ICP, SAP, CPP and PO_2 (time-plot)

The simplest computer evaluation is constituted by a time-lapse long-term representation of the measured values in the form of a time-plott (Fig. 2). Depicting the trend

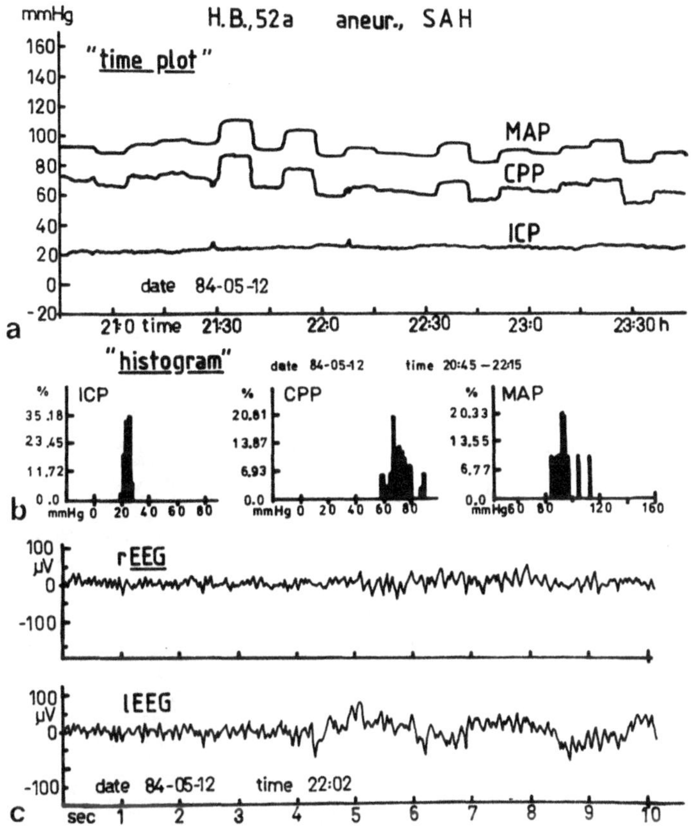

Fig. 2a–c. Computerized ICP, CPP and EEG evaluation: increased ICP after subarachnoid hemorrhage (vasospasm); therapy with Glycerosteril and HAES-steril, no further progression: CPP uncritical in time-plot **(a)** and histogram **(b)**, no ICP waves; stable α-rhythm in the EEG **(c)**. Recovery

(Figs. 3, 4) plotted or stored on floppy disc over 12 or 24 hours, this method replaces the voluminous documentation by analogous recording on paper. This is important in the case of dynamic measuring values which are characterized by wave formation, such as the ICP (Fig 3); here we distinguish between B-waves (frequency: 1 to 2 min^{-1}) which occur prior to ICP failure; the high A-plateau waves (duration: 5 to 20 min), which require immediate therapy; and slower background fluctuations (D-waves, Gaab 1981; Gaab and Heissler 1984). For resolving such waves in long-term depictions the time plot may be enlarged by up to 32 times on- and off-line on both screen and plotter.

It is not the ICP *per se* which is the significant intracranial risk factor but the so-called cerebral perfusion pressure (CPP). The CPP is the difference between SAP and ICP:

$$CPP = SAP - ICP \tag{1}$$

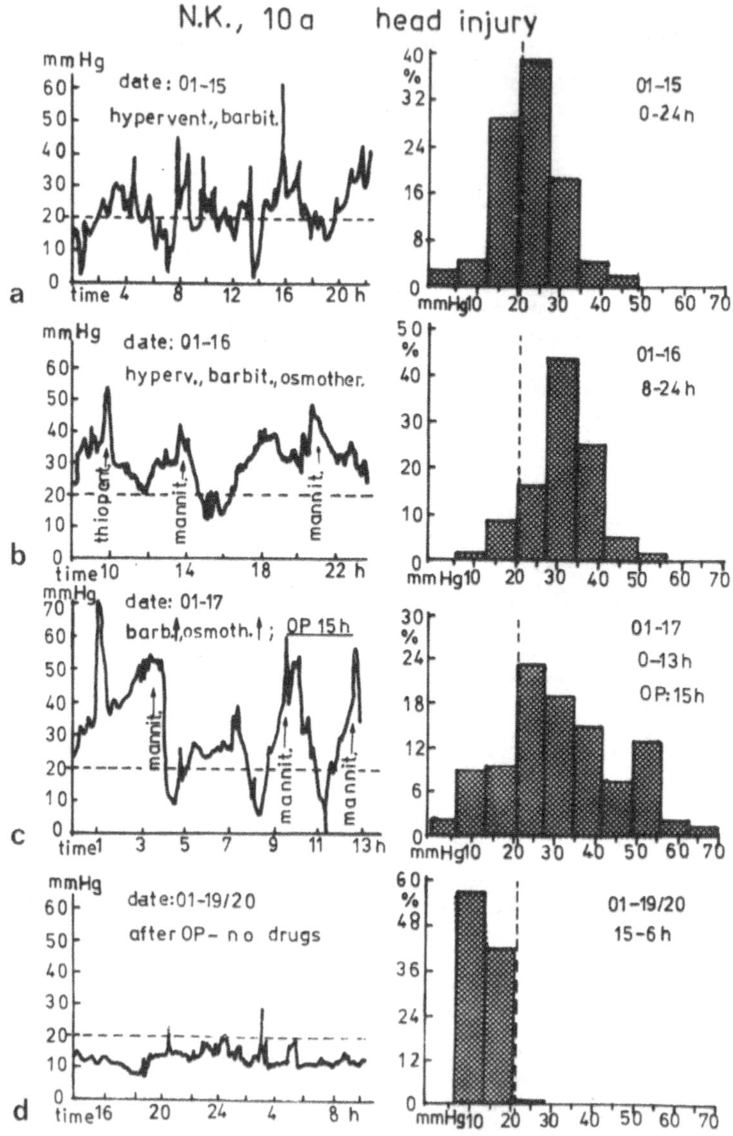

Fig. 3a–d. ICP decompensation, operative therapy: increasing ICP with plateau waves after trauma (time-plot, histogram, **a, b, c**). Normalization after decompression trepanation **(d)**. Outcome: moderately disabled

If the CPP drops and remains below 50 mmHg (30 mmHg in children) longer than a few minutes (Gaab 1981; Gaab and Heissler 1984; Marshall et al. 1979) irreversible cerebral lesions and finally brain death occur. If SAP and ICP are measured, the computer derives the CPP, and ICP, SAP, and CPP are plotted on the same time plot (Figs. 2, 4). The CPP has become our main parameter for therapeutic control of the ICP (Fig. 4) and may be used as an alarm parameter by the computer; even a closed-loop therapy for the ICP with a computer-controlled infusion pump is in preparation.

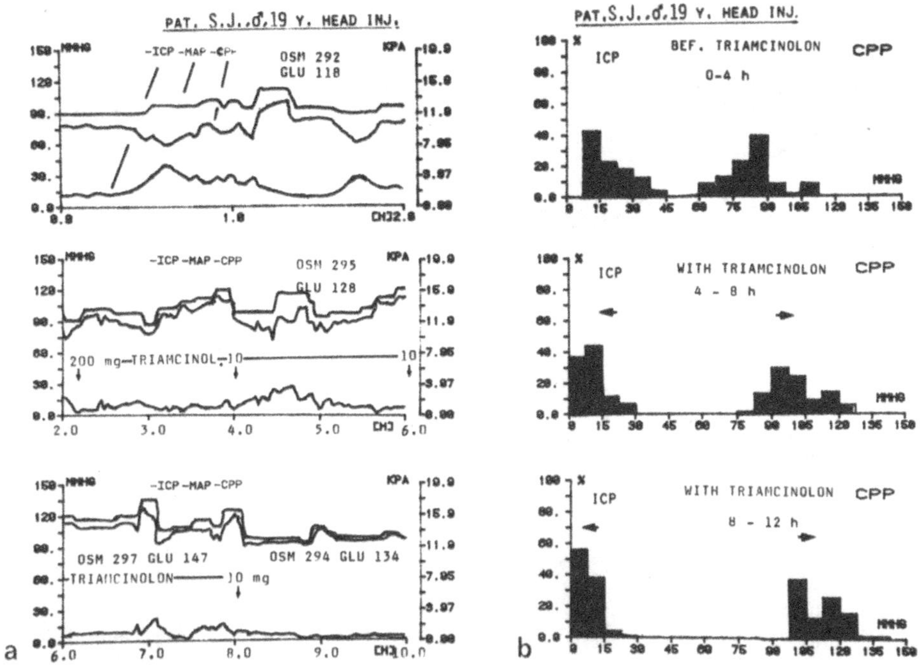

Fig. 4a, b. Effective ICP treatment. **a** The ICP normalizes during therapy with triamcinolon-acetonid; overproportional CPP increas clearly recognized in the histogram **b**

For parameters that are characterized by their amplitudes and fluctuations whose frequency is not above 1 to 2 min^{-1}, a time-plot depiction is suitable; some of these parameters are ICP, SAP, and CPP, as well as PO_2 measured by single sensors. In the intensive care unit and in intraoperative monitoring, e.g. operation for stenosis of the carotid, measuring the PO_2 in the upper conjunctiva has proved to be efficient (Fig. 5); this area is almost exclusively supplied by the a. carotis interna and therefore reflects the supply of oxygen to the brain via this artery. Measurement is possible over a maximum of three days without irritation of the conjunctiva. With the same, quite stable, sensor we can, after special sterilization, also measure the cortical O_2 tension after implantation (simultaneous with the ICP transducer). The time-plot allows, however, no quantification of the data; also it is useless in the case of data like that from EEG, which are characterized by higher frequency; here a mathematical frequency analysis is necessary.

Statistical Analysis of Amplitude Signals: The Histogram

The "amplitude signals" ICP, SAP, CPP and PO_2 can be quantified with the statistical methods used for independent variable special values (Hufenbeck 1983; Weber 1980). The histogram (amplitude-frequency histogram, frequency polygon, Figs. 2–4 Table 2) is a descriptive, graphical and mathematical, comparable depiction.

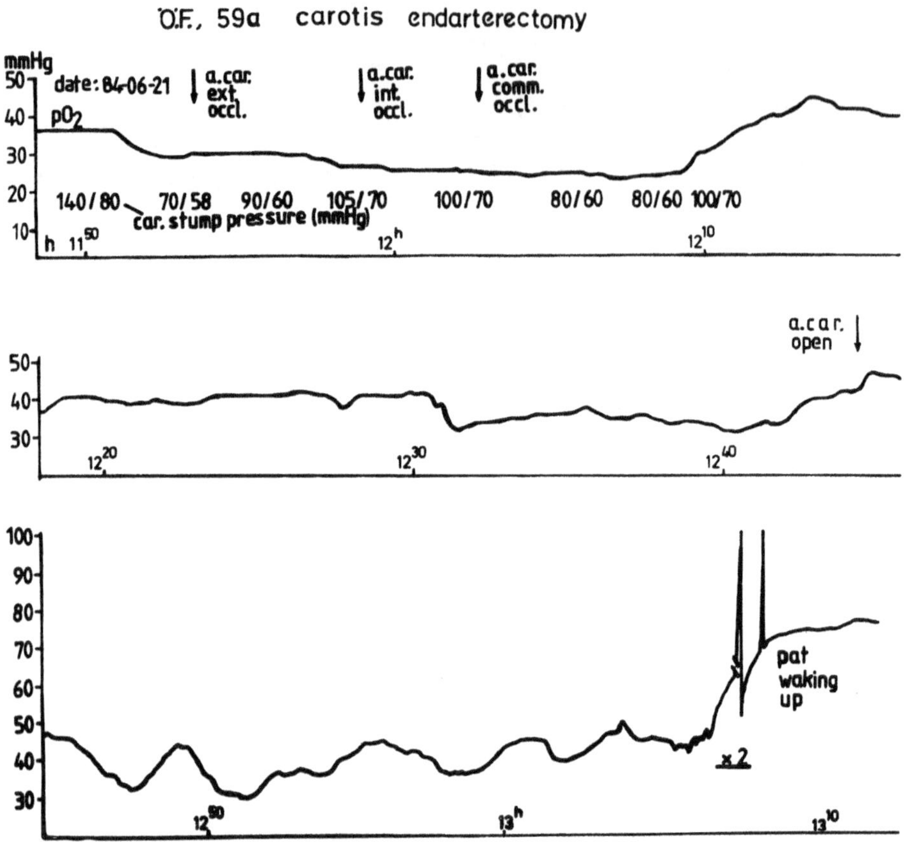

Fig. 5. Continuous conjunctival PO_2 record: ipsilateral PO_2 remains stable after carotid clamp for thrombendarterectomy; sufficient carotid stump pressure. No shunt required: occlusion occluded

The chronological input of data (scan rate of the neuromonitor: 1 kHz!) is distributed according to frequency (amplitude = input voltage) into classes; for graphical depiction the range of a class can be freely chosen and changed before or after the measurement. Additionally, smoothing functions are possible.

The graph alone makes a quick estimation possible: both ICP and SAP and CPP have not only maximal normal rates which can be cross-faded (Fig. 3), but also a standard distribution with about 95% of the measured data below the normal rate limit. Pathological distribution is not only documented by a clear *shift* to the right of the ICP and to the left of the CPP (Fig. 3, 4), but even more so by a deviation from the normal distribution: due to pressure waves the histogram is skewed to the right and finally double-peaked (Fig. 3) until in the end a collapse of the intracranial circulation leads to a very narrow normal distribution pattern of the ICP in the range of the SAP and thus a CPP of less than 20 mmHg (Gaab 1981, Hutenbeck 1983).

The sequential histogram not not only makes visual trend comparisons possible and documents thearapeutical effectiveness (Fig. 4), it can also be characterized quantita-

Table 2. Numerical statistics of a frequency polygon (histogram). Values belong to the histograms of Fig. 2b; ICP elevated, but CPP stable; arithmetic mean ARM, median and mode identical = no pressure waves, no further decompensation under therapy with Glycerosteril and HAES-steril; recovery

12-05-84	H.B.	52 A ANEUR., SAH	20^{45}–22^{15}
	ICP	SAP	CPP
ARM	24	95	72
MED	24	94	71
MOD	24	94	67
VABR	31	26	46
STABW	2.185	7.212	7.126

tively by the arithmetic mean ARM, median, modus, skewness, and curtoisis (Table 2). With the so-called normal pressure hydrocephalus (NPH), for example, this allows the determination of the activity, and thus indication for surgery, by the skewness to the right and characteristic dissociation between ARM, median, and modus (Gaab and Heissler 1984; Hufenbeck 1983).

When a multichannel PO_2 electrode is used, a histographic evaluation with only one input channel is possible, as the signal changes only slowly, thus allowing sequential input to the channels via a multiplexer. The changes which can consequently be computed, e.g., after successful neurosurgical bypass operations, are impressive (Fig. 6).

Frequency Analysis by FFT

Not only can the EEG be analyzed after a *Fourier transformation* (FFT) but also the pulse and respiration changes of the ICP. The given frequency mixture is resolved into basic frequencies, the result providing – with continuous analysis – the frequency trends and the intensity (power) in the frequency tape.

The usual way of representing the 3-dimensional result graphically is the peak spectrum (IFT spectrums, Fig. 7), in which chronologically defined power spectrums are recorded chronologically on the abscissa of the frequency scale, the ordinate representing at the same time intensity and time.

Our neuromonitor can depict on-line continuously spectrums with hidden line suppression, with time being freely selectable; an identical time scale of ICP/SAP/CPP and PO_2 time-plots and EEG spectrums makes a clear comparison of the interactions possible. For example, we did not find marked changes of the EEG until the CPP sank to below 60 mmHg; below 50 mmHg the EEG may collapse rapidily (Fig. 7); equally epileptic discharges of the EEG may provoke typical B-waves, a Grand Mal even plateau waves in the ICP (Gaab and Haubitz 1983; Knoblich et al. 1980).

For comparative representation a chronospectral (Gaab et al. 1982) EEG depiction by the neuromonitor has shown good results (Fig. 7): here the total power, the intensities in the individual EEG frequency tapes, and mean and predominant frequencies, are plotted above each other on the time axis. Usually we plot IFT spectra in on-line monitoring and print the chronospectral depiction off-line. The data of the chronospectrum may also be plotted in tables of quantities, which makes trend

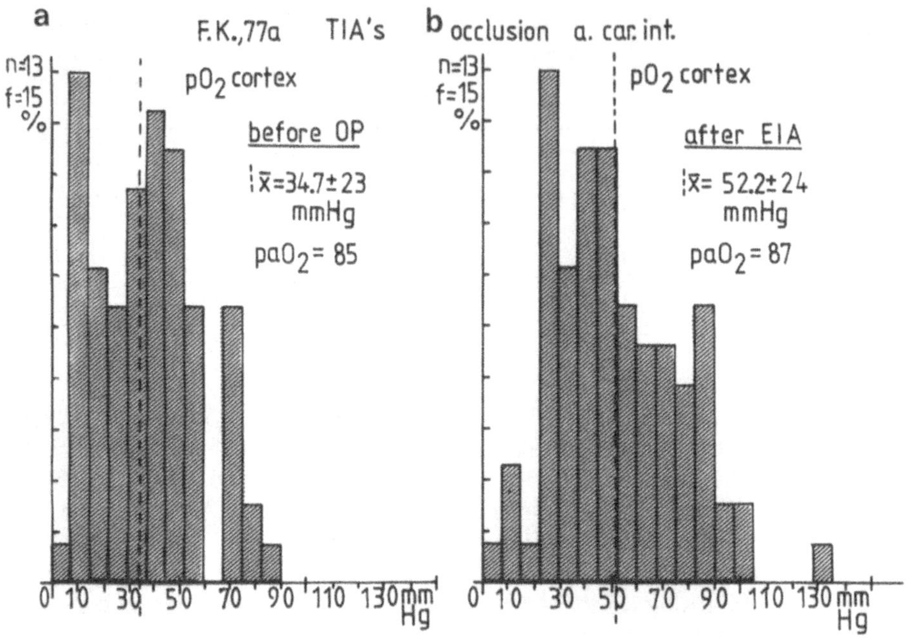

Fig. 6a, b. Cerebral PO_2 histogram before **a** and after **b** extra-intracranial anastomosis (EIA). Clear improvement. No recurrence of preoperativeley frequent TIASs. PaO_2 = peripheral arterierial PO_2

comparisons (e.g., summarizing EEG every 24 h) as well as statistical tests, e.g., with therapeutic checks possible (Gaab et al. 1984; Prior 1979). Another important aspect of the evaluation is the recognition of artifacts, which distinguishes between epileptic discharges and artifacts, provides the type of the artifact as alarm on the screen and controls the electrode impedance.

In ICP pulsation analysis the Fourier analysis makes the intensity of pulse and respiration fluctuations clearly visible (Fig. 8); this allows an earlier recognition of disturbances of the intracranial complicance and vasoregulation than the mean pressure (Brawanski et al. 1984; Gaab et al. 1983) in the case of intracranial space occupation the pulse amplitude increases rapidly, the mean pressure changing hardly at all initially, and the respiration amplitude decreases (Fig. 8); with cerebral vasospasm after subarachnoid hemorrhage, in contrast, the mean pressure rises, the pulse amplitude being small (Brawanski et al. 1984; Gaab 1981). The neuromonitor can plot the frequency analysis of the intracranial pulsation on-line and off-line in graphs or tables, the time-scale being optional.

Pulse Amplitudes-Mean Pressure Analysis of ICP, Pressure-Volume Diagram and CSF Dynamics

The above-mentioned changes of the ICP pulse amplitude as an early warning parameter can often be recognized better if the height of the pulse amplitude is plotted

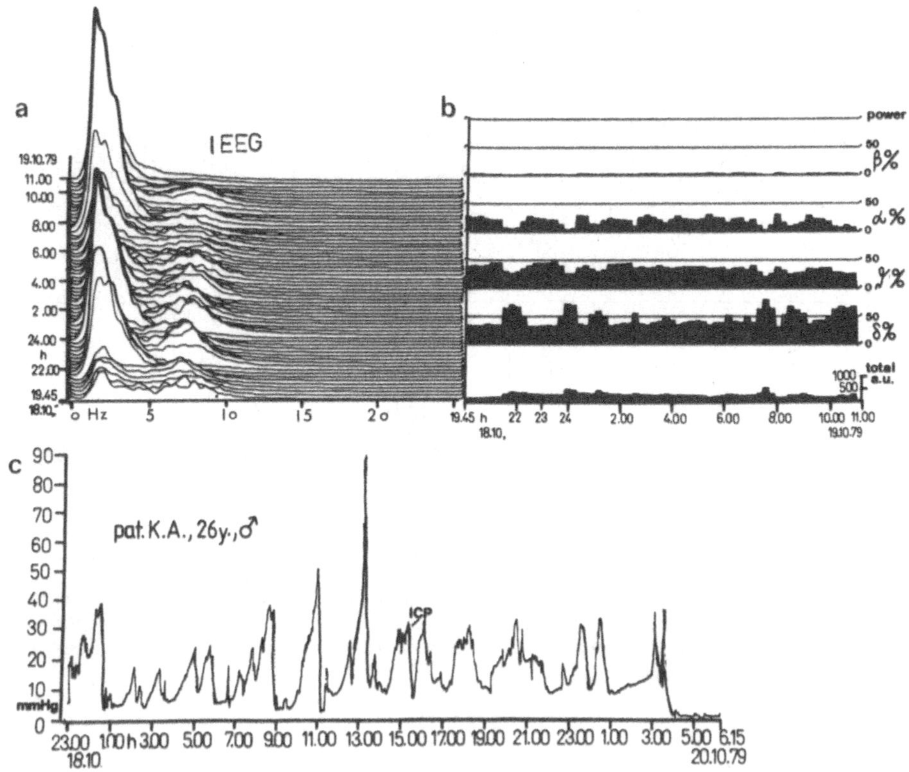

Fig. 7a–c. Simultaneous ICP and EEG analysis. The EEG depression due to ICP-waves **(c)** is better recognized in a chronospectral plot of the EEG power intensities **(b)** due to the hidden line suppression in a conventional IFT spectrum **(a)**. Herpes-encephalitis

above the mean ICP, the neuromonitor computing the linear regression (Fig. 8a). Vasoparalysis and space occupation lead to a steeper regression line. In the individual trend the steepness of these straight lines is a semiquantitative measure of the intracranial reserve space (Gaab 1981; Gaab et al. 1983).

The intracranial reserve space can be quantitatively determined by constructing the pressure-volume diagram (*P/V* diagram) and computing the PVI after the bolus test. For this purpose the initial pressure, volume of the bolus injection, and the resulting peak pressure (P_p) are fed into the computer via the keyboards. Simultaneously the pulse amplitude mean pressure diagram is provided; after the constant speed infusion of mock CSF resistance and conductance of the CSF are also computed and compared with normal value (Gaab 1981; Gaab et al. 1983). This method is particularly important in diagnosing the pressure activity, e.g., of hydrocephalus (Gaab 1981; Symon and Hinzpeter 1977); thus, besides the intensive care monitoring neurological diagnostics is another area for which the neuromonitor is indicated.

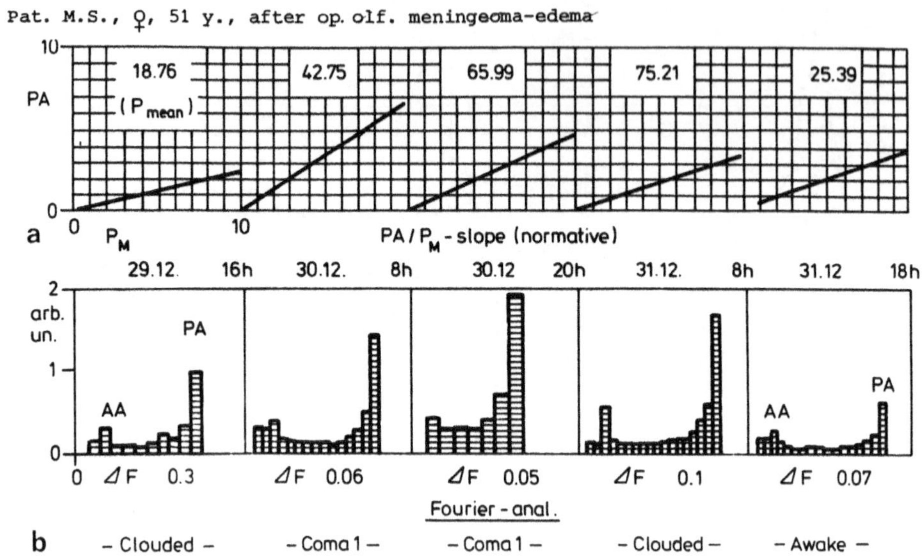

Fig. 8a, b. ICP analysis by pulse amplitude (PA) mean pressure regression **(a)** and Fourier transformation **(b)**. The increase of PA with steeper PA/mean ICP (PM) regression **(a)** and increasing PA/decreasing breath amplitude AA **(b)** clearly correlate with the clinical status (WFNS coma scale, Gaab 1984), Pm unchanged. Brain edema

Further Developments: Frequency Analysis with Transfer Function; EEG Back Transformation; Evoked Potentials; EMG

By merely observing the ICP pulsation no differentiation between an increase in intracranial volume and disturbances of the vasoregulation is possible; it is influenced by blood pressure changes (Hoffmann and Zierski 1982). If, however, the arterial blood pressure (SAP) and the central venous blood pressure (CVP) are taken into account as input data, parameters of the intracranial volume such as reserve space and vasoregulation can be determined according to the black-box-model. We are, therefore, at present working on complementary software with which a distinction is made between autoregulation and volume disturbances by means of the transfer function between SAP/CVP and ICP (transfer factor x_t, frequency and amplitude of the input signal being different), and even a quantitative marking line of the autoregulation results (Portnoy et al. 1982). Disturbed cerebral autoregulation is a sign of almost all brain swellings (Baethmann 1978), it occurs often prior to brain edema. Until now examination of the autoregulation has required measurement of the cerebral blood circulation and continuous examination was impossible; continuous analysis would provide pathophysiological insights and the development of novel methods of treatment. The treatment of brain swelling with hyperventilation, barbiturates and buffering probably improves autoregulatory disturbances (Gaab 1981; Gaab and Bushe 1981).

From the analysis of EEG signals further analytical methods are to be expected which will go beyond the Fourier method and which can be as easily integrated as complementary software into the neuromonitor as the FFT back-transformation, which allows reconstruction and plotting of the original EEG curves from the computed and stored spectra.

The analysis of evoked potentials (EVP) makes relatively modest demands on the computing capacity of the neuromonitor; averaging and correcting functions are simple to fulfill in view of the high scan rate; more important is the complementation of the hardware with adapted stimulation gadgets.

A further field of application of the neuromonitor is in quantitative EMG-analysis, for which first methods (Kopec and Hausmanova-Petrusewicz 1983) are provided, for which scan rate and storage capacity are adequate. As a result reliable sleep stage analysis can be achieved, which is very important in the prognosis of severe brain lesions and complements the EEG analysis (Alexandre et al. 1983; Gaab et al. 1982).

Clinical Use of Computerized Neuromonitoring

Without requiring additional personnel the bedside neuromonitor equipped with the functions described above makes first of all an improved signal input possible: the monitor recognizes disturbances of the signal transmittance; this is especially important for the EEG. It reduces the risk for the patient, both when the monitoring is interrupted by failure, and by the intelligent time- and datacontrolled alarm when a certain value reaches a critical level.

The time-plot, especially in combination with the histogram (Figs. 2, 3, 4), makes a clearly surveyable observation of trends possible, saving registration paper etc. while no loss of data occurs, as these are stored on floppy disks; later enlargements also allow the recognition of minute changes such as B-waves. This quantitative depiction makes early recognition of complications and therapy possible before brain damage becomes irreversible; the success of therapy is also checked (Fig. 3). This quantitative documentation also leads to new pathophysiological and therapeutic insights; thus we have been able to define clear age-dependent ICP limits (Fig. 9) from the statistics of ICP trends with traumatic head injury and clinical outcome, limits which indicate when consequent treatment of ICP increases is necessary (Gaab 1981; Gaab and Bushe 1981; Gaab and Haubitz 1983).

Longterm EEG-control must at any rate be computer-aided, which is of advantage for prognosis, therapy, and anesthetic control (Gaab and Haubitz 1983; Prior 1979). Of particular value in this connection is the clear comparison between EEG and ICP.

Analysis of the ICP pulsations allows an even earlier recognition of complications than the ICP mean pressure analysis (Brawanski et al. 1984; Gaab 1981); from a frequency transfer analysis between the input values of SAP/CVP and the resulting ICP, even a continuous quantitative analysis of the intracranial reserve space and the cerebral autoregulation can be expected, which opens up new dimensions of pathophysiological examination and therapy.

The possibilities of localizing lesions and establishing a prognosis via evoked potentials are well known (Alexandre et al. 1983; Chiappa and Yiannikas 1983); it is only by integration of the EVP measurement into a relatively inexpensive bedside

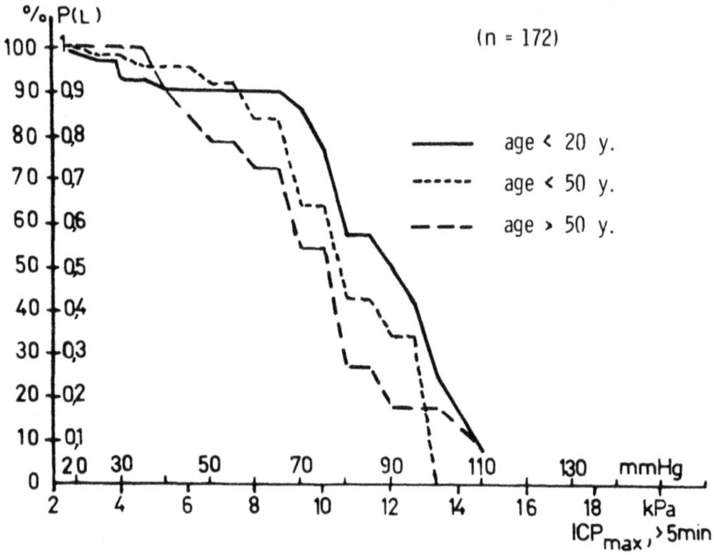

Fig. 9. ICP and prognosis after head injury. Age-dependent decrease of survival probability ((P(L)) with increasing ICP of only ≥ 5 min duration. ICP of > 30 mmHg must therefore be treated immediately

monitor, however, that routine clinical examination has become possible. Recognition of epileptic potentials and examination of the brain stem activity via analysis of the sleep stages improve the recognition of complications and also the prognostics (Alexandre et al. 1983) in the patient undergoing artificial respiration.

Finally, the latest development in intensive cerebral monitoring with PO_2, PCO_2, pH, lactate and selective ion sensors is only clinically usable when aided by a computer, as for examples the cerebral O_2 supply in not characterized by individual measured data but only by PO_2 distribution patterns in the histogram (Fig. 6, Heller et al. 1984).

Summary

In contrast to the control of vital functions, where computers are increasingly used in the intensive care unit, the control of cerebral functions is still based on inadequate clinical observation. We have therefore introduced a neuromonitor (Dr. Weiss Neuromonitor) based on microprocessors, which monitors continuously the intracranial pressure (ICP), systemic arterial pressure (SAP), and the cerebral perfusion pressure (CPP) computed therefrom, as well as the EEG, cerebral oxygen tension and clinical data (coma scale etc.). The computer-aided evaluation requires first of all a reliable signal, which is achieved by preamplification of the electrode in the EEG, polarographical microsensors in PO_2. The neuromonitor controls automatically the signal quality and reports artifacts.

The signal analysis varies according to the type of data: slowly variable data, such as pressure, are characterized by their amplitudes, and are computed as long-term depictions (time-plot) with optional enlargements, on- and off-line, as well as statistically with histographic analysis. The data are graphically depicted on the screen and/or 4-color plotter on- and off-line, stored on floppy discs, and can also be printed out in tables.

Data such as the EEG and ICP pulsation, characterized by frequencies, are evaluated online after Fourier analysis (FFT) parallel to the plotting; further representations at a later time are possible, either graphically as power spectra or chronospectra with intensity and frequency dat?, or in the form of tables. The ICP pulsation can also be analyzed via amplitude mean pressure regression. Fourier back-transformation of EEG/ICP, analysis of sleep stages and EMG, evoked potentials, as well as frequency trend analysis between SAP/CVP and ICP (making continuous quantitative control of the cerebral autoregulation and intracranial reserve volume possible) are in preparation. The methods of computerized neuromonitoring guarantee, without additional personnel, uninterrupted monitoring, early recognition of complications, therapeutic control and prognosis in cerebral risk patients; from the quantiative data new pathophysiological insights and therapeutical developments are gained.

References

Alexandre A, Colombo F, Nertempi P, Benedetti A (1983) Cognitive outcome and early indices of severity of head injury. Neurosurg 59: 751–716

Baethmann A (1978) Pathophysiological and pathochemical aspects of cerebral edema. Neurosurg Rev 1: 85–100

Bramm G, Koschke P, Novak O, Gaab MR (1982) Cavity resonator sensing system for monitoring and longterm registration of intracranial pressure. In: Bleifeld W, Harder D, Leetz HK, Schaldach M (ed) Proceedings of the world congress on medical phyiscs and biomedical engineering. MPBE, Hamburg, pp 7–27

Brawanski A, Gaab MR, Heissler HE (1984) Computer-analysis of ICP modulations: clinical significance and prediction of ICP dynamics. In: Ishii S, Nagai H, Brock M (ed) Intracranial pressure 5. Springer, Berlin Heidelberg New York Tokyo, pp 186–190

Brierley JB, Meldrum BS (1971) Brain hypoxia. Heinemann, London

Chiappa KH, Yiannikas C (1983) Evoked potentials in clinical medicine. Raven, New York

Dietrich K, Gaab MR, Knoblich OE, Schupp J, Ott B (1977) A new miniaturized system for monitoring the epidural pressure in children and adults. Neuropädiatrie 8: 21–28

Gaab MR (1981) Die Registrierung des intrakraniellen Druckes. Grundlagen, Techniken, Ergebnisse und Möglichkeiten. Thesis (Habil-Schr.), Julius-Maximilian University, Würzburg

Gaab MR (1985) Schädel-Hirn-Trauma: Wertigkeit von Überwachungskriterien. In: Hossli G (ed) Anaesthesiologie und Intensivmedizin. vol 175. Springer, Berlin Heidelberg New York (in press)

Gaab MR, Bushe KA (1981) The therapy of intracranial hypertension. Intensivbehandlung 6: 34–52

Gaab MR, Haubitz I (1983) Intracranial pressure, primary/secondary brain stem injury and prognosis in cerebral trauma. In: Ishii S, Nagai H, Brock M (ed) Intracranial pressure 5. Springer, Berlin Heidelberg New York Tokyo, pp 501–507

Gaab MR, Heissler HE (1984) ICP Monitoring. In: CRC critical reviews in biomedical engineering. CRC Press, Boca Raton (in press)

Gaab MR, Baumgarten F, Marquart I, Heissler HE, Hassel W, Brawanski A (1982) Intracranial pressure and EEG. Simultaneous long-time registration and analysis. In: Stefan H, Burr W (ed) Mobile long-term EEG monitoring. Fischer, Stuttgart, pp 179–192

Gaab MR, Haubitz I, Brawanski A, Faulstich J, Heissler HE (1983) Pressure-volume diagram, pulse amplitude and intracranial pulse volume. Analysis and significance. In: Ishii S, Nagai H, Brock M (ed) Intracranial pressure 5. Springer, Berlin Heidelberg New York Tokyi, pp 501–507
Gaab MR, Heissler HE, Haubitz I, Korn A, Czech T (1984) Steroide bei Schädel-Hirn-Trauma: Kontroversen und neue Ergebnisse. In: Grumme T (ed) Das Hirnödem. De Gruyter, Berlin, pp 115–128
Heller V, Poch B, Gaab MR, Sold M (1984) CBF, O_2-tension and O_2-metabolism in vasogenic brain edema and the effects of dexamethasone and nimodipine. In: Piotrowski W, Brock M, Klinger M (ed) Advances in neurosurgery, vol 12. Springer, Berlin Heidelberg New York Tokyo, pp 274–280
Hoffmann O, Zierski JT (1982) Analysis of the ICP pulse-pressure relationship as a function of arterial blood pressure. Acta Neurochir 66: 1–21
Hufenbeck B (1983) Quantitative Auswertung des intrakraniellen Druckverlaufs mit Rechnerhilfe. Methode und klinischer Wert. Thesis, Julius-Maximilian University, Würzburg
Knoblich OE, Gaab MR, Weber W, Dietrich K, Meyendorf R (1980) Intracranial pressure and electrical activity of the brain in various forms of experimental and clinical seizures. Neurosurg Rev 3: 243–249
Kopec J, Hausmanova-Petrusewicz I (1983) Computeranalyse des EMG und klinische Ergebnisse. Z EEG-EMG 14: 28–35
Marshall LF, Smith RW, Shapiro HM (1979) The outcome with aggressive treatment in severe head injuries. Part 1: The significance of intracranial pressure monitoring. J. Neurosurg 5: 20–25
Portnoy HD, Chopp M, Branch C, Shannon MB (1982) Cerebrospinal fluid pulse waveform as an indicator of cerebral autoregulation. J Neurosurg 56: 666–678
Prior P (1979) Monitoring cerebral function. Long-term recordings of cerebral electrical activity. Elsevier, Amsterdam
Symon L, Hinzpeter T (1977) The enigma of normal pressure hydrocephalus: Tests to select patients for surgery and to predict shunt function. Clin Neurosurg 24: 285–315
Toole JF (1984) Cerebrovascular disorders, 3rd edn Raven, New York
Weber E (1980) Grundrisse der biologischen Statistik, 8th edn Fischer, Jena
Wiener F, Weil MH, Carlson RW (1982) Computer systems for facilitating management of the critically ill. Comput Biol Med 12: 1–15

Computer-Assisted Monitoring of Intracranial Pressure in Stroke

A. Haass, T. Madler, and K. Schimrigk

In the past, double-blind studies were conducted to monitor the clinical course of cerebral stroke during drug therapy. It was remarkable to what extent these patients worsened during the first few days despite standard therapeutic procedures. This deterioration involved the entire neurological spectrum, including the level of consciousness, orientation, agnosia, degree of paralysis, and mixed brain stem symptoms. The development of cerebral edema is a significant, complicating factor in the precipitation of these neurological symptoms. A stroke is primarily accompanied by cytotoxic edema, which may then be followed by vasogenic edema. Cerebral edema causes an increase in intracranial pressure (ICP) and thus a decrease in the cerebral perfusion pressure (CCP) with a subsequent reduction in cerebral circulation. The tissue surrounding the site of infarction is damaged even further, which in turn leads to a worsening of the clinical symptoms.

In this regard, the major problem has been the fact that the clinical parameters for evaluating the course of cerebral edema and intracranial pressure are too imprecise to be useful. Such symptoms are headache, vomiting, psychomotor disturbances, a clouding of consciousness, coma, synergic stretching, and mydriasis. (Gobiet 1978). A therapeutic regimen as prophylaxis against the exponential rise in cerebral pressure after reaching the break point in the pressure-volume diagram cannot be sufficiently regulated by these criteria (Gaab and Bushe 1981).

The second major difficulty is that no uniform opinion exists what constitutes on adequate treatment of cerebral edema in stroke.

One possibility which could solve both problems is the continuous monitoring of intracranial pressure. Epidural pressure measurements are advantageous because the patient is not overburdened or exposed to a significant risk. We utilized a Gaeltec transducer which can be implanted in the epidural space under general or local anesthesia. The transducer is extremely reliable, its function can be tested externally, and the obtained values correspond to intraventricular pressures (Gaab et al. 1979). The transducer may remain implanted for days or weeks without danger of infection under careful maintenance. These pressure measurements will not hinder the routine care and treatment of the patient.

In addition, Dr. Weiss' neuromonitor, a computer-assisted device, was employed to project three pressure curves: the ICP, the SAP (systemic arterial pressure), and the difference between these two, which is known as the CPP (cerebral perfusion pressure). These pressures can be monitored for a short interval to assess individual pressure amplitudes or as trend curves over hours or days. This apparatus contains a computer-supported calculator which can evaluate pressure values according to specific programs. The frequency distribution of mean pressure values for ICP, SAP, and CPP can be calculated and projected with associated statistical data for different time intervals. The frequency distribution of the pulse amplitudes of all three pressures can also be obtained in histogram form. The ICP pulse pressure relationship was also analyzed as a function of the arterial blood pressure and represented as a curve (Hoffmann and Zierski 1982).

Continuous computer-assisted monitoring and evaluation of epidural and arterial pressure measurements allows rapid assessment of cerebral edema development and the effectiveness of therapeutic measures.

In some cases, the epidural pressure was monitored on the stroke side as well as on the nonaffected hemisphere of the brain in order to obtain a comparison. The indication for epidural pressure monitoring was the development of severe edema after recent stroke as evidenced by clinical and CCT findings. The patients were predominantly middle-aged and had suffered an acute, extensive media stroke. The monitoring was conducted 9–20 h after stroke. At this time, the stroke could not yet be detected in the CCT or only a slight hypodensity could be identified. The onset of edema could only be seen by a slight expansive tendency, particularly in the anterior horn. In this phase, a pressure difference was always found between both hemispheres. Nine to ten hours after stroke the pressure of the affected side was between 8 and 15 mmHg, whereas the nonaffected side had values between 0 and 10 mmHg. The higher pressure characteristically showed a greater amplitude. Despite various therapeutic regimens, the pressures of both sides often increased within the first 2–4 days. As the pressure rose to 30–40 mmHg, the values of the stroke side and the other hemisphere gravitated towards each other until both sides were equal. A dramatic intracranial pressure increase was frequently seen on the 2nd to 4th day. It began with peaks and plateau waves and could have led to vasoparalysis, with the cerebral pressure passively adopted the arterial pressure in the brain. These cerebral pressure crises were extremely difficulty or even impossible to treat. Thus, the emphasis of any therapy should be on early prophylaxis.

The positive effect of the following therapeutic procedures could be evaluated by the above-mentioned computer-assisted monitoring of intracranial pressure. The remarkable intracranial pressure reducing effect of mechanical measures was demonstrated. They decreased the pressure by reducing the cerebral blood volume. Posi-

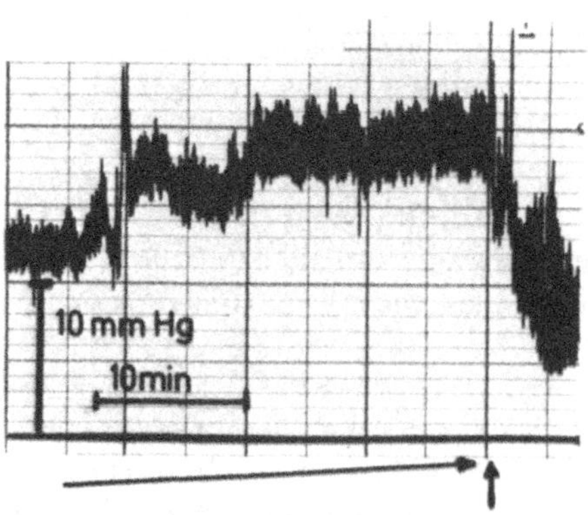

Fig. 1. Conventional registration of the increasing intracranial pressure as a result of turning the head (→) and decreasing pressure in the straight forward position (↑)

tioning of the patient such as elevating the torso by 30–45° and keeping the head in a "straight forward" position led to a hydrostatic effect and improved venous return, resulting in a marked decrease in intracranial pressure (Hulme and Cooper 1976). Fig. 1 shows an increase in the intracranial pressure if the patient was in a supine position and a decrease if the patient was reelevated. In this case, the mean value increased from 30 to 40 mmHg and returned to the baseline value after reelevation. If the ICP curves showed homogeneous mean values using the conventional measurement, the assessment of therapeutic measures was not difficult. However, computer-assisted evaluation was very helpful when waves of increasing pressures predominated. An example of this is given in Fig. 2, which demonstrates the effect of a "head-up" position. The pressure increased to 17 mmHg and the pulse amplitude to 5 mmHg when the head was turned. Both decreased to 13 and 3 mmHg respectively when the head was placed straight forward. The statistical values are provided in the lower half of the figure. The histograms showed this positive effect in the frequency distribution of the mean pressures and of the pulse amplitudes calculated over a period of 30 min.

Hyperosmolar solutions such as mannitol and sorbitol were very useful for decreasing ICP. However, this reduction was short-lived, possibly being canceled out by a rebound effect. Therefore, frequent low dosages are recommended, although a continuous reduction of ICP was difficult to attain over a period of several days. Glycerol alone could sufficiently reduce intracranial pressure if the dosage was high enough and if osmolality was controlled to avoid hemolysis. In combination with mannitol or sorbitol, glycerol prolonged the pressure-reducing effect over hours. This effect was terminated at the end of the infusion due to its rapid metabolism. The pressure-reducing effect after infusion was related to the degree of cerebral swelling and the initial cerebral pressure values. These data must be considered if an adequate assessment is to be made. Since computer-assisted analysis allows a more objective

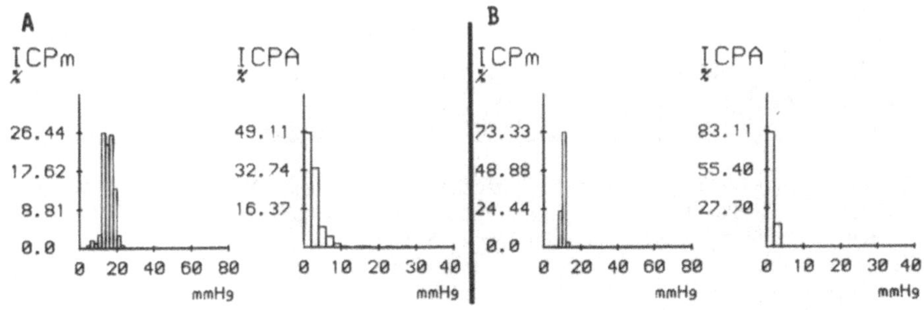

Statistics		ICPm	ICPA
Mean	:	17	5
Median	:	17	4
Mode	:	16	4
Range	:	18	27
Stand. dev.	:	2.009	2.022

Statistics		ICPm	ICPA
Mean	:	13	3
Median	:	13	3
Mode	:	13	3
Range	:	4	4
Stand. dev.	:	0000.237	0000.095

Fig. 2a, b. Computer-assisted evaluation of **A** increased intracranial pressure as a result of turning the head and **B** the decreased pressure in the straight forward position. The frequency distribution of the mean intracerebral pressure *(ICP_m)* and its amplitudes *(ICPA)* is plotted in the upper part of the figure. The corresponding statistical values are given below

and detailed evaluation of these parameters, this method offers a more precise estimation of the true situation.

Although corticosteroids successfully reduce the edema of cerebral tumors, their edema-reducing effect in stroke is still a matter of controversy (Hartmann 1983). Preliminary results indicate a positive effect in the treatment of cerebral hematoma.

Conclusion

The extent of cerebral edema development in severe stroke is crucial for the prognosis. Only continuous monitoring of intracranial pressure allows adequate care and treatment of these high-risk patients. Epidural pressure measurements are easier on the patient and relatively risk-free. Computer-assisted analysis of ICP, SAP, and CPP and their amplitudes allows a rapid and precise evaluation of the patient's progress and the effect of therapeutic measures. This study found support for the importance of elevating the torso, straight forward positioning of the head, and early ventilation in reducing intracranial pressure. Osmotic substances such as mannitol and sorbitol significantly lower the pressure but are inadequate for the long-term pressure reduction necessary in the case of stroke. Glycerol offers an alternative, particularly when given in high dosages while controlling osmolality. The effect of cortisone remains controversial even though a positive trend was observed. It is expected that this method for evaluating intracranial pressure will lead to generally acceptable therapeutic regimens.

References

Gaab MR, Bushe KA (1981) Die Behandlung der intrakraniellen Drucksteigerung. Intensivbehandlung 1: 34–52

Gaab M, Knoblich OE, Dietrich K (1979) Miniaturisierte Methoden zur Überwachung des intrakraniellen Druckes. Langenbecks Arch Chir 350: 13–31

Gobiet W (1978) Diagnostik and Therapie der akuten Hirnschwellung. Intensivbehandlung 4: 121–129

Hartmann A (1983) Die medikamentöse Behandlung des Hirnödems. Nervenarzt 54: 277–293

Hoffmann O, Zierski JT (1982) Analysis of the ICP pulse-pressure relationship as a function of arterial blood pressure. Acta Neurochir (Wein) 66: 1–21

Hulme A, Cooper R (1976) The effects of head position and jugular vein compression (JVC) on intracranial pressure (ICP). A clinical study. In: Beks JwF, Bosch DA, Brock M (eds) Intracranial pressure III. Springer, Berlin, pp 259–263

Microprocessor-Controlled Registration and Evaluation of Respiratory Pressure-Volume Diagrams in ICUs

W. KELLERMANN, Y. SUMMA, and K. PETER

Introduction

The work of breathing required for adequate gas exchange depends much on the elastic and flow-resistive properties of the lung and thorax. According to Peters and co-workers (Peters et al. 1969, 1972), respiratory work is an important determinant in evaluating the patient's ability to breathe spontaneously i. e., in deciding whether the patient must be artificially ventilated or whether he can be weaned from the respirator.

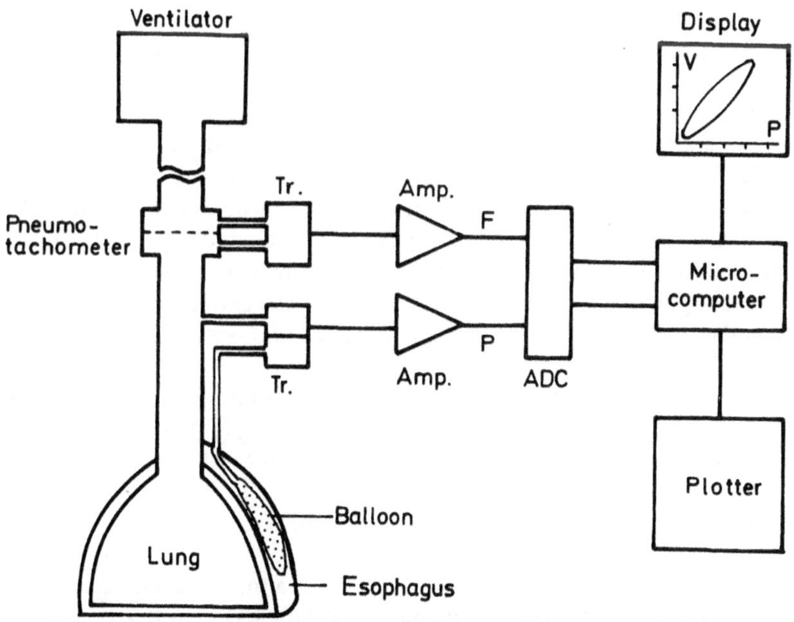

Fig. 1. System set-up. The difference between mouth pressure and esophageal pressure is measured by a differential pressure transducer *(Tr.)*. Flow is measured by a pneumotachometer (Fleisch). After passing through an amplifier *(Amp.)* and analog-to-digital conversion *(ADC)* the signals are transmitted to the computer

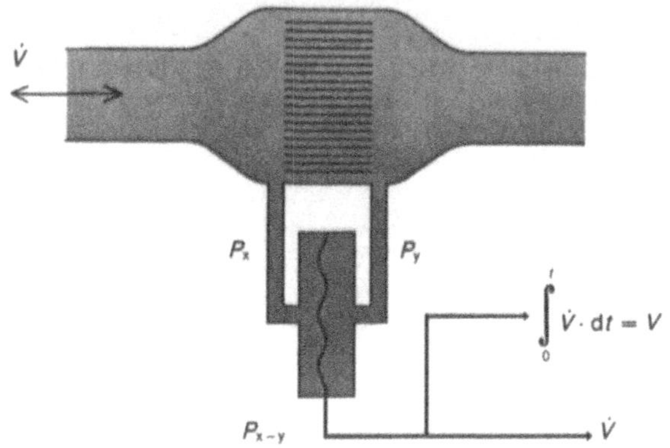

Fig. 2. Fleisch pneumotachograph

To measure work and other variables of lung mechanics at the ICU bedside, based on the considerations above we developed a measuring system for these parameters. In order to analyze the measured data in a reasonably short time, the use of a microcomputer was planned from the beginning (Bone 1976, Peters et al. 1972; Turney and Blumenfeld 1973).

In Fig. 1 the set-up of the system is displayed schematically. The arrangement on the left-hand side is used to measure pressure and flow. A Fleisch pneumotachograph, connected to the endotracheal tube or to a mouthpiece, serves as a flow-measuring device (Fig. 2). The gas flowing through the tube produces a pressure drop of a certain number of millimeters in the water column across a defined small resistor. This drop in pressure is proportional to the flow. It is measured by a differential-pressure transducer. Volume is computed by integrating the flow.

To determine the elastic and resistive properties of the lung, the transpulmonary pressure is used. It is equivalent to the difference between the mouth pressure and the intrathoracic or pleural pressure. For a good approximation of the intrathoracic pressure, the esophageal pressure measured via an esophageal balloon is used.

The balloon is placed in the lower third of the esophagus, as described, for example, by Milic-Emili et al. (1964), and thereafter the position is varied until the maximum amplitude of pressure is reached. The absolute values depend on the filling volume of the balloon, as shown in Fig. 3. Clinically a volume of 0.2–0.4 ml is appropriate. At this filling, measured pressures differ from those extrapolated to "zero filling" only slightly. The measurement is done in the supine position, with the chest elevated about 30°.

After amplifying and analog-to-digital conversion, the measured values are transferred to the microcomputer for further processing (Fig. 1).

Figure 4 shows the time-course of measured pressure in solid lines and of flow in dotted lines. These measurements have to be refined further through use of some software in order to analyze and to display these graphically on the screen.

A flow-chart of the computer program for data acquisition and processing developed by ourselves is shown in Fig. 5. In a menue-controlled manner the logic subprograms – here marked by arrows – may be selected by function keys. Calibrating and zeroing the measuring instruments makes up the first step. That is done by software support. Subsequently the measured signals are filtered by a 4-point moving

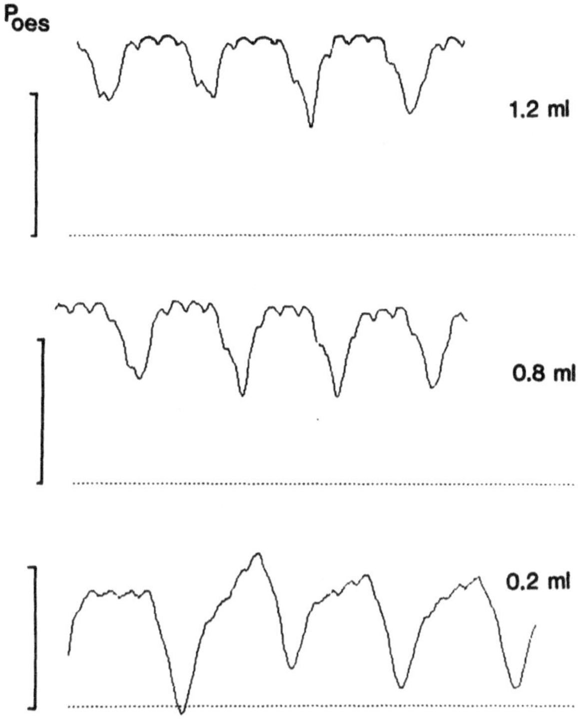

Fig. 3. Esophageal pressure recording at different balloon volumes. The abscissa represents time, the ordinate represents esophageal pressure in relative values. The distance from zero pressure *(dotted line)* as well as the pressure drop in inspiration varies due to the filling volume of the balloon (1.2, 0.8, and 0.2 ml in this example)

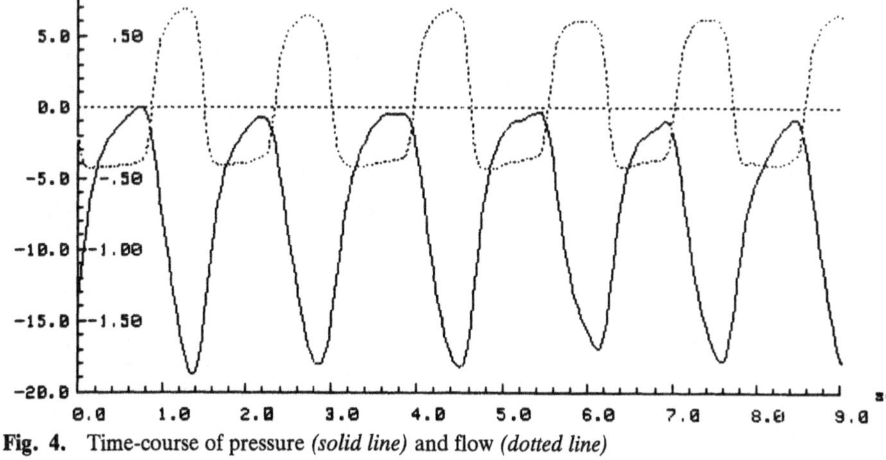

Fig. 4. Time-course of pressure *(solid line)* and flow *(dotted line)*

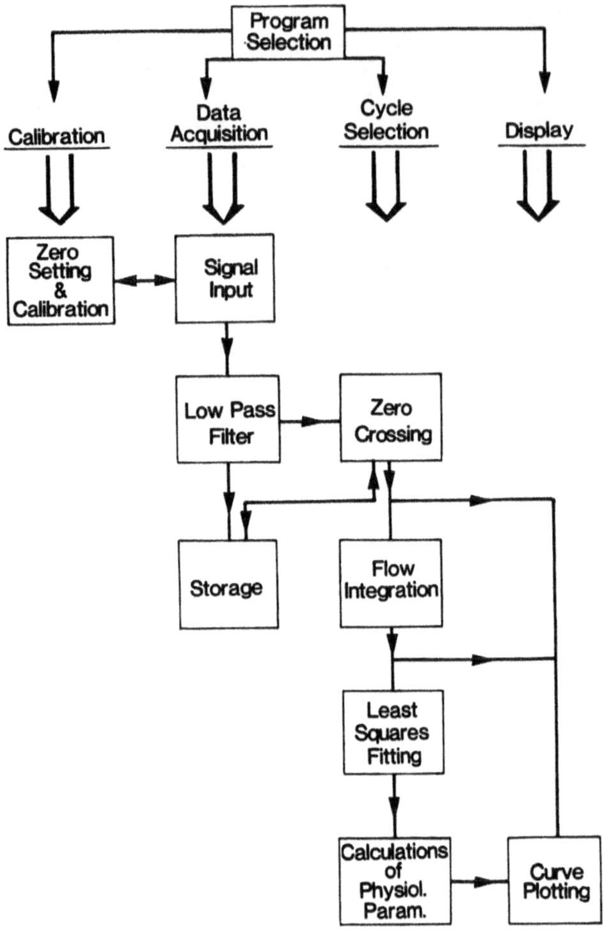

Fig. 5. Flow-chart of the computer program for data acquisition and processing

window average filter, transformed to physiological values, and converted to BTPS conditions.

In the program section "cycle selection" a respiration cycle appropriate to further computing is chosen. In this step, the zero crossing of the flow curve is detected and the beginning and the end of inspiration and the cycle termination are fixed. Integrating the flow yields the inspiratory and expiratory tidal volumes.

The transpulmonary pressure consists of elastic, resistive, and inertial components, as shown in the upper formula in Fig. 6. The inertial component as well as components

$$P_L = P_{ao} - P_{pl} = P_{el} + P_{res} + P_{in}$$

$$P_L = \frac{1}{C_{dyn}} \Delta V + R \cdot F$$

Fig. 6. Simplified mathematical model of lung mechanics. P_L, transpulmonary pressure; P_{el}, elastic pressure component; P_{res}, resistive pressure component; P_{in}, inertial pressure component; C_{dyn}, dynamic compliance; V, tidal volume; R, resistance; F, flow

		Inspiration		Expiration
Time				
Time	sec	2.22		2.35
Frequency	1/min		13.14	
Ratio (I:E)			.95	
Volume				
Tidal	L	.84		.85
Minute	L/min	11.10		11.16
Mechanics				
Compliance	L/cm H2O	.14		.14
Spec.Compliance	1/cm H2O	.17		.17
Resistance	cm H2O/L/sec	1.37		3.58
Work (Joule)				
Elastic	Wel		.25	
Viscous	Wvis		.30	
Total	Wtot		.55	
Wel/Wvis			.82	
Wel/Wtot			.45	
Wvis/Wtot			.55	
Work/L (J/L)				
Wtot/L			.65	
Power (J/min)				
Elastic	Pel		3.24	
Viscous	Pvis		3.96	
Total	Ptot		7.20	

Fig. 7. Tabular printout (example)

of second order in flow may be ignored on account of their relative smallness (Mead and Agostoni 1964; Mead 1961; Wilson 1976). Accordingly, a linear equation results, in which the pressure depends only upon volume and its time derivative, i.e., flow (lower formula in Fig. 6). Using this equation a least-squares fitting has been applied to the measured values of pressure and flow, for inspiration and expiration separately (see Fig. 5). This method yields the dynamic compliance (C) and the resistance (R) for both inspiration and expiration. As expected, the inspiratory and expiratory compliances differ only slightly.

Additional physiological parameters, such as respiration frequency, tidal volume, and work of breathing are calculated and presented graphically or in tabular form. An example of the tabular printout is presented in Fig. 7.

The triangle (horizontal lines in Fig. 8) built by the line representing the compliance, i.e. the linear dependence of volume and pressure, and the volume axis gives the elastic respiratory work. In the absence of dissipative forces, this area equals the total work of breathing. The convexity of the inspiration branch is due to the resistance. The inspiratory flow-resistive work is given by the area shown by longitudinal lines in Fig. 8. The whole area (horizontal and longitudinal lines) corresponds to

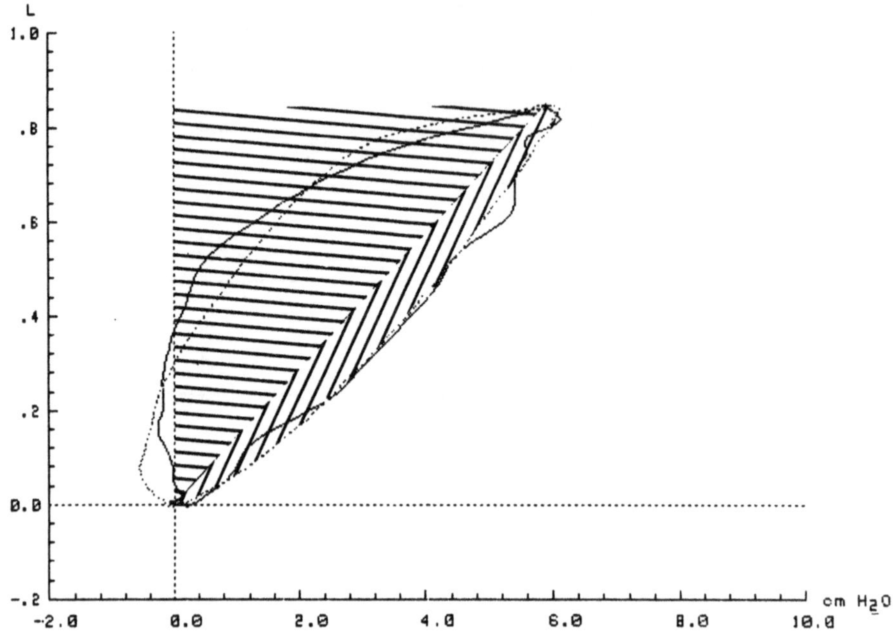

Fig. 8. Components of respiratory work. The elastic work is represented in the triangle by *horizontal lines*, the inspiratory flow-resistive work by *longitudinal lines*. *Solid lines* represent measured and *dotted lines* extrapolated loop values

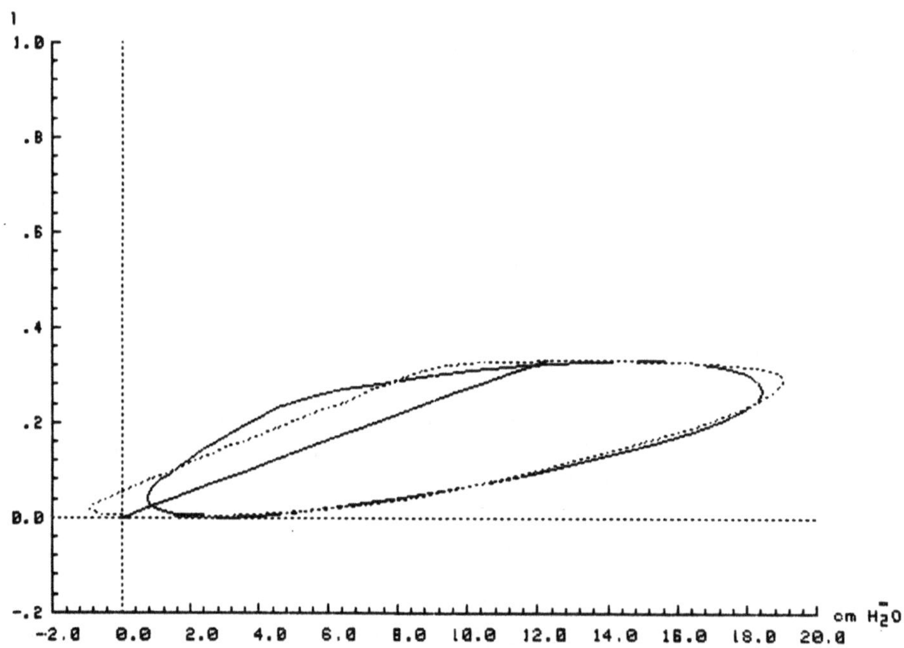

Fig. 9. Pressure-volume loop at forced ventilation after laparotomy in a patient with peritonitis

the total work done by inspiration. The loop area represents the flow-resistive work of both inspiration and expiration (Mead and Agostoni 1964).

At rest the flow-resistive work is small in healthy persons; under this condition it amounts to about 40% and the elastic work to about 60% of the total work. At forced ventilation the ratio is reversed (Peters et al. 1969; Proctor and Woolson 1973; Wilson 1976). The relationship between work and compliance, resistance, frequency, and ventilated volume is far from simple (Nunn 1977).

Examples of clinical measurements are given in Fig. 9 and 10. In Fig. 9 a pressure-volume loop is presented, obtained from a patient breathing spontaneously after laparatomy for peritonitis.

Minute ventilation (13 l) and work of breathing (24 J/min) are markedly elevated because of the impaired mechanics of respiration. The work exceeds the critical value for ventilatory support (18 J/min) as described by Peters et al. (1969). Analog values are given by Proctor and Woolson (1973). The compliance is reduced to about 30 ml/cm H_2O, the inspiratory resistance is raised to 13 cm H_2O/l/s. At this time the resistive work of breathing exceeds the elastic work substantially (by about 2.5 times). During attachment to the CPAP system (Fig. 10) the respiratory work per cycle and the work per minute decrease (by 30 and 43% respectively). The entire ventilation is reduced simultaneously (by 11.6%). This is probably due to decreased resistance (up to 75% in inspiration) as a result of distending airway diameters. At this stage the compliance only slightly increases and the elastic work does not change essentially. The ratio of elastic to viscous work is nearly reversed to almost "normal" values.

In summary, our system makes possible the bedside registration, processing, and analysis of lung mechanics parameters, such as compliance, resistance, and work of

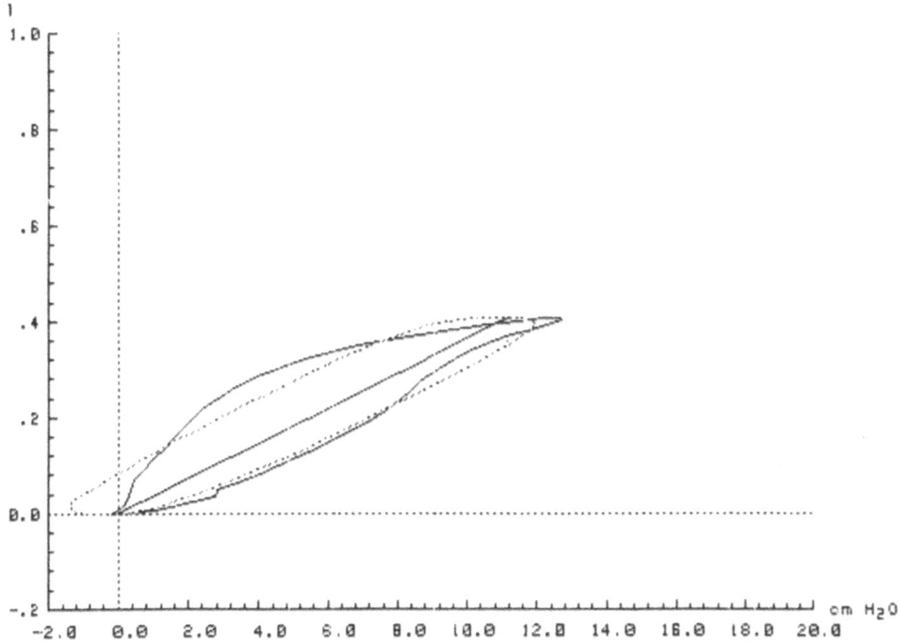

Fig. 10. Pressure-volume loop; same patient as in Fig. 9 after application of CPAP

breathing, in ICUs. More importantly, the latter parameter could be clinically applied to estimate the patient's ability to breathe spontaneously and serve as an objective parameter for weaning from the ventilator. In addition, indication and procedure selection of artificial ventilation, e.g., CPAP, may be facilitated.

References

Bone RC (1976) Diagnosis of causes for acute respiratory distress by pressure-volume curves. Chest 70: 740

Mead J (1961) Mechanical properties of lungs. Physiol Rev 41: 281

Mead J, Agostoni E (1964) Dynamics of breathing. In: Handbook of physiology. Respiration. Am Physiol Soc, Washington DC 3, I: 411

Milic-Emili J, Mead J, Turner JM, Glauser E-M (1964) Improved technique for estimating pleural pressure from esophageal balloons. J Appl Physiol 19: 207

Nunn JF (1977) Applied respiratory physiology. Butterworth, London

Peters RM, Wellons HA, Htwe JM (1969) Total compliance and work of breathing after thoracotomy. J Thorac Cardiovasc Surg 57: 348

Peters RM, Hilbermann M, Hogan JS, Crawford D-A (1972) Objective indications for respirator therapy in post-trauma and postoperative patients. Am J Surg 124: 262

Proctor HJ, Woolson R (1973) Prediction of respiratory muscle fatigue by measurements of the work of breathing. Surg Gynecol Obstet 136: 367

Turney SZ, Blumenfeld W (1973) Online respiratory-waveform analysis using a digital desk calculator. Med Biol Eng: 275

Wilson RS (1976) Monitoring the lung: mechanics and volume. Anesthesiology 45: 135

NAPROS

A semiautomatic and easy to use anaesthetic record system

D. WINTER, P. M. OSSWALD

During the past years a series of computer based systems have been developed in order to improve documentation of haemodynamic and pulmonal parameters during anaesthesia, to standardize and at the same time automate anaesthetic records. At the Department for Anaesthesiology and Reanimation of the Clinic of Mannheim a similar system had been developed in 1980 and introduced on a trial base. The breathtaking development in the field of microcomputer technique resulting in greater efficiency of the systems together with declining prices inspired to reconsider that project taking into account the experiences gained.

Former experiences

The computer based monitoring system for patients being in operation at our department for some years offers the possibility to sample parameters from up to 16 sensors on-line which can be completed by manual off-line data. Experience has shown that above all immediate graphic presentation of registered parameters on screen means a great help to the anaesthetist to evaluate the course of anaesthesia. At the same time the testing phase revealed weak points which at all rates should be avoided in future development of such systems.

For example a partial use of digit-codes lead to a limitation of users to a small circle of insiders. It could clearly be demonstrated that a high acceptance of such systems, which is a necessary pre-condition for the use in every day routine, can only be achieved if the handling is clear and simple, no computer-specific knowledge is required and if it will be less laborious than manual record-keeping.

It has proved to be a problem that the former system was planned as part of a network. The entered anaesthetic record data was to be transferred after a short-termed storage in the microprocessor to a central minicomputer. There a concentration and final storage of the data was planned for later scientific/statistic analysis as well as for output of a final anaesthetic record via plotter or printer-plotter at the end of anaesthesia.

This concept already failed due to comparatively "small" problems such as the very expensive installation of data-transmission lines from the sterile operating theatre to the minicomputer, a problem many old clinics will have to deal with in one way or another. Moreover, such a concept requires a high reliability of the minicomputer, because failure of the central unit would cause a break-down of the entire system.

On the other hand, the anaesthetic record represents an important document [7], being essentially needed after anaesthesia for adequate treatment of the patient in the recovery room or on the ward. Delayed printing or partial loss of data cannot be accepted. As long as for security-reasons a parallel manual record has to be kept, this means additional unacceptable work.

NAPROS

Hardware and Software

For realization of the system we chose an ACORN (BBC-ModelB) microcomputer with diskdrive to store data and programs and a matrix printer EPSON RX-80 to print the anaesthetic record. For our purposes this machine offers the following advantages:

1. extremely efficient and fast BASIC which allows structured programming
2. very good and fast graphic with high resolution on screen
3. inbuilt AD-converter with 4 channels for on-line sampling from as many sensors
4. a good and efficient disk-filing-system for quick saving/loading to/from disk
5. possibility for expansion of the system with respect to:
   - addition of a slave processor to increase processing speed
   - connection of various similar computers for communication in a network
6. good price/efficiency relation. On the German market the computer is sold for about 6.000 DM, disk drive and printer included.

All system programs are computed in BBC-BASIC.

System description

The system consists of a BBC-micro, a disk drive, a matrix printer linked to a non-invasive arterial pressure monitor (DINAMAP 845 a) and an inhalation narcotic monitor (Engstroem EMMA) for measurement of the inspired concentration of narcotic inhalation agents (Fig. 1).

The inbuilt 4-channel AD-converter monitors automatically records cardiovascular parameters (AP-syst., AP-diast., HR) as well as the inspired concentration of narcotic inhalation agents. Parameters are registered automatically within short time intervals, graphically demonstrated on screen and finally stored. Moreover, manually sampled parameters may be inserted via keyboard of the terminal.

Great importance has been attached to the fact that even a complete system breakdown does not lead to loss of any data concerning stored parameters infusions, drugs, administrative data etc. In such a case it is possible to reconstruct the entire anaesthetic record, and graphic presentation of cardiovascular parameters within a few seconds by a key-stroke.

At intervals of a few minutes a preliminary anaesthetic record is printed by NAPROS including all registered data (parameters, drugs, infusions). Automatically recorded parameters are printed out time scheduled in form of a diagram. At the time of input into the computer, administered drugs are printed on the anaesthetic record

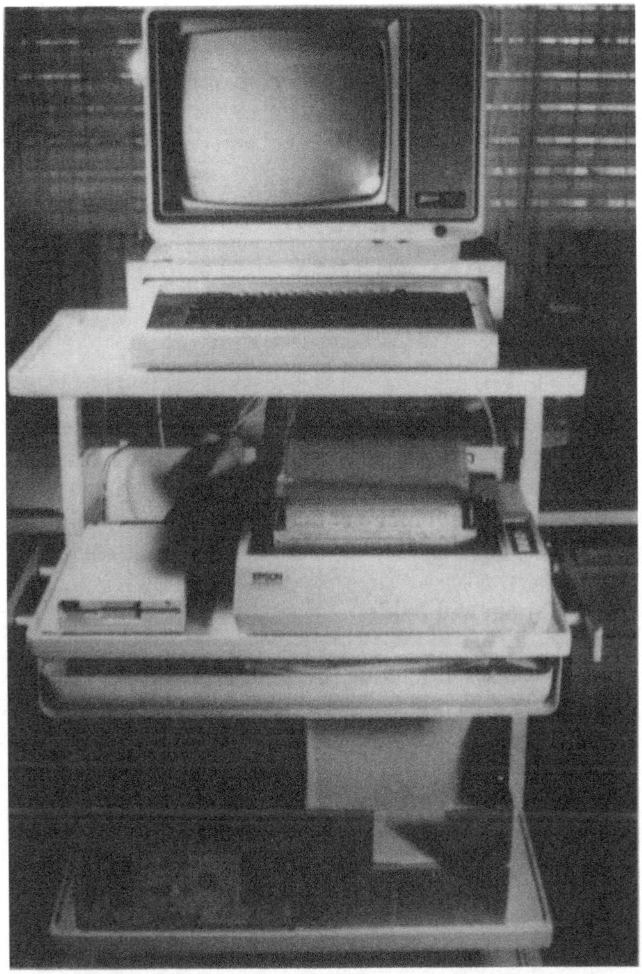

Fig. 1. Shows the arrangement of the microcomputer with screen, keyboard, diskdrive and printer as a functional unit on a trolley. The Dinamap arterial blood-pressure monitor and an inhalation narcotic monitor (not to be seen in this picture) are also grouped on the same trolley

stating exact time of application. This may lead to time discrepancies on the chart if data is entered retrospectively, i.e. if a drug is administered at 8.00 o'clock but entered at 9.00 o'clock. At the end of anaesthesia however all entered data is sorted according to time indexes and printed exactly time scheduled on a final anaesthetic record.

Functions of the anaesthetic record system

Following functions have been implemented in NAPROS
- automatic registration of cardiovascular data and concentration of narcotic inhalation agents
- input of drugs and fluids

- input of any event and particularities
- input of laboratory and ventilatory parameters
- automatic registration and graphic or numeric representation of fluid-balances
- survey of all or selected drugs that have been administered up to that time
- collection of administrative data and data concerning the preoperative state of the patient
- possibility for recalling dosage information for drugs and drops
- parallel printing of all collected data as a preliminary anaesthetic record
- printing of a final anaesthetic report at the end of anaesthesia.

Choice of particular functions

The choice of functions is done by menue technique. All available functions are presented on screen as a menue and the corresponding function key is indicated.

Fig. 2 shows the screen divided into two parts representing cardiovascular parameters graphically in the upper and the basic menue in the lower part of the screen.

Input of drugs and fluids

Input of administered drugs or fluids is done by first pressing the respective function key and then identifying the drug or fluid by a number. The numbers for routine-drugs/fluids are well-known after a short period. However, all numbers can be recalled from the system by function key, so that the user always has all lists at his disposal. Furthermore time of administration and quantity of the administered drug or fluid have to be fed into the computer.

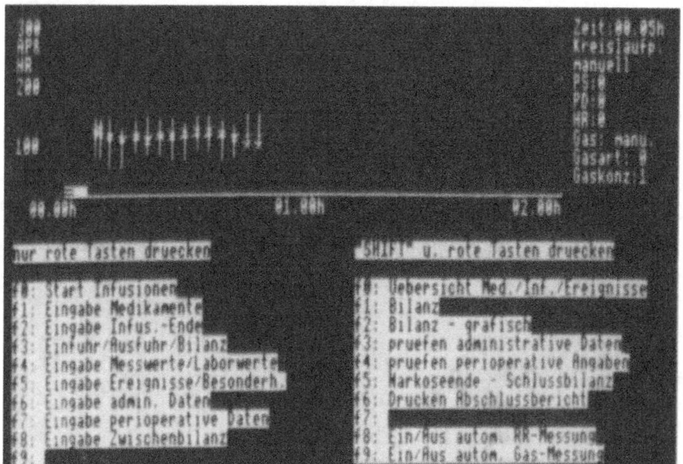

Fig. 2. Shows the graphical representation of the cardiovascular parameters in the upper part, and the basic menue in the lower part of the screen

To relieve the user from keyboard entries the system offers in many cases so-called "default-values" which only have to be confirmed by key-stroke, if true. The computer inserts for example the actual time for all time data which is only to be corrected if input for drugs/fluids is done retrospectively. Correspondingly, most infusions are registered as fluid-input of 500 ml, concentrated erythrocytes as 250 ml. In case of deviations the user may correct these values.

Finally, after all data of an administered drug/fluid have been collected, there is a request to check if the entered data is correct. In case of error, corrections are still possible. After confirmation the data finally is stored on disk.

Recall of dosage information for drugs

NAPROS offers the possibility to include dosage information for drugs and drips as well as short informations concerning drugs. There is a beep-signal on drug input to signal that the system is keeping information available to be called by function key. All this information may be updated easily using a service-program.

Fluid-balance

There is an automatic fluid balance according to the administered infusion therapy for all input fluid data. Comments of the anaesthetist on blood losses, urine production or other intraoperative fluid losses (ascites, gastric secretion) are automatically balanced.

At any time it is possible to obtain an interim balance in numeric or graphic form (see Fig. 3 and 4).

If there had been information about the patient's preoperative fasting period the system will calculate the fluid loss according to the formula for basic fluid requirements. Evaluation of this value is up to the anaesthetist, of course, who will have to judge the actual situation following his clinical experience.

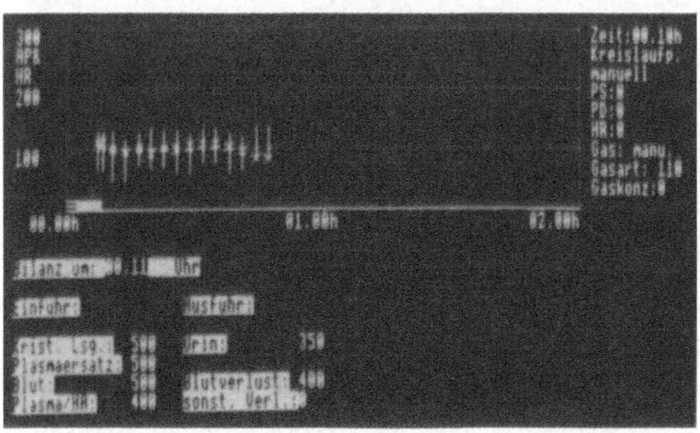

Fig. 3. The lower part of the screen shows the output of the interim fluid-balance at 00.11 h

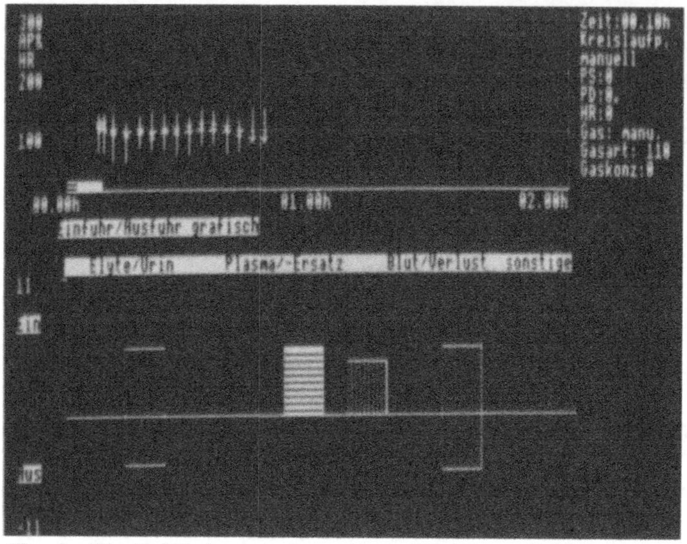

Fig. 4. The fluid-balance is shown in graphical form. Fluid-inputs are represented as a column towards the top, fluid-outputs as a column towards the bottom of the screen

Survey of administered drugs or fluids

If the anaesthetist needs a survey of all drugs or fluids that have been administered up to that time for example or if another collegue takes over, the system is able to deliver such a list at any time.

This list may sum up all or selected drugs. In the latter case the administer volumes are added up and given as a sum. Fig. 5 shows such a survey for Alloferin.

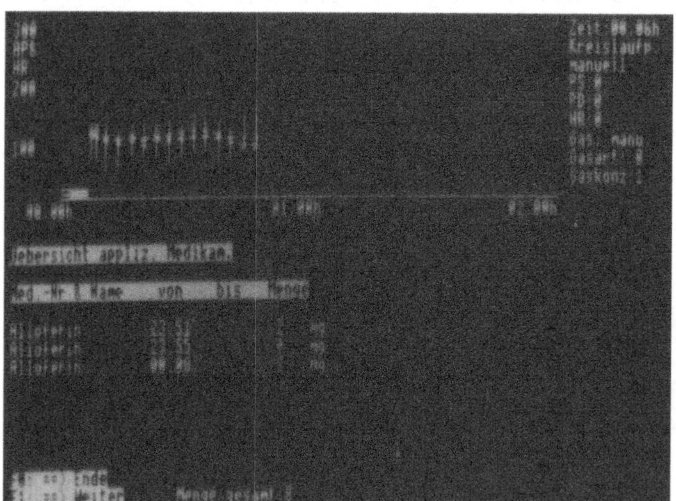

Fig. 5. Gives a survey for Alloferin. Three times Alloferin has been given at dosages of 2, 4 and 6 mg and at the bottom the total amount of 8 mg is shown

Input of events and particularities

Besides measured parameters or administered drugs a series of certain incidents have to be documented on an anaesthetic record (such as in/extubation, onset or end of operation etc.). This is done in the above mentioned way of menue technique, whereby common incidents are programmed and chosen by function key only, whereas special events, an anaesthetist wants to document, may be inserted by input of a free text.

Input of administrative and perioperative data

Input of administrative data such as name, date of birth, date and time of operation, duration of anaesthesia etc. naturally is very time-consuming and is done in steps in form of a dialog via keyboard. The same way of input applies to perioperative data concerning the preoperative state of the patient, applied anaesthesia, complications etc.

The concerning data input may be interrupted at any time and completed at a later stage if the anaesthetist has to devote his concentration on the course of anaesthesia. There is also always the possibility to complete and update erroneous or incomplete data (for example in the case of an unknown casulty patient).

Adjustment of the system to any particularities of a clinic

Current preparations introduced in our clinic have been taken into consideration primarily on introduction of the code for drugs and fluids.

But a procedure has been chosen on programming that allows a simple adjustment to specific requirement of any clinic. That means, that without changes in program further drugs may be inserted or certain numbers may be identified with other drugs or fluids.

Such changes are performed with the help of an additional service program and do not require specific programming knowledge. However, these service programs are only at the disposal of selected users, who are entitled to do these changes. The same principle applies to asked administrative and perioperative data thus simplifying accommodation to local conditions.

Discussion

For seven months NAPROS has been on clinical test in our clinic. It could be shown that it is possible to reliably and objectively document automatically important cardiovascular parameters. The anaesthetist is completely relieved from that task of documentation. Simultaneously, the graphic representation on screen as well as the printed documentation gives a survey of the circulatory conditions from the moment anaesthesia started. Especially in critical moments, requiring full attention of the anaesthetist, a release of the task for documentation is a helpful device not to be underestimated.

On the other hand, the dialog with the computer for input of data, drugs, fluids and events means a certain psychological barrier which however, if overcome, is rewarded by the convenience of automatic balances, the possibility of recalling interim fluid-balances at any time, survey of the administered drugs and dosage information.

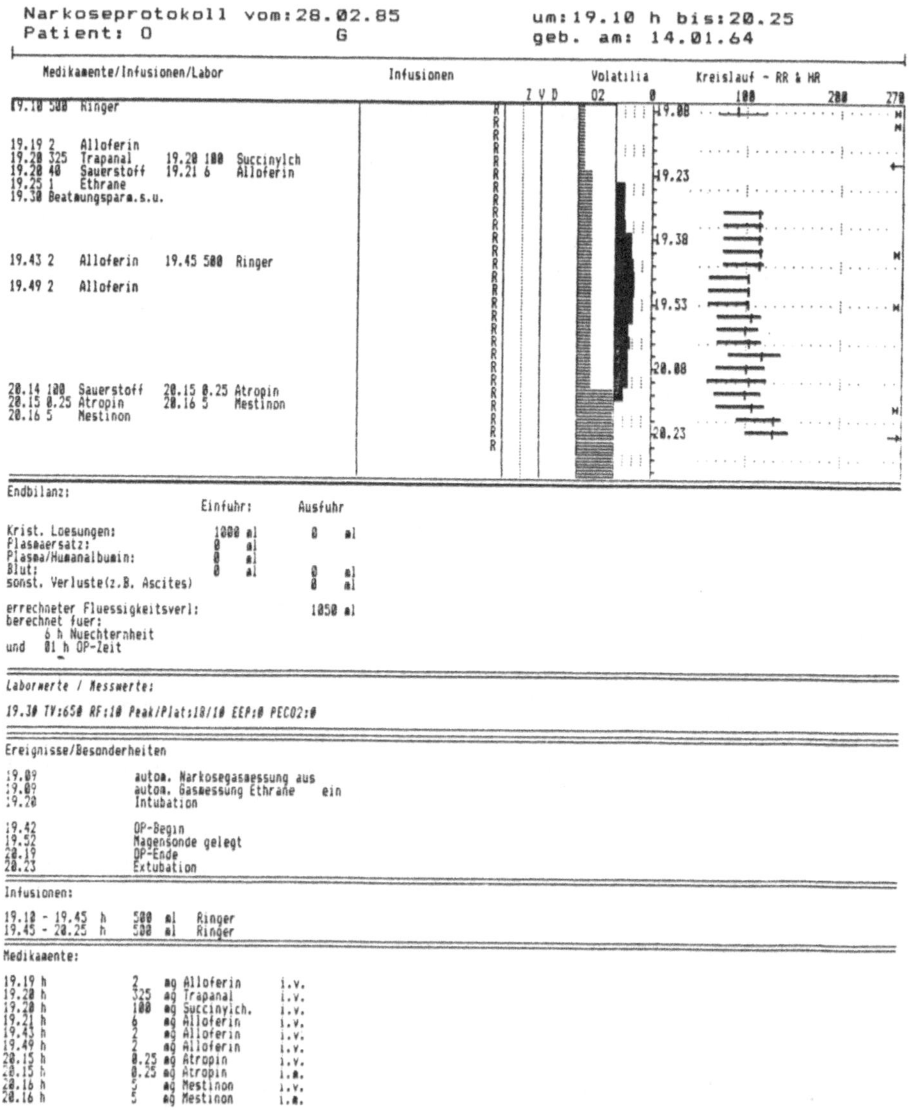

Narkoseprotokoll vom:28.02.85 um:19.10 h bis:20.25
Patient: O G geb. am: 14.01.64

Medikamente/Infusionen/Labor | Infusionen | Volatilia | Kreislauf - RR & HR

19.10 500 Ringer

19.19 2 Alloferin
19.20 325 Trapanal 19.20 100 Succinylch
19.20 40 Sauerstoff 19.21 6 Alloferin
19.25 1 Ethrane
19.30 Beatmungsparam.s.u.

19.43 2 Alloferin 19.45 500 Ringer
19.49 2 Alloferin

20.14 100 Sauerstoff 20.15 0.25 Atropin
20.15 0.25 Atropin 20.16 5 Mestinon
20.16 5 Mestinon

Endbilanz:

	Einfuhr:	Ausfuhr
Krist. Loesungen:	1000 ml	0 ml
Plasmaersatz:	0 ml	
Plasma/Humanalbumin:	0 ml	
Blut:	0 ml	0 ml
sonst. Verluste(z.B. Ascites)		0 ml
errechneter Fluessigkeitsverl:		1050 ml

berechnet fuer:
6 h Nuechternheit
und 01 h OP-Zeit

Laborwerte / Messwerte:

19.30 TV:650 RF:10 Peak/Plat:18/10 EEP:0 PECO2:0

Ereignisse/Besonderheiten

19.09	autom. Narkosegasmessung aus
19.09	autom. Gasmessung Ethrane ein
19.20	Intubation
19.42	OP-Begin
19.52	Magensonde gelegt
20.19	OP-Ende
20.23	Extubation

Infusionen:

19.10 - 19.45 h	500 ml	Ringer
19.45 - 20.25 h	500 ml	Ringer

Medikamente:

19.19 h	2 mg	Alloferin	i.v.
19.20 h	325 mg	Trapanal	i.v.
19.20 h	100 mg	Succinylch.	i.v.
19.21 h	6 mg	Alloferin	i.v.
19.43 h	2 mg	Alloferin	i.v.
19.49 h	2 mg	Alloferin	i.v.
20.15 h	0.25 mg	Atropin	i.v.
20.15 h	0.25 mg	Atropin	i.m.
20.16 h	5 mg	Mestinon	i.v.
20.16 h	5 mg	Mestinon	i.m.

Fig. 6. Shows an anaesthetic record printed by NAPROS with the on-line registered parameters (cardiovascular data and concentration of narcotic inhalation agents) on the right side. On the left side all off-line data concerning type, time and amount of administered drugs as well as laboratory values and comments of the anaesthetist are printed. At the end of the record the final fluid-balance and summary of all drugs and infusions, laboratory-values and comments of the anesthetist are printed

Implementation of high modern technology does not allow to present all relevant data on one screen. To get further information the user has to be active. This is considered to be a disadvantage and irritates the need for immediate survey of all information. On the other hand, the anaesthetist would need more time to calculate interim fluid-balances and dosages in the conventional way.

Concerning system break-down, NAPROS has proven to be reliable enough to use the computer based anaesthesia record instead of manual record-keeping. After stabandoning double record-keeping the system enjoys great acceptance among our staff. There are hardly any user problems. A short introduction was only needed to

```
Name                      O
Vorname                   G.
Geb.-Datum                14.01.64
Strasse & Nr
Plz & Ort

Narkose-Nr.               10799
Prot. vom                 28.02.85
Anf. Vorber.              19.00
Operat. von               19.43
Operat. bis

Anaesth. bis
Station                   CH8B
Op-Tisch                  4
Oper. Klin                CH
Betten Klin.              CH

Anaesthesist              WINTER
Anaesth.-Nr               80
von                       19.00
bis
Supervis.&Nr

Diagnose                  APPENDICITIS
Diag2                     akute !!
Diag3
Diag4
Diag5

Operation                 APPENDEKTOMIE
OP2
OP3
OP4
OP5

Operateur                 SCHWALL
Operateur2                WESCH
Operateur3                HERRMAN
Operateur4                SPRINGER=BIRGIT
Operateur5

Anaesth-Abl1
Abl1 I-Nr
Abl1 von
     bis

Anaesth-Abl2
Abl2 I-Nr
Abl2 von
     bis

WP ja/nein                NEIN
Anz. Zugaeng              1
Narkoseger.               SERVO 900 B
Anaesth.Sr                PETER
Blutgruppe
==========================================
Perioperative Angaben:

   weiblich
       nicht schwanger
   ohne Arztwahl
   Ber.D    16.00-08.00h
   bed.  dringlich
   keine Vorerkr.
   ITN
       orotrach.  Tubus
   RR & Puls
   EKG
   Ruecken
   Laborwerte im Normb.
   intraab.   ohne Get.
Ende der perioperativen Angaben
```

Fig. 7. Shows the print-out of the administrative and perioperative data

learn the system handling. Nevertheless, there were and there still are reactions of disapproval, based on sceptic opinions concerning the use of microcomputers in general.

This might be due to the fact that microcomputers of all kind always submit the user to structural patterns thus undermining own spontaneous behaviour. In comparison with the conventional manual record-keeping the computer based system, without any doubt, delivers a more objective documentation. In case of great discrepancies between the manual record keeping and the automatic recording of parameters the automatic data input may be switched off or the manually recorded parameter may be inserted into the system additionally.

After adaption to the different form (see Fig. 6 and 7) the automatically produced record surely is better readable than the individual handwriting of a conventional anaesthetic record.

Time analyses have shown that time, spent on documentation, takes about 10% of the duration of anaesthesia for both systems of record-keeping. There is no direct time-saving effect by semi-automation. It has to be taken into consideration though, that data recorded by NAPROS are directly suitable for statistic/scientific analysis as well as for accountancy purposes. Thus, part of the data registration, normally done at a later stage, has already been done in the operating theater. Despite additional possibilities offered by NAPROS there is no extra time spent.

Facing tight financial sources, we deliberately limited ourselves to the main cardiovascular parameters representing the main "pillars" of anaesthesia monitoring for on-line data input. At times it may for example be desirable to record automatically ventilatory parameters of modern respirators. Memory capacity as well as system-design allow such an option but expensive hardware extension would be required. As suitable respirators are not available in most cases we have put great importance on an inexpensive secure system which is easy to handle with great acceptance by the users.

This aim could be achieved by the here presented system.

References

Bender HJ (1981) Implementierung eines rechnergestützten Patientenüberwachungssystems. Diss. Mannheim

Bender HJ, Osswald PM, Hartung HJ, Lutz H (1982) Online-Erfassung hämodynamischer und respiratorischer Größen in der Anästhesie. Anästh. Intensivther Notfallmed 18

Cushman J, Bushman JA (1983) The semiautomatic production of anaesthetic records. Br J Anaesth 55: 240 P

Hartung HJ, Bender HJ, Osswald PM, Lutz H, Olsson SG (1983) Entwicklung und Einsatz eines computergestützt erstellten Anaesthesieprotokolls. Anaesthesist 32: 205–213

Lutz H, Kunze I (1980) Autonome rechnergestützte Anästhesiedokumentation. Anasth Intensivther Notfallmed 15: 494

Naqvi NH (1983) Computer-based automatic anaesthetic records. Br. J. Anaesth., 55: 916 P

Osswald PM, Hartung HJ, Winter D, Bender HJ, Lutz H (1984) Das Narkoseprotokoll. Anaesthesist 33: 395–401

Prakash O, Meij S, Zeelenberg C, Borden v. d. SG (1982) Computer-based patient monitoring. Crit Care Med 10/12

Prentice JW, Kenny GNC (1984) Microcomputer-Based anaesthetic record system. Br J Anaesth 56: 1433

Whitesell R, Jablonski J, Burgos L (1979): Microprocessor automation of anesthesia records. Anesthesiology 51: 333

A Real Time Pattern Recognition Program for Continuous Processing of Cardiovascular Biosignals

M. MAIWALD

Introduction

Continuous monitoring of electrocardiograms is routine practice in intensive care units. Much effort has been devoted to the development of automatic systems capable of processing ECGs. Template matching, thresholding, or syntactic pattern detection are used to identify the characteristic ECG waves. However, many of these programs are designed to produce an ECG diagnosis from limited time spans of standard lead ECG registrations. The digitized raw signal must be stored on a mass storage device prior to processing. Such programs do not conform to real time requirements.

The introduction of microprocessor technology, although reducing the hardware costs, imposes considerable restrictions on the size of the extraction algorithms. This is due to the conflicting demands of real time processing and the limited number crunching properties of the widely distributed 8 bit single board CPUs.

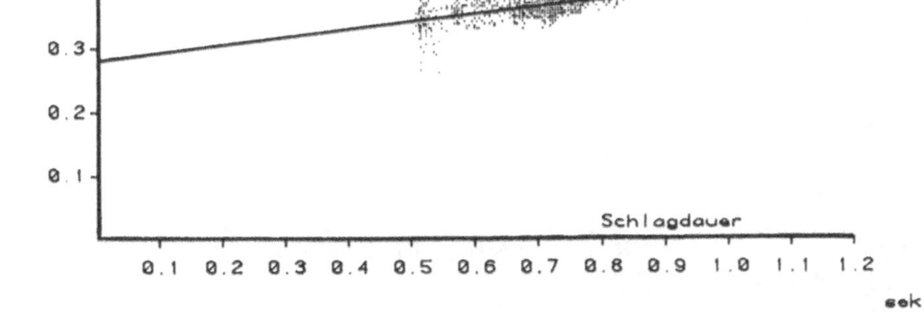

Fig. 1. Scatter diagram: Interbeat interval (IBI) vs. QT interval (QT). Number of beats: 867; regression coefficients: J = 0.28 + 0.12 ×

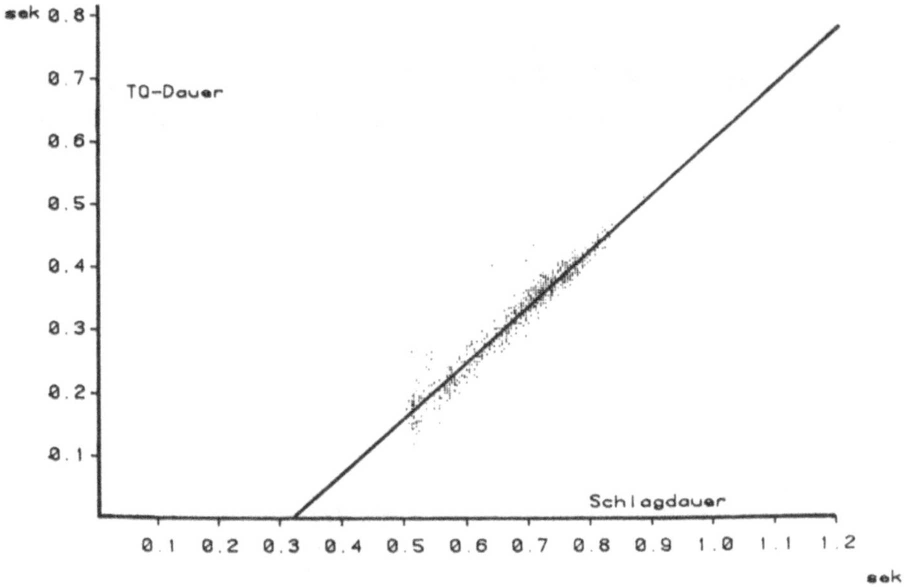

Fig. 2. Scatter diagram: Interbeat interval (IBI) vs. TQ interval (TQ). Number of beats: 867; regression coefficients: J = −0.28 + 0.88 ×

This report is intended to outline the hard- and software requirements of a newly developed program system. The system is based on a real time pattern recognition algorithm for ECG and other cardiovascular signals. For the development, a fast minicomputer has been used. A transfer to smaller computers is possible.

Technical details, a block diagram, and a list of the parameters extracted from the raw signals are given below. The Figures illustrate the relationship of interbeat intervals (heart rate) and ventricular diastole (Fig. 1) and ventricular systole (Fig. 2). The data were collected in a 5-min period by ECG telemetry and processed on line. This 5-min period included a rest phase and knee bending exercise.

Technical specifications

Hardware

Processor system	Digital Equipment PDP 11/70
Processor unit	KB11-B CPU
Clock frequency	30 MHz
Cache memory	1 kW
Memory (Core)	160 kW
AD conversion	Laboratory Peripheral System (LPS-11) 16 AD-, 2 DA channels
Disks	4 RK05 (2.5 MB), 2 RP05 (40 MB)
Graphic display	DEC VT55
Plotter	Tektonix 4662

Software	
Operating system	RSX-11M
Compiler	DEC FORTRAN IV
Library	FORTRAN callable subroutines for interrupt service
Program Specification	
Size	Approximately 25 kW
Voltage resolution	12 bit
Voltage range	+/− 1 volt
Time resolution	4 ms dwelltime
Sampling frequency	250 Hz
Signal conditioning	Digital smoothing
QRS detection	Digital differentiation
Buffer types	a) Two alternating buffers for raw data b) Work buffer
Buffer size	a) 3 s b) Variable
Processing time/buffer	< 1 s

List of Parameters

A) *Intervals in ms:*

Atrial activity:

1. PP interval
2. Duration of P-wave
3. PQ interval (beginning of P- to beginning of Q-wave)
4. PQ distance (end of P- to beginning of Q-wave), isoelectric baseline

Ventricular activity:

5. QR interval (intrinsic deflection)
6. QS interval
7. Length of ST segment
8. QX interval (intersection of ST segment with baseline marks X-point)
9. QT interval (ventricular systole)
10. QTc (corrected QT interval according to Bazett)
11. QX/QT relation
12. Duration of T-wave
13. TQ interval (ventricular diastole)
14. Interbeat interval (RR distance)
15. Heart frequency

B) *Amplitudes in mV:*

16. P-wave
17. Baseline (PQ distance)
18. Q-wave
19. R-wave
20. S-wave
21. Junction point (end of S-wave)
22. ST segment (60–80 ms after junction point)

C) *Spatial velocities:*
23. Maximal slope of R-wave
24. Slope of ST segment over 1-period

D) *Integrals*
25. Area enclosed between ST segment below baseline
26. Area enclosed above baseline and ST segment
27. Area below QS complex

E) *Cross correlation:*
28. Match between template and PQRST complex

Additional parameters extracted from impedance cardiogram and peripheral pulse signal (finger or ear lobe) by ONL3S2-program:

E) *Systolic time intervals in ms:*
29. Preejection period (PEP)
30. Left ventricular ejection time (LVET)

F) *Derived parameter:*
31. Stroke volume
32. Cardiac output

G) *Pulse intervals:*
33. Pulse propagation time (PPT)

H) *Pulse amplitudes:*
34. Maximum of dicrotic wave [pulse volume amplitude (PVA)]
35. Minimum of dicrotic wave

Acknowledgment. This work has been supported in part by the German Federal Ministry for Research and Technology (BMFT) under contract 01 VD 235-B13-TAP 0011.

Block Diagram for EKGP5 Program

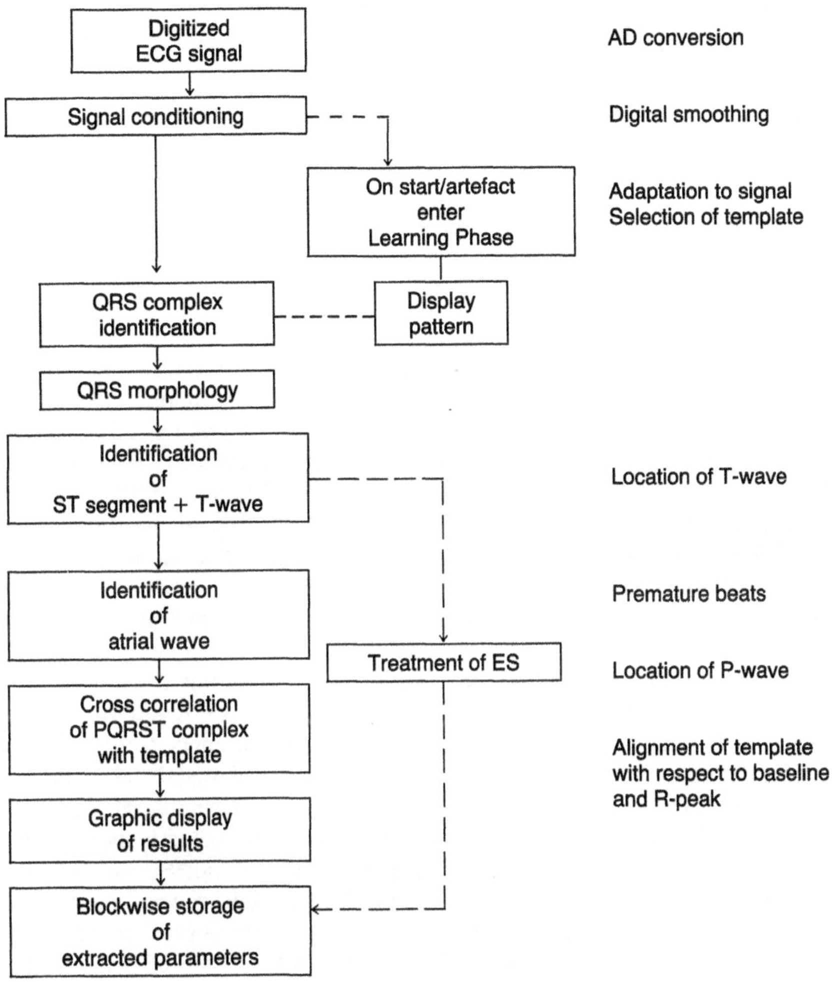

Microcomputer-Assisted ICP Monitoring in Neurological Patients

G. Schmieder, C. Garner, K. M. Einhäupl, K. Siegl, and G. Kufner

In patients with potentially increased intracranial pressure (ICP), continuous monitoring of ICP is a commonly used diagnostic procedure in intensive care units. Conventional chart recordings or isolated computer analyses are of limited use unless they can easily be correlated with other factors which might affect the ICP signal [e. g., arterial blood pressure (SAP), central venous pressure (CVP), and ventilation parameters]. A monitoring system should provide on-line information and be able to store data from different biological parameters economically for later evaluation.

We developed a microcomputer system which allows on-line monitoring of up to 16 parameters simultaneously and storing of them on a single data base. Further, the ICP signal contains more information than that expressed by the mean value. Often the mean ICP level remains normal, whereas an increased intracranial elastance (E) indicates an impending decompensation (Szewczykowski et al. 1977; van Eijndhoven and Avezaat 1980). Therefore an estimation of intracranial elastance yields valuable clinical information in addition to that provided by the ICP signal. The volume/pressure test (VPT) is widely used to measure intracranial elastance. However, in patients with a high intracranial elastance the addition of extra volume may provoke secondary rises in pressure, sometimes even plateau waves (van Eijndhoven and Avezaat 1980). As reported by others (Friden and Ekstedt 1980; Szewczykowski et al. 1977; van Eijndhoven and Avezaat 1980), the intracranial pulse pressure (CSFPP) gives the same information as the VPT. The CSFPP (relationship of pulse-related amplitude and mean ICP level) can be calculated continuously and without any danger for the patient. In addition to the CSFPP, we calculate cerebral perfusion pressure (CPP) and the histogram of the ICP signal.

To give this on-line information a high sampling rate is required. When sampled with other signals, this results in an accumulation of a mass of data. Reduction of these data is necessary in order to store them conveniently for later statistical analysis. We have solved this problem by storing reduced data in a single computer data-base coordinated in realtime. We consider that this low-cost microcomputer system allows practical clinical ICP monitoring.

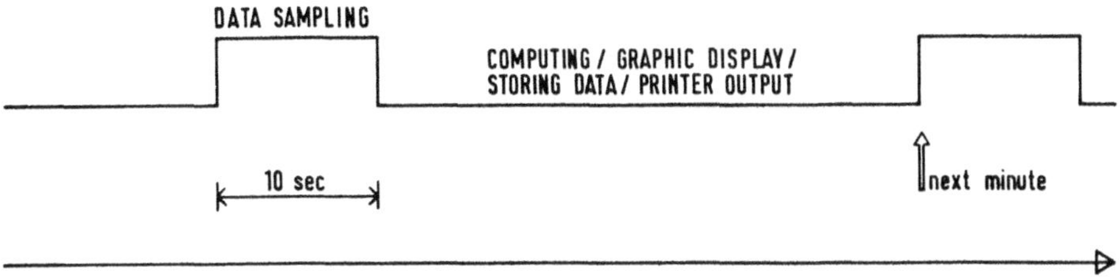

Fig. 1. Time intervals of tasks

Methods

We use a 16-channel analog-to-digital converter which allows the simultaneous acquisition of ICP and other physiological parameters. The scale of each channel is independently adjustable. Six of the channels are sampled at 100 per second for a period of 10 s (e. g., ICP, SAP, CVP). Up to ten channels are sampled at 1 per minute (e. g., temperature, heart rate). Mean values and computed parameters are stored on floppy disk at 1-min intervals (Fig. 1).

Depending on the patient's individual situation, the following parameters can be monitored and recorded in addition to ICP:

- Systemic arterial blood pressure (SAP), heart rate (HR), temperature
- Ventilation parameters in patients with artificial respiration
- Central venous pressure (CVP) in patients with central venous catheters

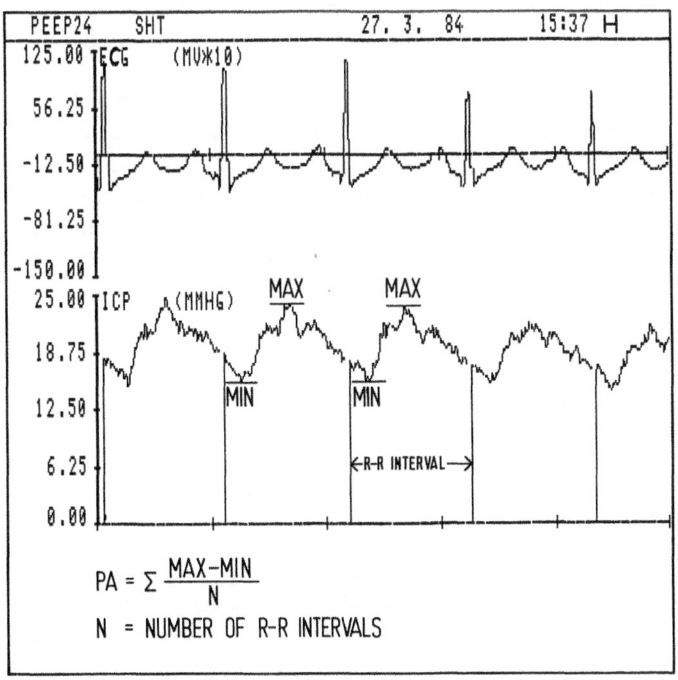

Fig. 2. Method of computing pulse-related amplitudes of ICP

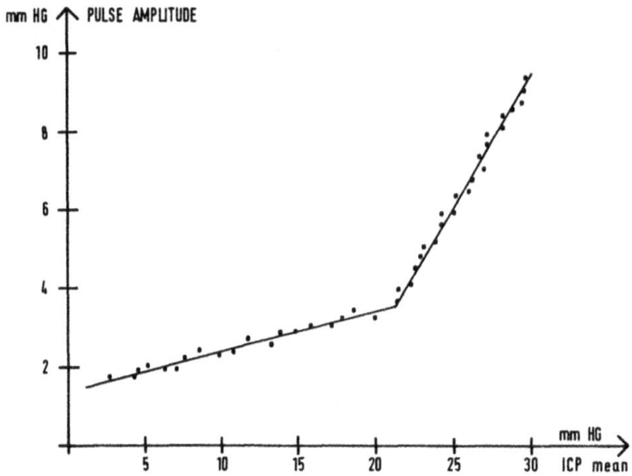

Fig. 3. PA-ICP mean curve

- Pulmonary artery pressure (PAP) and pulmonary wedge pressure (by manual intervention) in patients with Swan–Ganz catheters

For on-line information regarding intracranial elastance we use the relationship of pulse-related amplitude (PA) and the mean level of ICP (Friden and Ekstedt 1980). An analog-filtered electrocardiogram is used for R-wave detection, and the pulse amplitude of ICP signal is computed for each R-R interval. Mean pulse amplitude and mean ICP are calculated for the sampled interval of 10 s (Fig. 2). At variable time intervals (15–30 min), the regression line of consecutive PA and mean ICP is calculated. The regression line is displayed on the graphic monitor, and the slope and intercept are printed.

Figure 3 shows a schematic PA–ICP mean curve which consists of two straight lines with different slopes. A small slope is found in the state of compensation. At a "breakpoint" the slope is increasing, indicating the state of pathological decompensation. In addition we compute statistical parameters and frequency distribution. The histograms are updated every minute and displayed on the graphic terminal at preset time intervals (Fig. 7). For hard copy of graphics the matrix printer is used.

Software

The programs are written in FORTRAN. Assembly language subroutines are used for interrupted data sampling, for graphic display, and for hard copy to matrix printer. The package consists of several overlay modules. MODUL 1 does the major operations for on-line analysis of sampled data and performs the following tasks:

- Data acquisition and graphic display of sampled data (Fig. 6)
- Computing of mean values and storing them on floppy disk
- Updating of histograms and graphic display (Fig. 7)
- Printer output of mean values and computed parameters
- Calculation of the relationship between the ICP pulse amplitude and CSFPP

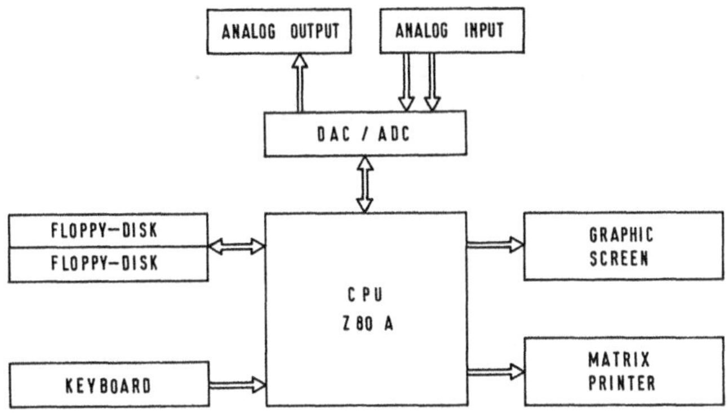

Processor/CPU:	Z80 A, 4 MHz, 64 kByte RAM, CP/M
Mass storage:	2× Floppy disk, 2× 600 kByte
Printer:	Matrix printer
Screen:	24 lines × 80 characters, 512×256 pts.
Real-time clock:	battery-buffered
Analog inputs:	16 channel to 12 bit ADC / 28 µs conv.
Input voltage:	−5 V to +5 V
Analog output:	1 channel from DAC / 7 µs conv.

Fig. 4. Block diagram of microcomputer system

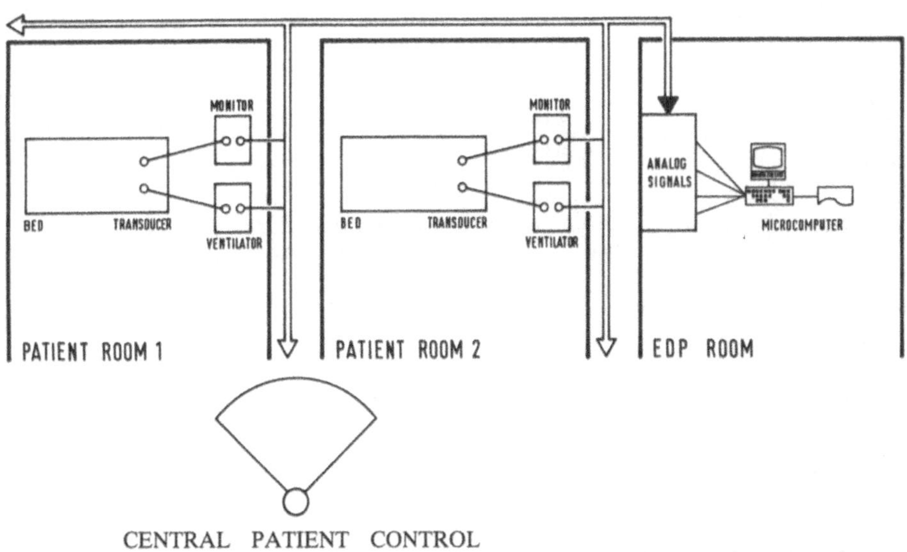

Fig. 5. Block diagram of intensive care unit. The system is placed in a separate room in the neurological intensive care unit. Analog signals are accessed from each normal bedside monitor and ventilator

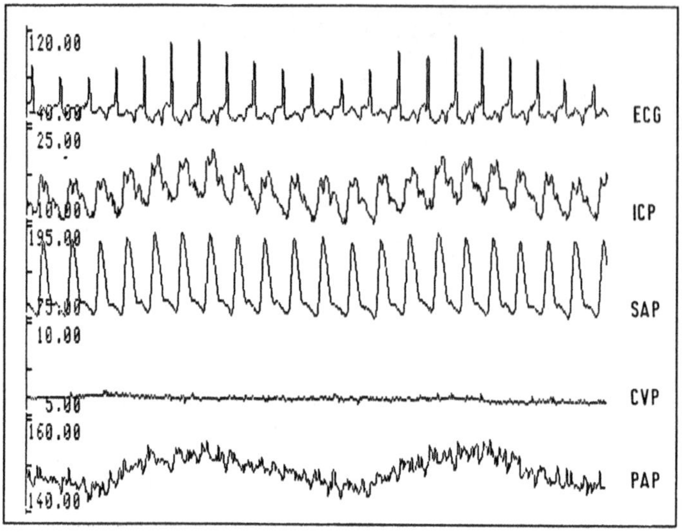

Fig. 6. Plot of sampled data (10-s interval)

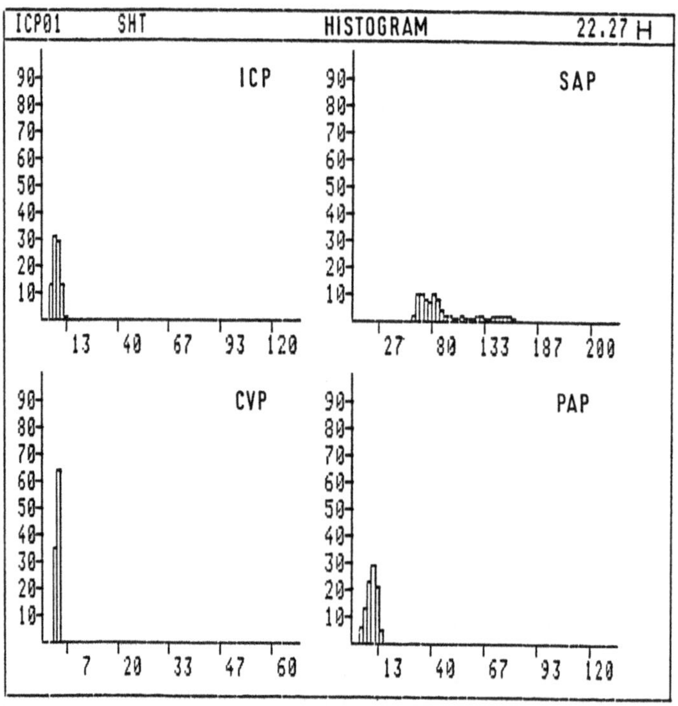

Fig. 7. Histograms of ICP, SAP, CVP, and PAP for a 10-min period

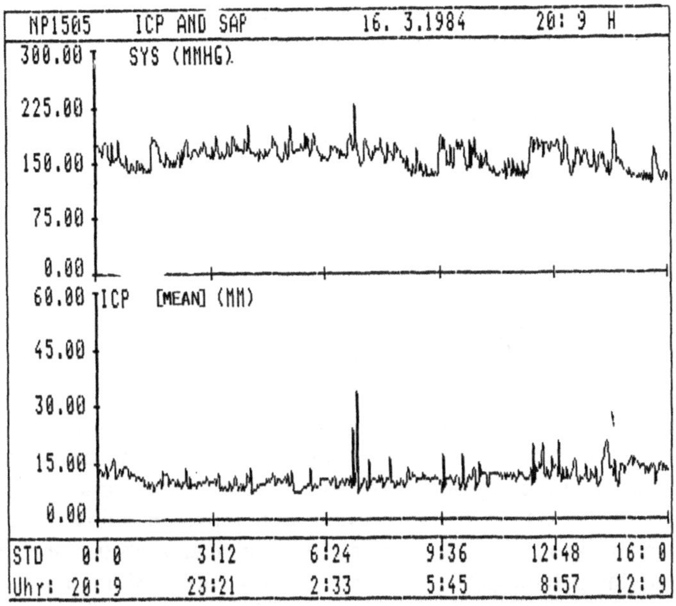

Fig. 8. Display of stored mean values. ICP and SAP were recorded with other signals over 16 h

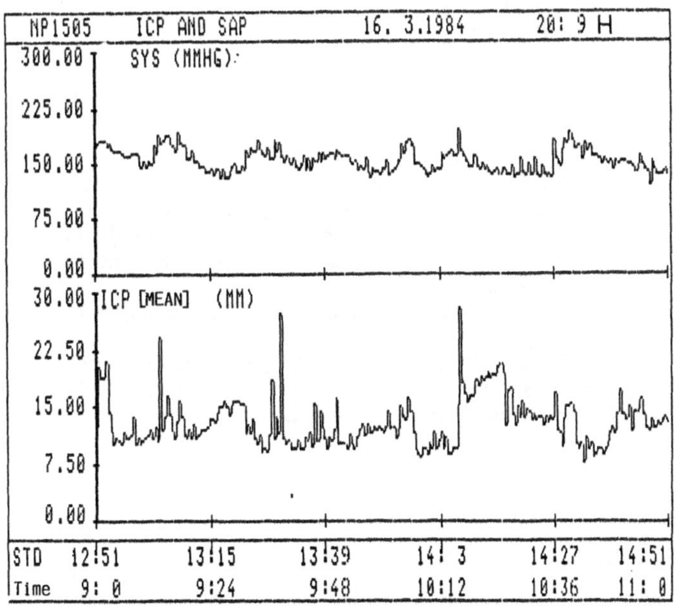

Fig. 9. A 2-h period from Fig. 8, plotted to provide more detailed information

Other modules allow off-line operations to be performed on stored data. For example, MODUL 2 will give a graphic display of the whole or selected portions of stored mean values of the monitored period (Figs. 8, 9).

MODUL 3 does detailed statistical calculations for the whole recording period or sequentially for any preset time interval. At any time the program can be interrupted by keyboard in order to get a hard copy of graphic terminal.

Discussion

A low-cost microcomputer system has been developed which enables ICP data to be integrated with other analog signals. The system is used in normal clinical situations and analysis of ICP signal was done in a limited number of patients.

In individual patients on-line computed CSF pulse pressure was found to be a reliable parameter in monitoring alterations in intracranial elastance. The CSFPP is based on the transient increase in cerebral blood volume per cardiac cycle (dV). At subsequent time intervals variations in the slope of this relationship are caused either by intracranial elastance or by dV. Both increased elastance and increased dV relate to the pathological situation of autoregulation failure and the occurence of progressive vasoparalysis (Avezaat et al. 1979).

In the course of ICP monitoring, dV may be affected by factors changing cerebral hemodynamics, such as arterial carbon dioxide tension, blood pressure, and arterial pulse pressure (Avezaat et al. 1979). This makes it difficult to compare CSFPP values from patient to patient, and to calculate reference values (Friden and Ekstedt 1980).

However, the possibility of store these factors in a convenient data base for detailed statistical calculations enables us to study their influence on the relationship between the ICP signal and the CSFPP. This complex correlation will be dealt with in a subsequent study.

References

Avezaat CJJ, van Eijndhoven JHM, Wyper DJ (1979) Cerebrospinal fluid pulse pressure and intracranial volume-pressure relationship. J Neurology Neurosurg Psychiatr 42: 687–700

Friden H, Ekstedt J (1980) CSF pressure-volume relation and pulse related CSF pressure variations in man. In: Shulman K, Marmarou A, Miller JD (eds) Intracranial pressure IV. Springer, Berlin Heidelberg New York, pp 93–95

Szewczykowski J et al (1977) A fast method of estimating the elastance of the intracranial system. J Neurosurg 47: 19–26

van Eijndhoven JHM, Avezaat CJJ (1980) The analogy between CSF pulse pressure and volume-pressure response. In: Shulman K, Marmarou A, Miller JD (eds): Intracranial pressure IV. Springer, Berlin Heidelberg New York, pp 173–176

GPSR Compliance

The European Union's (EU) General Product Safety Regulation (GPSR) is a set of rules that requires consumer products to be safe and our obligations to ensure this.

If you have any concerns about our products, you can contact us on ProductSafety@springernature.com

In case Publisher is established outside the EU, the EU authorized representative is:

Springer Nature Customer Service Center GmbH
Europaplatz 3
69115 Heidelberg, Germany

Batch number: 10704763

Printed by Printforce, the Netherlands